Challenging Cases in Respirology and Critical Care

Gurmeet Singh

Challenging Cases in Respirology and Critical Care

Springer

Gurmeet Singh
Division of Respirology and Critical Illness,
Department of Internal Medicine
Cipto Mangunkusumo Hospital,
Universitas Indonesia
Jakarta, Indonesia

ISBN 978-981-96-5001-9 ISBN 978-981-96-5002-6 (eBook)
https://doi.org/10.1007/978-981-96-5002-6

This Springer imprint is published by the registered company Springer Nature Singapore Pte Ltd.
The registered company address is: 152 Beach Road, #21-01/04 Gateway East, Singapore 189721, Singapore

This book is dedicated to My Family. They had a decisive influence on the course of my life. To the memory of my late grandfather, Harchand Singh, my late grandmother, Jaswant Kaur, my late mother, Kuljit Kaur. To my father, Manmohan Singh; my wife, Simarjeet Kaur; my daughters, Milandeep Kaur and Harshavin Kaur; my son, Shanndeep Singh. To my sister, Hardeep Kaur, and my brothers, Bhupinder Singh and Jadbinder Singh.

Preface

It is my pleasure to present to you the *Challenging Cases in Respirology and Critical Care*. In this book, the topic is presented in a case-based study format.

This area of medicine includes the diagnosis and treatment of respirology and critical care diseases. Approaching a patient with respirology and critical care disorder has always been challenging partly because the patient is often either a poor historian or present in a late stage of the respirology and critical care complication.

The target audience of this book comprises educators and clinicians in the field of respirology, critical care, fellows-in-training, residents of internal medicine, and allied health providers.

The book consists of 25 challenging complicated cases. The unique style comprises a short abstract, followed by case presentation, some medical intervention, working diagnosis, data, final diagnosis, and discussion. In addition, to stimulate the reader's thought process, we added a total of five multiple-choice questions and answers.

I would like to express my gratitude to the executive editor who has supported this book, and the entire editorial and publishing staff at Springer.

I hope the readers find the collection of 25 cases in this book as a valuable and helpful resource. Furthermore, I will be happy to hear your comments and use them in future editions. I can be reached at: gurmeet.singh01@ui.ac.id.

Several individuals contributed to the writing of this book. I am especially grateful to: the multidisciplinary physicians team who were also involved in the treatment and surgical intervention of the patients, including Adityo Susilo, Adi Basuki, Adi Wijaya, Adhrie Sugiarto, Anne Dinna Subroto, Ardhi Rahman Ahani, Arif Sejati, Cleopas Martin Rumende, David Hutagaol, Denio Adrianus Ridjab, Dita Aditianingsih, Erika Marfiani, Hadian Setia, Hariadi Hadibrata, Hartanto Wijaya, Hasan Maulahela, Iwan Rivai Alam Siahaan, Ivan Banjuradja, Jeffry Beta Tenggara, Kemal Fariz Kalista, Lie Khie Chen, Jordan Sardjan, Meisa Putri Maharani, Muhammad Arza Putra, Muhammad Kurniawan, Nadia Ayu Mulansari, Ralph Girson Gunarsa, Ray Bryan Charles Rattu, Rajesh Kalwani, Resultanti, Reza Prabowo, Robiatul Adawiyah, Rr. Dyah Purnamasari Sulistianingsih, Robert Shinto, Sidharta Kusuma Manggala. The Radiologist and Pathologist for their support in the contributions of the images in all clinical cases.

I'm grateful to my Research Assistants, namely, Cipta Mahendra, Ersananda Arlisa Putri, Muhammad Rizki Triono, Steffi Cong Andi Nata and Nova Bornida

Fauzi, for their invaluable contribution in facilitating the proof of my ideas and thoughts, as well as providing the relevant reference materials and papers.

I would like to thank all the patients and/or their families for permitting the inclusion of their cases in this book.

I would also like to thank members of Cipto Mangonkusumo Hospital, including the director, the head of Internal Medicine department, the staff of Respirology and Critical Illness division, and allied health professionals. I'm grateful to the staff of Mochtar Riady Comprehensive Cancer Centre Siloam Hospital, including the director and allied health professionals, as well as the Dean of Medical Faculty Universitas Indonesia for all their support in the completion of this book.

Jakarta, Indonesia Gurmeet Singh

Contents

Mediastinoscopy in Spontaneous Pneumomediastinum

1

1.1 Case Illustration

A 23-year-old male patient came to the hospital emergency room with a chief complaint of shortness of breath causing restricted physical activities. The shortness of breath had become worse 2 days before hospital admission. In addition, the complaint was accompanied by chest pain during inspiration. The patient had a history of asthma with no routine control, and the condition was managed with the use of only a *short-acting beta-2 agonist (SABA) inhaler* 2–3 times a day. The complaint experienced was also accompanied by feeling tense on the right and left sides of the neck, but a history of chest trauma and a fall were denied.

The patient appeared short of breath with a respiratory rate of 24 per minute, and the pulse increased to 104 times per minute. The saturation level was 99% with nasal cannula oxygen at 4 lpm. Examination of the lungs revealed bronchial breath sounds, wheezing, and prolonged expiration, with cardiac assessment showing a positive Hamman sign. Laboratory examination showed increased levels of leucocyte (13.1), CRP-Hs (3.1), and Immunoglobulin E (275.0). The chest X-ray (Fig. 1.1) revealed fibrosis in the upper field of the right lung, pneumomediastinum, and subcutaneous emphysema. The patient was then nebulized with a combination of SABA and anticholinergic every 4 h, steroid intravenous, antibiotic intravenous, and drip MgSO4 20%.

Based on clinical findings and initial laboratory results, the patient was diagnosed with *Spontaneous Pneumomediastinum in Moderate Acute Asthma*. On the admission day, there was still severe complaint of breathing difficulties. The blood oxygen saturation was measured at 99% with cannula nasal oxygen supplementation at 4 lpm. CT thorax was performed to confirm the diagnosis, and the results showed extensive pneumomediastinum and subcutaneous emphysema, along with ground glass opacity of the apicoposterior segment and anterior segment of the superior lobe of the left lung. In addition, abnormalities suggestive of interstitial lung abnormality or pneumonia were observed in the middle

G. Singh, *Challenging Cases in Respirology and Critical Care*,
https://doi.org/10.1007/978-981-96-5002-6_1

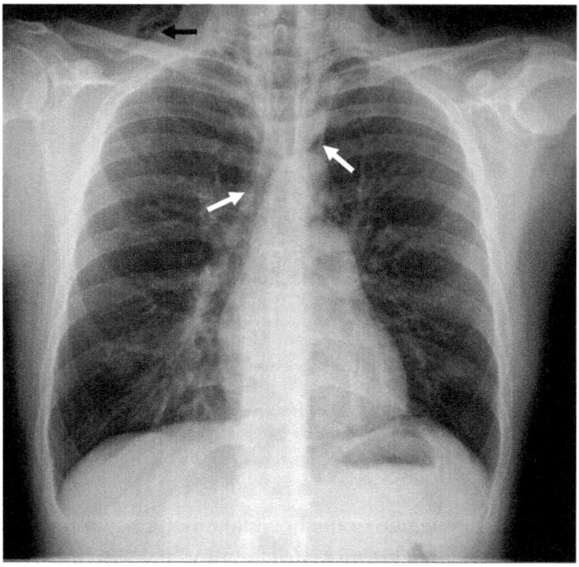

Fig. 1.1 The chest X-ray showed linear lucency outlining the mediastinum and paratrachea (pneumomediastinum) (white arrow) and subcutaneous emphysema in the supraclavicular–lower region of the neck (black arrow). (Image Courtesy: Dewi Tantra MD)

lobe of the right lung. Mosaic attenuation of the right middle lobe and the lingula of the left lung indicated possible small airway disease, while no pneumothorax or pneumoperitoneum was observed (Fig. 1.2). Subsequently, the patient was consulted in the department of cardiovascular and thoracic surgery and was scheduled for mediastinoscopy.

On the second day of hospitalization, a mediastinoscopy was performed to evacuate air in the mediastinum (Fig. 1.3), leading to significant improvement of complaints. Oxygen supplementation was reduced to 2 lpm, a Combivent nebulizer was administered four times each day, and other therapies were continued. A post-operative CT thorax (Fig. 1.2) was carried out on the patient, and the results showed a relative reduction of pneumomediastinum and subcutaneous emphysema. Ground glass opacity in segments 4–5 of the right lung and segment 5 of the left lung was also relatively reduced, along with laminar atelectasis in the lingula (segment 4–5) of the left lung.

The following day, there were no complaints of shortness of breath, and no sign of respiratory distress was found. The patient was given formoterol corticosteroid inhalation therapy and was planned for discharge, with follow-up scheduled at the Outpatient Department. Another CT thorax examination was carried out 2 months after mediastinoscopy (Fig. 1.4).

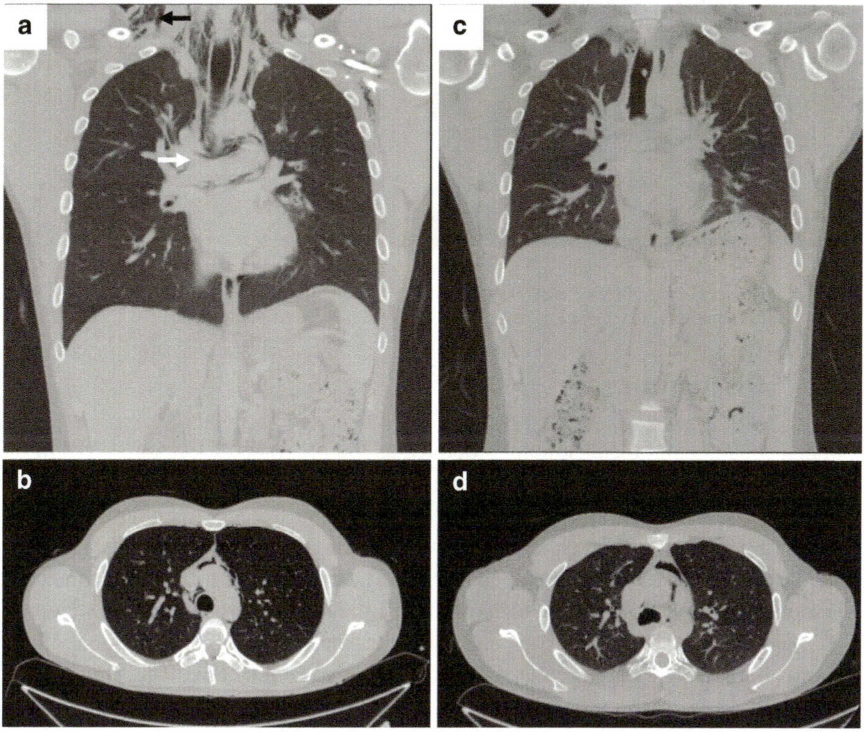

Fig. 1.2 CT Thorax before mediastinoscopy showed air in the mediastinum (white arrow) and subcutaneous (black arrow) (**a**, **b**). CT Thorax after mediastinoscopy showed air in the mediastinum and subcutaneous relatively reduced (**c**, **d**). (Image Courtesy: Dewi Tantra MD)

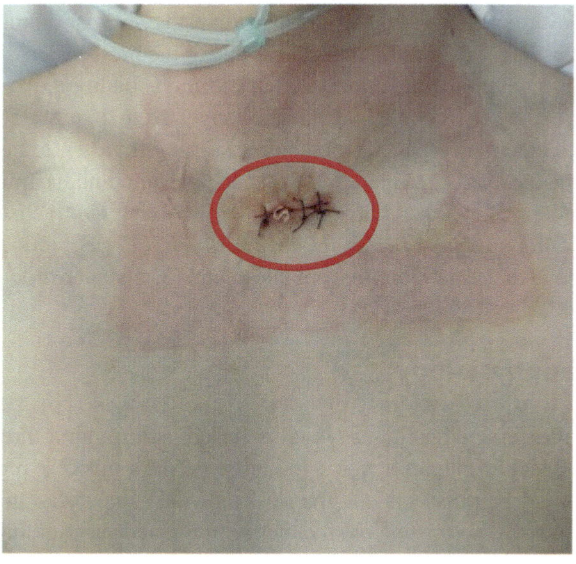

Fig. 1.3 Mediastinoscopy was performed to evacuate air in the mediastinum

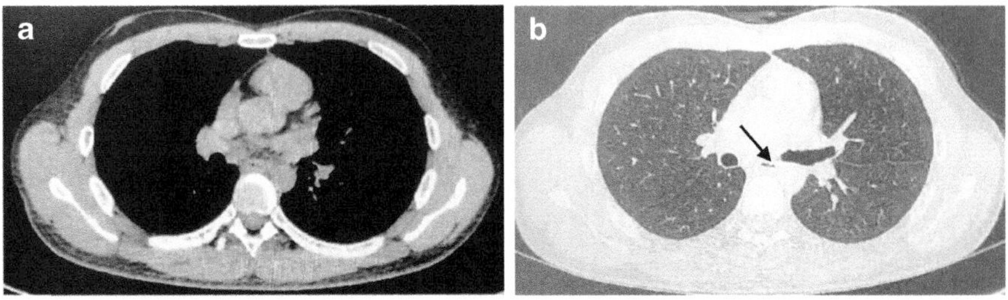

Fig. 1.4 (**a**) CT-Thorax showed almost complete resolution after mediastinoscopy. (**b**) small air in the right lower paratracheal (black arrow). (Image Courtesy: Dewi Tantra MD)

1.2 Discussion

Spontaneous pneumomediastinum is defined as the presence of free air or gas in the mediastinum without an identifiable cause, such as chest trauma. Several studies have highlighted its association with various conditions and triggers, including bronchial asthma, diabetic ketoacidosis, strenuous physical exertion, drug inhalation, and other activities involving the Valsalva maneuver [1]. The condition is primarily attributed to the rupture of the alveolar tree, which results in a sudden increase in intra-alveolar pressure. The escaped alveolar air then dissects centripetally through the pulmonary interstitium along the bronchovascular sheaths, ultimately reaching the mediastinum [1].

1.3 Prevalence

Spontaneous pneumomediastinum is a rare but underreported complication of asthma in recent years. Severe asthma exacerbations and obstruction of the smaller airways often result in overexpansion of distal airspaces, causing alveolar rupture. The escaped air then migrates into the extraluminal spaces due to the pressure gradient [2].

Spontaneous pneumomediastinum is an uncommon condition that predominantly affects young males. Its reported prevalence ranges from 1 in 8005 to 1 in 42,000 among hospital emergency and accident admissions. According to previous studies, three distinct mechanisms can lead to spontaneous pneumomediastinum: (1) disruption of a cutaneous or mucosal barrier, typically involving the tracheobronchial tree or esophagus, allowing gas to enter the mediastinum; (2) gas production by organisms within the mediastinum or adjacent chest; and (3) alveolar rupture [1].

1.4 Pathophysiology

Spontaneous pneumomediastinum typically develops through a three-step process known as the Macklin phenomenon: (1) increased intra-alveolar pressure leads to alveolar rupture, (2) air dissects into the peribronchial and perivascular sheaths, and (3) the air progressively spreads into the mediastinum and surrounding tissues [3, 4].

Another possible explanation for spontaneous pneumomediastinum is an abnormal increase in mediastinal pressure, which is typically low and negative. This pressure change allows air to dissect between the mediastinal structures that support the mediastinal organs. A significant decrease in intravascular pressure can also create a relative pressure gradient in the perivascular spaces. Consequently, air may dissect into the neck, upper abdomen, or skin via the loose alveolar fat tissue, resulting in subcutaneous emphysema. Additionally, air can traverse the pleura, leading to pneumothorax, or the peritoneum, causing pneumoperitoneum [5, 6].

1.5 Clinical Symptoms

Common symptoms of spontaneous pneumomediastinum include chest and neck pain, dyspnea, subcutaneous emphysema, hypotension, dysphagia, and cough. Chest pain is typically sudden, pleuritic in nature, and may radiate to the back and shoulders. Subcutaneous emphysema, which occurs when intrathoracic air escapes into the soft tissues following pneumothorax or pneumomediastinum, has a reported prevalence of 40–100%. Another notable clinical feature is Hamman's sign, first described by Hamman as crepitation detected during the apex beat on cardiac auscultation. This sign is often characterized as a crunching or rasping sound synchronized with the heartbeat, best heard in the left lateral decubitus position [5].

1.6 Diagnosis

The diagnosis of spontaneous pneumomediastinum is confirmed in approximately 90% of cases through chest radiography, which typically reveals linear lucencies traversing the mediastinum. However, studies indicate that these radiographic signs can be subtle and are often overlooked. Pneumothorax may accompany the condition in up to 10% of cases. Computed tomography (CT) of the thorax is widely regarded as the gold standard for diagnosis, as it provides detailed visualization of mediastinal air and identifies associated conditions, such as lung parenchymal abnormalities. Furthermore, contrast-enhanced CT offers additional value in excluding secondary causes, such as esophageal rupture [6].

Recent reports suggest that a chest CT scan is a routine diagnostic tool used to evaluate the extent of pneumomediastinum confirm the diagnosis in cases with inconclusive chest X-rays, and identify potential causative factors or underlying pathologies. CT scans are also instrumental in distinguishing between pneumomediastinum and pneumopericardium, the latter being air within the pericardium rather than the prepericardial fat, which may have a less favorable clinical course and require specific treatment. Additionally, when pneumomediastinum is missed on plain chest X-rays, particularly in cases with severe subcutaneous emphysema, CT scans are often used to confirm the diagnosis [5].

Bronchoscopy, esophagoscopy, or esophagography is not routinely needed in cases of spontaneous pneumomediastinum, unless an underlying pathology is suspected or has been identified through clinical presentation and medical history. Obtaining a thorough understanding of the patient's previous health status and events is crucial and cannot be overstated [5].

Ultrasound of the mediastinum is increasingly used in the accident and emergency department to quickly identify pneumomediastinum in cases requiring immediate attention [5]. Pneumomediastinum is typically a benign condition with a favorable clinical outcome. Clinical sequelae are generally related to the underlying cause, such as in cases of esophageal rupture with accompanying mediastinitis [7].

1.7 Management

The management of spontaneous pneumomediastinum is generally conservative and focuses on addressing the underlying cause. Invasive interventions, such as needle aspiration or surgical decompression, are typically reserved for life-threatening cases where there is significant hemodynamic or respiratory compromise due to the compression of mediastinal structures [7].

Several reports have shown that placing bilateral intercostal drains using transthoracic mediastinoscopy, despite the absence of a pneumothorax, can help achieve a reduction in the trans-pulmonary pressure gradient, leading to a decrease in intra-alveolar pressure and preventing alveolar rupture. This can subsequently lead to a reduction in pneumomediastinum and facilitate the weaning process. The option of placing a mediastinal drain is often kept in reserve for cases that experience further deterioration. This strategy is adopted, as chest drains are simpler to place and generally associated with fewer complications compared to mediastinal drains [4].

1.8 Mediastinoscopy

Mediastinoscopy is a thoracic surgical procedure performed using a mediastinoscope to examine the mediastinum—the space in the thoracic cavity between the lungs—for various purposes, including diagnostic tissue sampling, mediastinal lymph node biopsy, and TNM (tissue, nodes, and metastasis) staging. Cervical mediastinoscopy provides access to the pre-tracheal, paratracheal, and anterior subcarinal lymph nodes [8].

Malignant pneumomediastinum is a life-threatening condition characterized by an excessive presence of air in the mediastinum. In such cases, subcutaneous aspiration and incisions may be necessary to evacuate the excess air. Cervical mediastinotomy can also be performed if aspiration proves insufficient. This type of decompression is often lifesaving in many pneumomediastinum patients, providing greater efficacy compared to conservative management. Predictions suggest that the use of cervical mediastinotomy is expected to rise in the future [3].

1.9 Complication Mediastinoscopy

During the procedure, insertion of the mediastinoscope can lead to compression of the innominate artery. This compression may result in a decrease in the pulse oximeter signal and blood pressure when the device is placed in the right upper extremity, due to reduced blood flow to the extremity. Compression of the innominate artery can also cause intracerebral hypoperfusion, leading to cerebral ischemia and, in severe cases, stroke [8].

Intraoperative complications during mediastinoscopy are relatively common, with bleeding being the most frequent. Injury to the great vessels can lead to significant hemorrhage, which may be life-threatening. In such cases, an emergent thoracotomy or median sternotomy may be required to control the bleeding while simultaneously using the mediastinoscope to tamponade the site of hemorrhage [8].

In patients with a large mediastinal mass, superior vena cava (SVC) syndrome may also be present. Obstruction of the superior vena cava leads to facial swelling, distension of the neck, and the development of collateral venous drainage along the thoracic wall. This syndrome is frequently associated with symptoms such as dyspnea and dysphagia. Diagnostically, SVC syndrome can be identified on imaging, often accompanied by a positive Pemberton's sign [8].

1.10 Prognosis

The prognosis of spontaneous pneumomediastinum is typically favorable, with resolution occurring within a few days in most cases. The recurrence rate is generally low. However, spontaneous pneumomediastinum cases require hospitalization to monitor for potential complications [3].

Key Points

Spontaneous pneumomediastinum has been linked to various conditions and triggers, including bronchial asthma. The management of this condition is usually conservative and focuses on addressing the underlying cause. In some cases, cervical mediastinotomy may be performed, and decompression through this procedure can be more effective in saving lives for many patients with pneumomediastinum compared to conservative approaches.

Question

1. Spontaneous pneumomediastinum can be induced by these conditions, except:
   (a) Chest Trauma
   (b) Asthma Bronchial
   (c) Diabetic Ketoacidosis
   (d) Forceful Straining During Exercise
   (e) Inhalation of Drugs

2. A crepitation detected at the time of the apex beat during cardiac auscultation is called:
   (a) Musset's sign
   (b) Muffled Heart Sound
   (c) Pounding Heartbeat
   (d) Gallop
   (e) Hamman Sign
3. The gold standard of pneumomediastinum diagnosis?
   (a) Chest X-Ray
   (b) MRI
   (c) CT scan
   (d) Bronchoscopy
   (e) Thoracoscopy
4. Below are clinical manifestations of spontaneous mediastinum, except:
   (a) Chest and neck pain
   (b) Dyspnea
   (c) Subcutaneous Emphysema
   (d) Hypotension
   (e) Hypertension
5. A chest X-ray sign found in spontaneous mediastinum?
   (a) Cavitas
   (b) Demonstrates linear lucencies traversing the mediastinum
   (c) Air within the pericardium
   (d) Fibrosis
   (e) Atelectasis

Answer Keys

1. A
2. E
3. C
4. E
5. B

Acknowledgment **Ersananda Arlisa Putri, MD,** Department of Internal Medicine, Respirology and Critical Illness Division, Universitas Indonesia, Dr. Cipto Mangunkusumo General Central National Hospital, Jakarta, Indonesia.

Hariadi Hadibrata, MD, Department of Cardiovascular and Thoracic Surgery, Mochtar Riady Comprehensive Cancer Center (MRCCC) Siloam Hospital, Jakarta, Indonesia.

References

1. Murayama S, Gibo S. Spontaneous pneumomediastinum and Macklin effect: overview and appearance on computed tomography. World J Radiol. 2014;28(6):850–4.
2. Covanţev S, Mazuruc N, Uzdenov R, Corlateanu A. Spontaneous pneumomediastinum – a rare asthma complication. Folia Med Plovdiv. 2019;61:472.

3. Iteen AJ, Bianchi W, Sharman T. Pneumomediastinum. In: StatPearls; 2023. http://www.ncbi.nlm.nih.gov/books/NBK557440/. Accessed 23 Jan 2024.
4. Singh BP, Shetty GS, Vijayan PA, Gopalakrishna U, Chandan G, Santini A. Management of pneumomediastinum associated with H1N1 pneumonia: a case report. J Crit Care Med. 2019;5:28–33.
5. Kouritas VK, Papagiannopoulos K, Lazaridis G, Baka S, Mpoukovinas I, Karavasilis V. Pneumomediastinum. J Thorac Dis. 2015;7:S44–9.
6. Tezel C, Varer P, Baysungur V, Okur E, Halezeroglu S. Spontaneous pneumomediastinum: report of two cases. Turk J Trauma Emerg Surg. 2011;17:368–70.
7. Gleeson M, McEnery T, Gaine S. Pneumomediastinum complicating acute asthma. QJM Int J Med. 2023;117:229–30.
8. McNally PA, Arthur ME. Mediastinoscopy. StatPearls [Internet]; 2023.

Electrocautery and Snare in a Tuberculosis Complicated Pleural Effusion

2

2.1 Case Illustration

A 68-year-old male presented to the hospital with a chief complaint of shortness of breath, which was accompanied by fever and lack of appetite. During assessment, symptoms of coughs, chest pain, night sweats, weight loss, and leg or abdominal swelling were denied. Medical intervention was initially received at a primary healthcare facility, where antibiotics were administered, but no improvement was observed. The patient was then referred to the current hospital's outpatient ward and given dyspepsia medications. However, the symptoms still persisted, leading to an eventual transfer to the hospital's emergency room (ER). The patient had a history of daily smoking for over 20 years as well as hypertension. Medications had been previously prescribed to treat the underlying hypertension but were not routinely consumed.

On physical examination, hypertension (152/82 mmHg) and high respiratory rate (32 times/min) were found, while no sound was heard at the left hemithorax during lung auscultation. Laboratory examination showed declining kidney function (eGFR = 68.6 mL/min/1.73 m^2), as well as an increase in aspartate transferase (AST) (67 units/L) and alanine aminotransferase (ALT) (150 units/L) values. In addition, chest X-ray revealed inhomogeneous consolidation of the left hemithorax (Fig. 2.1), suggesting a massive left lung pleural effusion. The patient was then scheduled for a chest tube insertion procedure.

An ultrasonography (USG) examination was performed on the patient, and the results were presented in Fig. 2.2.

After thoracocentesis, the patient still had complaints of shortness of breath, with a low-pitch sound of the left hemithorax being heard. The left lung X-ray imaging was found to be improved after the procedure (Fig. 2.3), and a chest tube insertion procedure was scheduled.

The complaint of shortness of breath still persisted after the chest tube insertion procedure, with the chest X-ray imaging showing the absence of improvement

G. Singh, *Challenging Cases in Respirology and Critical Care*,
https://doi.org/10.1007/978-981-96-5002-6_2

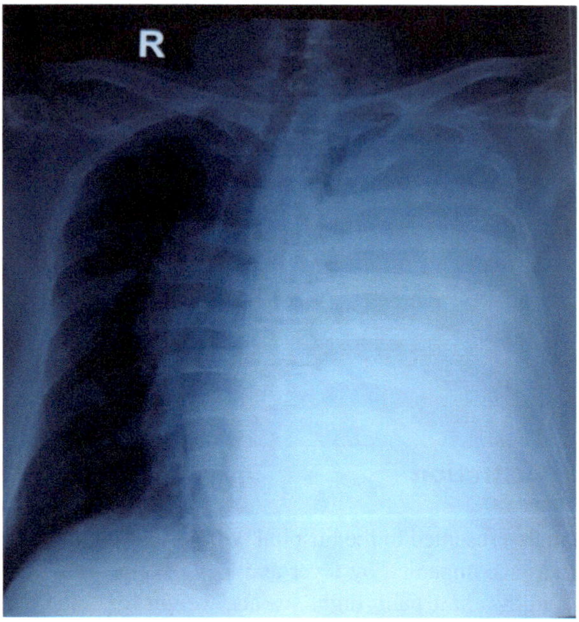

Fig. 2.1 Inhomogeneous consolidation of the left lung, suggesting a massive pleural effusion. (Image Courtesy: Marcel Prasetyo MD DM)

(Fig. 2.4). The patient was then subjected to a chest CT scan with a contrast (Fig. 2.5) (Image Courtesy: Marcel Prasetyo MD DM).

Pleural fluid analysis showed the following results, namely a cell count of 1038/μL, a protein ratio of 0.76, exudative consistency, and negative acid-fast bacilli (AFB) testing. Gram staining examination and culturing of the fluid did not show the presence of microorganism growth. However, cytological testing showed numerous cells, consisting of mesothelial cells, macrophages, and lymphocytes. Based on these findings, the patient was diagnosed with complicated pleural effusion caused by TB and was given the category I anti-TB drugs (according to body weight) and steroids. A chest CT scan was performed on November 11th, 2019, and the results were presented in Fig. 2.5.

The patient was finally feeling relieved of dyspneic symptoms 4 days after the thoracoscopy and electrocautery procedures. The left lung's auscultatory sound was restored, and chest tube production was measured at 150 mL/day. Subsequently, serial chest X-rays were obtained to monitor the treatment's progress (Figs. 2.7 and 2.8).

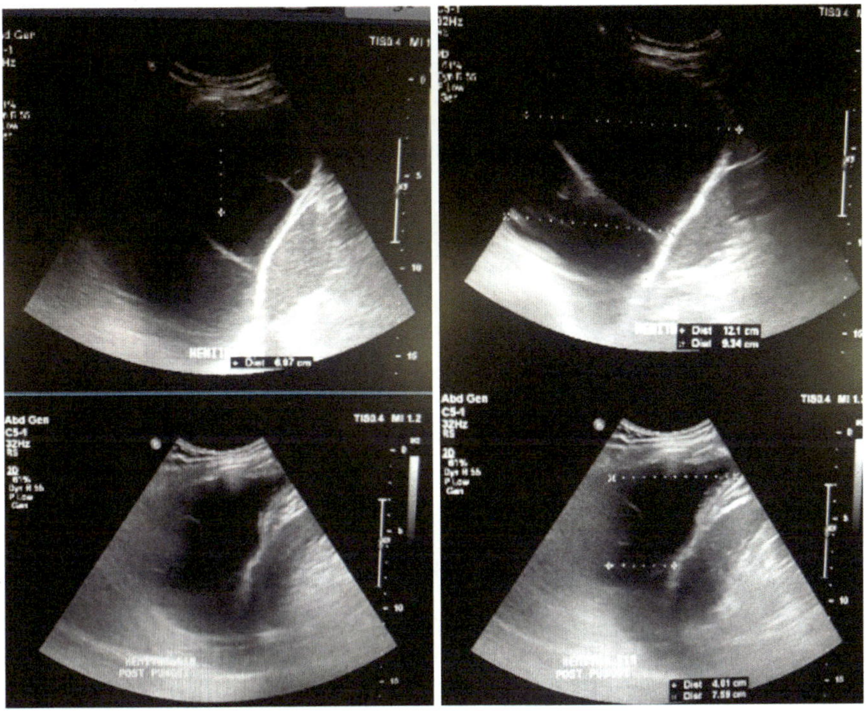

Fig. 2.2 Anechoic fluid with a septal component fills the left hemithorax with a volume estimation of 1500 mL. Thoracocentesis was performed; 800 mL of serous fluid was obtained. (Image Courtesy: Marcel Prasetyo MD DM)

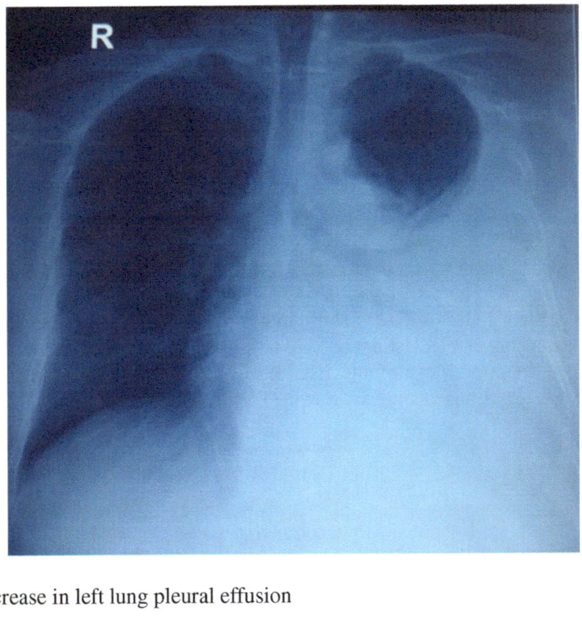

Fig. 2.3 A decrease in left lung pleural effusion

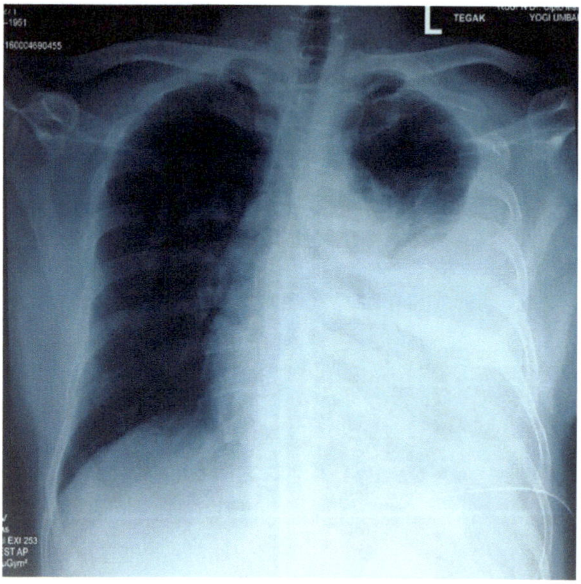

Fig. 2.4 No change in the chest X-ray imaging of the left lung pleural effusion. A chest tube tip was inserted into the left hemithorax at the tenth left posterior intercostal space. No sign of pneumomediastinum or subcutaneous emphysema was observed. (Image Courtesy: Benny Zulkarnaien MD DM)

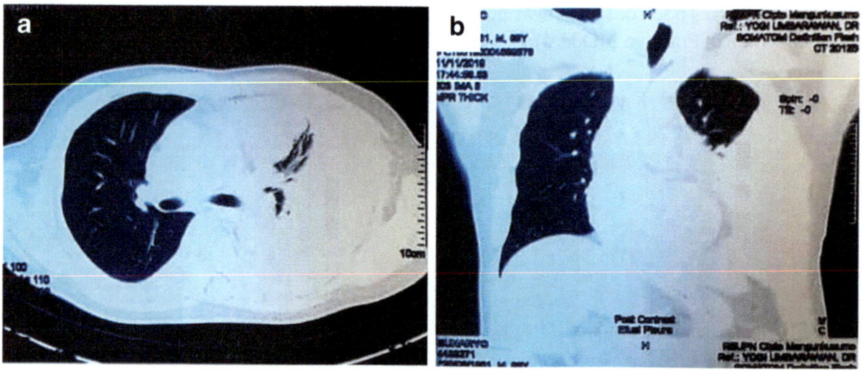

Fig. 2.5 (**a**) The patient's chest CT scan shows a hypodense lesion of the left anterior mediastinum (suspected empyema or mediastinal abscess), (**b**) left hemithorax pleural effusion with collapsed inferior and superior lobes of the left lung. The patient underwent thoracoscopy and electrocautery (Fig. 2.6). (Image Courtesy: Sawitri Darmiati MD DM)

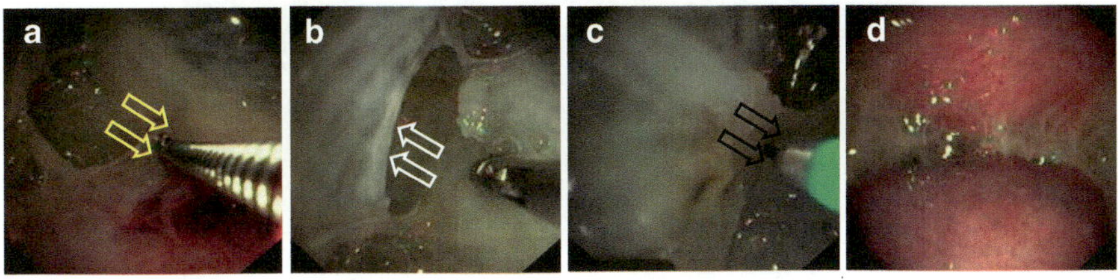

Fig. 2.6 Thick fibrin covers the patient's left lung. (**a**) Fibrin covers the patient's left lung and biopsy forceps (yellow arrow). (**b**) Thick Fibrin (white arrow). (**c**) Electrocautery (black arrow). (**d**) Collapses lung. (Image Courtesy: Gurmeet Singh MD DM PhD)

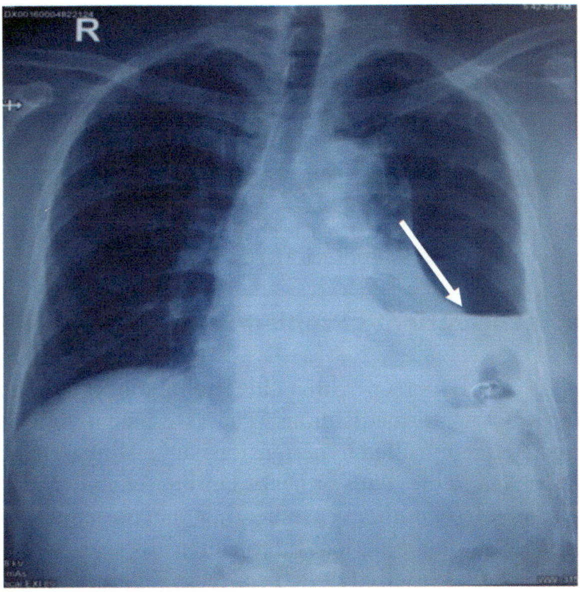

Fig. 2.7 Improvement of the left lung hydropneumothorax and subcutaneous emphysema. (white arrow). (Image Courtesy: Marcel Prasetyo MD DM)

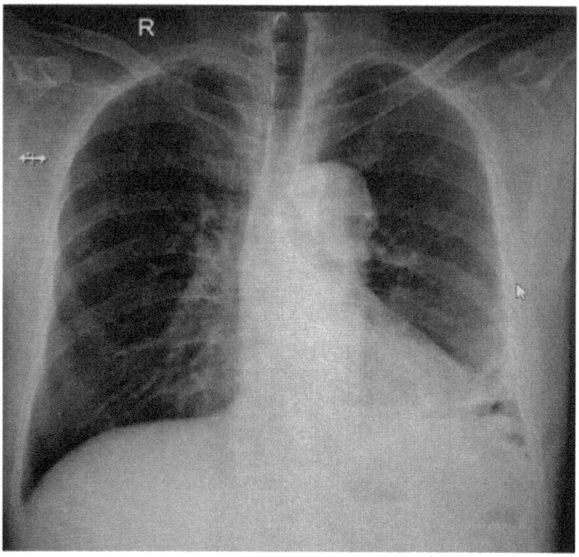

Fig. 2.8 Further improvement of the left lung hydropneumothorax. Fibrosis was observed on the left lung. (Image Courtesy: Benny Zulkarnaien MD DM)

2.2 What Is the Patient's Problem, and Why?

The patient is an elderly person with a chief complaint of persistent shortness of breath and refractory to medications. The assessment showed a history of active smoking and uncontrolled hypertension, suggesting potential underlying medical issues related to the lungs or heart. During lung auscultation, no sound was heard on the left hemithorax, indicating the presence of fluids in the lung(s). On chest X-ray examination, full opacity was seen on the left hemithorax, and a chest tube was inserted due to concerns regarding the extent of pleural effusion.

2.3 Discussion

According to the British Thoracic Society (BTS) guideline, patients with suspected pleural effusion must be asked and assessed for disease and medication histories.

2.4 Pleural Effusion

Pleural effusion is defined as the excessive accumulation of fluids in the pleural space due to an imbalance between production and absorption. In addition, it serves as a manifestation rather than a standalone diagnosis, indicating an underlying disease. Various conditions can lead to pleural effusion, emphasizing the importance of determining the exact underlying disease for appropriate management. The effusion can be categorized as either exudative or transudative based on its contents, which reflects the pathogenesis mechanism. To differentiate between the two types, most clinicians typically use the Light criteria [1].

In normal subjects, the pleural cavity is filled with only a small amount of fluid, totaling approximately 0.3 mL/kg. The majority of cases have elusive etiologies; hence, pleural fluid analysis, clinical manifestations, and radiological findings were essential in establishing the diagnosis. Pleural fluid analysis usually includes protein and glucose levels, pH, lactate dehydrogenase (LDH) levels, cytology, and microbiology examination [2].

2.5 Radiology

Radiological examination is the most common modality used to confirm the presence of pleural effusion. However, a minimum fluid amount of 250 mL is necessary for the accumulated fluid to be visible.

- Chest X-ray

In chest X-ray examination, pleural effusion typically presents with specific visual characteristics on the film. These include opacity on most or both hemithorax, blunted costophrenic and cardiophrenic angles, meniscus, and mediastinal shift to the contralateral side in massive cases.

- Thoracic USG

Thoracic USG can be used to recognize the minimal volume of pleural effusion. In thoracic USG, pleural effusion gives an echo-free image of the space between the visceral and parietal pleura. The effusion's characteristics as observed on the USG image can differentiate between transudate and exudate effusion. Based on its echogenicity, effusion can be classified as anechoic, either with or without septation, or homogeneous echogenic. A thick echogenic pattern is usually due to empyema or hemorrhagic effusion [3].

- Thoracic CT scan

A thoracic CT scan can detect pleural effusion when it is not recognized in a chest X-ray or the thoracic USG. This imaging modality can differentiate between the pleural fluid and tissue proliferation, which may provide a hint of the origin. Therefore, it is recommended to repeat the thoracic CT scan procedure after an initial thoracocentesis [4].

2.6 General Management of Pleural Effusion

The purpose of pleural effusion management is to alleviate the symptoms through fluid elimination from the pleural cavity and to manage the underlying causal disease. The treatment depends on its nature, phase, and the underlying disease. Transudative effusion is considered a noncomplicated variant and can be resolved using conservative approaches or antibiotics. Meanwhile, exudative or high-volume effusion is considered complicated. This indicates that draining out the fluid is necessary to restore the lung's parenchymal functional capacity and to establish a favorable prognosis. Some interventions for managing the complicated effusion include thoracocentesis, catheter drainage, fibrinolytic therapies, pleurodesis, or surgery.

2.7 Complicated Lung TB

Lung TB is caused by inhalation of droplets containing *Mycobacterium tuberculosis*. Several studies have shown that TB predominantly affects the lungs but can spread to or infect other body organs (extrapulmonary TB). In patients with comorbidities or unmanaged TB, a myriad of lesional complications (sequelae) can develop, including parenchymal (including tuberculoma, cavities, cicatrix, end-stage lung destruction, aspergilloma, and bronchogenic carcinoma), airway (bronchiectasis, tracheobronchial stenosis, and broncholithiasis), vascular (arteritis, pulmonary and bronchial thrombosis, bronchial artery dilatation, and Rasmussen aneurism), mediastinal (lymph node calcification, esophagobronchial fistula, pericarditis, and mediastinitis), pleural (chronic empyema, fibrothorax, bronchopleural fistula, and pneumothorax), and chest wall lesions (spondylitis and malignancies stemming from chronic empyema) [5].

Pleural effusion caused by TB infection is the most common inflammatory pleural condition encountered in TB-endemic countries. This condition frequently occurs 3–6 months after the primary infection phase. The effusion can ensue when the caseous cavities and foci on the pleura's parenchyma break out and infiltrate the pleural cavity. A direct hematogenous spreading can also induce pleural effusion, with clinical manifestations including dry cough, fever, chest pain, and dyspnea. In chronic infections, reduction in body weight, fatigue (malaise), and dyspnea are often experienced. On physical examination, breath sounds are not heard, with dull or faint sounds being found during chest percussion [6].

2.8 Pleuroscopy/Thoracoscopy

Pleuroscopy, also known as thoracoscopy, is a medical procedure comprising the insertion of a flexible scope into the thoracic compartment [7]. In addition, there are two major types, namely medical thoracoscopy and video-assisted thoracoscopy surgery (VATS). Table 2.1 shows the difference between the two methods.

Table 2.1 Comparisons of medical thoracoscopy and video-assisted thoracoscopy surgery (VATS)

	Medical thoracoscopy	Video-assisted thoracoscopy surgery (VATS)
Performing room	Procedure room	Operating room
Use of sedation	Local anesthesia, mild to medium sedation level	General anesthesia
Ventilation	Spontaneous	One-lung ventilation
Indication	Diagnostic (biopsies), therapeutic (pleurodesis, adhesiolysis)	Minimally invasive surgery (lobectomy, pneumonectomy)
Operator	Respirologist, pulmonologist, pediatrist	Cardiothoracic surgeon
Technicality	Minimally invasive, low-cost	Invasive

Pleuroscopy is the second most performed procedure after bronchoscopy for treatment. In cases of pleural disease, it is frequently performed in combination with ablative therapies, such as electrocautery. Several indications for thoracoscopy include:

1. Diagnostic indication
   (a) Pleural effusion with unknown etiologies
   (b) Staging determination of lung cancers
   (c) Staging determination of malignant mesothelioma
   (d) Diffuse lung diseases
   (e) Tuberculosis bacterium culturing
   (f) Presence of hormone receptors for breast cancer cases
2. Therapeutic indication
   (a) *Talc poudrage* (pneumothorax, massive and chronic pleural effusion)
   (b) Parapneumonic effusion
   (c) Empyema

2.9 Snare Electrocautery

Snare electrocautery is an ablative method that uses electrical currents to produce heat and cauterize body tissues (Fig. 2.9). The components of this method include a snare, a blade, a blunt probe, and hot forceps, each with their individual functions.

- Snare acts to bind the lesion at its base (useful in pedunculated airway lesions).
- An electrocautery blade is used to cut tissues and is very effective at inhibiting the formation of benign stenotic nets.
- The blunt probe is in direct contact with the lesion and causes tissue coagulation and destruction.
- Hot forceps conduct heat during biopsy and can be used in transbronchial or endobronchial cases.

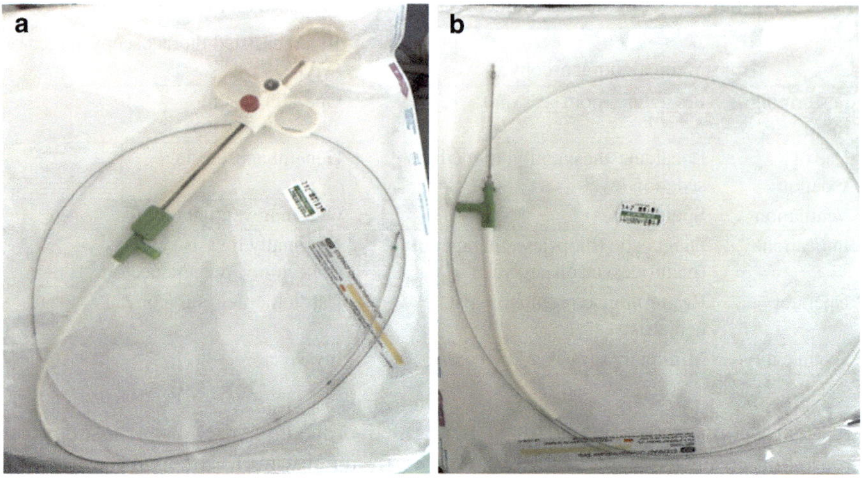

Fig. 2.9 Snare (**a**) and electrocautery (**b**)

Snare electrocautery is cost-effective, easier to perform, and widely available in many hospitals. This method is still underused in complicated pleural effusion cases but is predicted to achieve a high success rate and safety level for the treatment of central airway obstruction [8].

Key Points
In complicated pleuritis tuberculosis cases, interventional modalities such as snare and electrocautery may be an option besides conservative treatments, for a better patient outcome.

Questions

1. The following are parameters involved in the analysis of pleural fluids, except:
   (a) pH
   (b) Protein
   (c) Glucose
   (d) Lactate dehydrogenase (LDH)
   (e) Immunohistochemistry (IHC)
2. In pleural effusion, the level of echogenicity produced by CT scans can be classified as the following, except:
   (a) Anechoic
   (b) Complexes without septation
   (c) Complexes with septation
   (d) Homogenous echogenic
   (e) Heterogeneous echogenic

3. One of the clinical manifestations of tuberculosis-induced pleural effusion is
   (a) Wet cough
   (b) Chest pain
   (c) Night sweat
   (d) Muscle pain
   (e) Hemoptysis
4. The following are features of electrocautery, except:
   (a) Cold forceps
   (b) Snare
   (c) Blunt probe
   (d) Blade
   (e) Hot forceps
5. Which of the following is a diagnostic indication of a thoracoscopy procedure?
   (a) *Talc poudrage*
   (b) Empyema
   (c) Pedunculated tissue biopsy
   (d) Staging determination of malignant mesothelioma
   (e) Parapneumonic effusion

Answer Keys

1. E
2. E
3. D
4. A
5. D

Acknowledgment **Nova Bornida Fauzi, MD,** Department of Internal Medicine, Respirology and Critical Illness Division, Universitas Indonesia, Dr.s Cipto Mangunkusumo General Central National Hospital, Jakarta, Indonesia.

References

1. Porcel JM, Light RW. Diagnostic approach to pleural effusion in adults. Am Fam Physician. 2006;73:1211–20.
2. Mercer RM, Corcoran JP, Porcel JM, Rahman NM, Psallidas I. Interpreting pleural fluid results. Clin Med. 2019;19:213–7.
3. Karkhanis VS, Joshi JM. Pleural effusion: diagnosis, treatment, and management. Open Access Emerg Med. 2012;4:31–52.
4. Jany B, Welte T. Pleural effusion in adults-etiology, diagnosis, and treatment. Dtsch Arztebl Int. 2019;116:377–86.
5. Kim HY, Song KS, Goo JM, Lee JS, Lee KS, Lim TH. Thoracic sequelae and complications of tuberculosis. Radiographics. 2001;21:839–58.
6. Devi G. Complications of pulmonary tuberculosis. Concept TB, Book Chapter; 2019.
7. Alraiyes AH, Dhillon SS, Harris K, Kaphle U, Kheir F. Medical thoracoscopy, technique, and application. Pleura. Sage. 2016;3.
8. Wahidi MM, Unroe MA, Adlakha N, Neyea M, Shofer SL. The use of electrocautery as the primary ablation modality for malignant and benign airway obstruction. J Thorac Oncol. 2011;6:1516–20.

Return of Spontaneous Circulation Seven Times Post-cardiac Arrest

3

3.1 Case Illustration

An 80-year-old male presented with a chief complaint of breathing difficulty, which was experienced consistently for 24 hours, a day before hospital admission. The patient had to use a head pillow while sleeping to ease the difficulty. Symptoms of whole-body weakness, face paleness, and decreased appetite were also experienced, while the occurrence of fever, cough, history of seizure, and one-sided body weakness was denied.

The patient reported experiencing black stools twice daily when defecating for 5 days before admission. Instances of bloody vomiting or digestive tract bleeding were denied, while there was a history of prolonged painkiller consumption. Approximately 2.5 weeks before admission, the patient underwent herniotomy and hernioplasty with bilateral MESH surgery for bilateral inguinal hernia. After the surgery, there were no significant medical complications, such as major bleeding or hematoma. Following discharge, normal daily life activities resumed without any difficulty, and the surgical wound was tolerable.

On physical examination, the patient appeared severely ill, with symptoms of hypotension (85/62 mmHg) and high respiratory rate (30 times/min). Lung auscultation showed the presence of rough, wet crackles on both lungs and bilateral lower extremity pitting edema. In addition, laboratory examination showed various abnormalities, including low levels of hemoglobin (4.2 g/dL), declining kidney function (blood urea: 483 mg/dL; blood creatinine: 12.9 mg/dL; eGFR: 3.2 mL/min/1.73 m^2), hyperkalemia (6.3 mEq/L), high levels of procalcitonin (1.5 ng/mL), D-dimer (2100 ng/mL), hypoproteinemia (albumin: 2.7 g/dL; globulin: 1.3 g/dL), and hyperglycemia (332 mg/dL). The nasopharyngeal swab test for the presence of SARS-CoV-2 infection was shown to be negative. The presence of hepatitis B surface antigen (HBsAg), anti-hepatitis C virus (anti-HCV), and anti-human immunodeficiency virus (anti-HIV) in the blood was also negative. Chest X-ray showed cardiomegaly and bronchopneumonia, as presented in Fig. 3.1.

G. Singh, *Challenging Cases in Respirology and Critical Care*,
https://doi.org/10.1007/978-981-96-5002-6_3

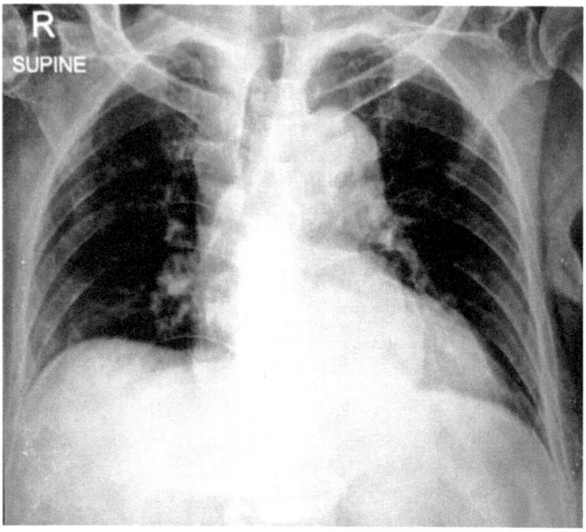

Fig. 3.1 Chest X-ray showing signs of cardiomegaly and bronchopneumonia. (Image Courtesy: Rahmad Mulyadi MD DM PhD)

Table 3.1 Management plans of the patient

Intervention	Group/type	Drugs/fluids
Medicamentosa/Fluids	Medical gas	Oxygen
	Blood products	Packed red cells
	Intravenous (IV) fluids	NaCl 0.9% Bfluid[a] Amino acids Natrium bicarbonate
	Proton pump inhibitor	Omeprazole
	Antifibrinolytic	Tranexamic acid
	Antibiotics	Azithromycin Cefuroxime
Devices/Tools	Tubes/Catheters	Nasogastric Tube (NGT) Central venous catheter (CVC)

[a]Contains electrolytes, vitamin B_1, glucose, and proteins

Based on the initial clinical and laboratory findings, the patient was diagnosed with septic shock and multiorgan dysfunction syndrome (MODS) due to severe community-acquired pneumonia (CAP), anemia, hyperglycemia, and malnutrition. Consequently, the patient was first administered oxygen, 10 lpm through a nonrebreathing mask (NRM). Several initiatives were then planned to improve the clinical condition and correct the abnormalities found on the laboratory examination, as shown in Table 3.1.

The patient was hospitalized, and a subclavian central venous catheter (CVC) was inserted the next day (first day in the hospital). Another chest X-ray examination was carried out to monitor the lung condition. The X-ray results are depicted in Fig. 3.2, showing right lung pneumothorax with the impression of the heart pressed to the left side of the thorax. On inspection and auscultation, the right thoracic wall's rise was lagging, and the right lung's sound intensity was blunted. Needle thoracocentesis and chest tube insertion (with water-sealed drainage (WSD) system) were then scheduled, but cardiac arrest was experienced during the procedures. Intubation and resuscitation efforts were then successfully performed to return the patient to a return of spontaneous circulation (ROSC) state.

After the needle thoracocentesis and chest tube insertion, the patient underwent another chest X-ray examination to observe the progress (see Fig. 3.3), and there was no sign of pneumothorax on the imaging. However, heterogeneous opacity of the right lung was found, and signs of subcutaneous emphysema were observed on the right hemithorax. The imaging results also showed the absence of changes in the other hallmarks.

On the second day in the hospital, the patient was still intubated and unconscious. The nasogastric tube (NGT) yielded reddish (presumably blood) production, leading to the administration of standard post-ROSC management protocols. On lung auscultation, bilateral rough wet crackles were still heard. The chest tube was also still installed, and expiratory bubbles were positive on the WSD system. Subsequently, blood samples were obtained for interleukin-6 (IL-6) determination, and a level of 7953 pg/mL was obtained (normal range: 3–12.5 pg/mL). Urine examination results suggested the presence of infection (cloudy appearance, leukocytes: 38–40 cells/field, erythrocytes: >70 cells/field, bacterial cells: +, leukocyte esterase: +++). The patient experienced five episodes of cardiac arrests during the day, with resuscitation attempts (by request

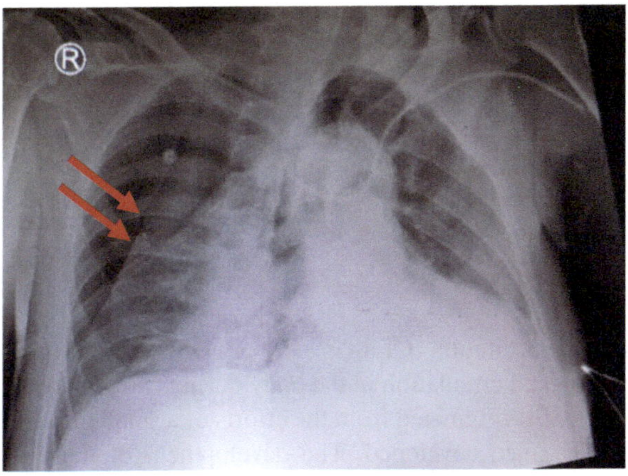

Fig. 3.2 Follow-up chest X-ray imaging, showing pneumothorax of the right lung (orange arrow) and suspected left pleural effusion. The tip of the double-lumen central venous catheter (DLCVC) was inserted into the central vein. (Image Courtesy: Sahat Matondang MD DM)

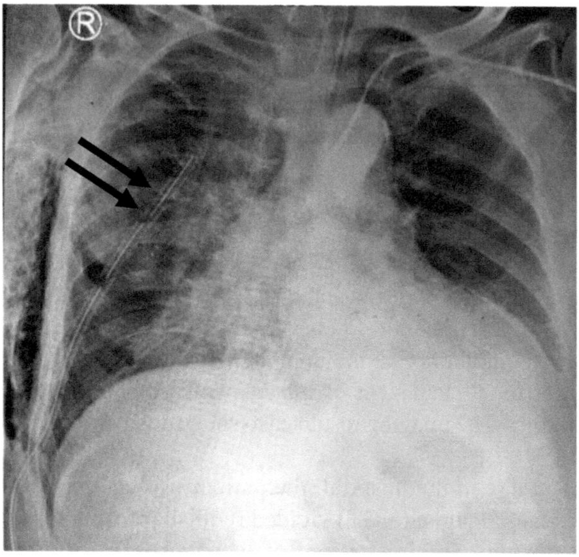

Fig. 3.3 Post-needle thoracocentesis chest X-ray examination. No sign of pneumothorax was found. Heterogeneous opacity of the right lung was found. The chest tube's tip is located at the 5th intercostal space of the posterior right hemithorax (black arrow). (Image Courtesy: Sahat Matondang MD DM)

from the patient's family) being performed each time to the ROSC state. Post-ROSC management protocols were always implemented and adjusted according to the current clinical conditions.

The next day (the third day in the hospital), the patient was still intubated, and reddish production was observed on NGT, along with black feces. The blood pressure was measured to be 73/37 despite the administration of the maximum dose of vasopressors. During the day, three additional cardiac arrests occurred, and the last arrest was not resuscitated by the family's request. The patient was finally declared dead, with the main cause identified as septic shock due to severe CAP and MODS.

3.2 Discussion

Cardiopulmonary resuscitation (CPR) is a set of medical procedures carried out to restore oxygenation and circulation in the body during cardiac arrests. The contemporary method for CPR originated from the efforts of a small group of physicians in the 1950s and has since developed. The development of the method is further explored in this discussion section. The American Heart Association (AHA) standards are widely accepted in North America. In addition, these standards are often released quinquennially following the International Liaison Committee on Resuscitation (ILCOR) conference [1].

3.3 Etiology

Annually, approximately 350,000 individuals in the United States succumb to heart disease. Among this number, 50% often experience abrupt cardiac arrests outside of a medical facility, leading to the rapid termination of organized cardiac activity. In this context, ventricular fibrillation has been reported to be the primary cause in adults. Despite ongoing advancements in emergency cardiac care, sudden cardiac arrests remain a prominent cause of mortality in various regions worldwide. In the United States, heart diseases remain the primary cause of mortality as of 2016 [2].

3.4 Epidemiology

The majority (70%) of cardiac arrests occurring outside of a medical facility typically take place in residential homes, with 50% of these events happening without any witnesses present. Despite the significant progress in emergency medical services, the rate of survival remains low. Several studies have shown that only 10.8% of adult victims of non-traumatic cardiac arrests who undergo resuscitation attempts by emergency medical personnel survive until discharge from the hospital. Meanwhile, adult patients who suffer from cardiac arrests while in a hospital have a survival rate of up to 25.5% until discharge [2].

3.5 Other Issues

Cardiopulmonary resuscitation (CPR) is an immediate medical intervention used during cardiac arrests to partially reinstate the circulation of oxygenated blood to the brain and heart. This invention was originally developed in the 1960s for post-operative care following heart surgery and has now become standard practice for all individuals undergoing cardiac arrests, except in cases of predetermined exemption. Building on this idea, several studies have investigated pre-resuscitation factors and outcomes following CPR, such as death rates, to gain a deeper understanding of the associated advantages and disadvantages [3]. However, there is a scarcity of studies examining its effects in critically ill patients who are receiving mechanical ventilation. Findings have also shown a paucity of evidence regarding the long-term survival of this specific patient cohort. Understanding these aspects is crucial for patients, families, and intensive care unit (ICU) clinicians when making decisions on CPR preferences [4, 5].

In a study conducted by Al-Alwan et al., ventilated patients in hospitals had a 52% reduced likelihood of survival compared to those who were non-ventilated. Another study was conducted in 2010 on a total of 49,656 patients who were critically ill. These patients were selected from the National Registry of Cardiopulmonary Resuscitation (NRCPR), with 24,522 being subjected to mechanical ventilation. The results showed that the survival rate until departure from the hospital was 11.2%, and the odds of survival were 0.60 when compared to those who did not receive ventilation [3]. Previous reports have also revealed that the chances of survival following in-hospital CPR are greater when CPR is administered in settings where monitoring is carried out. The discovery of unfavorable results in monitored ventilated patients was because previous reports did not limit their analysis to ventilated patients, who generally exhibited a significantly more severe state of illness compared to those who were non-ventilated. The percentage of individuals who were discharged home after receiving CPR while being ventilated and surviving until discharge was only 26.2%, while a percentage of 44.5% was recorded in the non-ventilated group. However, the findings of a previous NRCPR study differed from these figures. Building on this idea, the results revealed that 50% of critically ill patients who received CPR and survived to be discharged from the hospital were sent to an extended care facility or rehabilitation center instead of their homes. Despite the outcome, it is important to note that the previous study included ICU patients who did not need mechanical ventilation. These findings on long-term survival could also be significant data for patients and clinicians. Patients who require mechanical ventilation, undergo CPR, and manage to survive until discharge from the hospital, often have a mean survival period of only 6 months. The duration is less than one-third of the mean survival period of 19.1 months observed in those who do not require mechanical ventilation. The shorter life expectancy, along with a significant probability of spending a portion of that time in a care facility, may lead numerous patients and families to opt against CPR. A recent analysis using NRCPR data revealed that the likelihood of survival with CPR increased from 2000 to 2009 [3].

Another study showed that patients suffering from several chronic conditions, including congestive heart failure (CHF), chronic obstructive pulmonary disease (COPD), chronic kidney disease (CKD), cirrhosis, diabetes, and cancer, experienced considerably reduced long-term survival after surviving CPR and being discharged from the hospital. Individuals who have severe CHF, any level of COPD, malignancy, or cirrhosis with CPR while in the hospital, experience reduced chances of surviving their hospital stay compared to others without the chronic conditions. Patients who have undergone CPR and have pre-existing conditions, such as COPD, CHF, and diabetes, have a significantly lower probability of being returned to their homes and are more prone to have recurrent hospitalizations following the procedure [6].

Key Points

Individuals who after receiving CPR while being ventilated and have pre-existing conditions such as COPD, CHF, and diabetes have a significantly lower probability of being returned to their homes and are more prone to have recurrent hospitalizations following CPR. Having this knowledge is crucial for making decisions on CPR preferences.

Questions

1. What organ is targeted in cardiopulmonary resuscitation?
   (a) Brain
   (b) Skeletal
   (c) Skin
   (d) Ren
   (e) Gaster
2. What is the most common cause of sudden cardiac arrest in adults?
   (a) SVT
   (b) Atrial Fibrillation
   (c) Atrial Tachycardia
   (d) AV block
   (e) Ventricular Fibrillation
3. These chronic diseases have significantly shorter long-term survival after in-hospital CPR, except?
   (a) CHF
   (b) Diabetes
   (c) Malignancy
   (d) CKD
   (e) Pneumonia
4. In cardiopulmonary resuscitation, which of the following has the highest survival rate?
   (a) At home
   (b) In out of hospital
   (c) Hospital setting
   (d) Hospital setting on ventilated
   (e) Hospital setting without ventilated
5. The survival rate of adult patients who received CPR during cardiac arrest is:
   (a) 25.5%
   (b) 10.8%
   (c) 11.2%
   (d) 70%
   (e) 52%

Answer Keys

1. A
2. E
3. C
4. E
5. B

Acknowledgments Cipta Mahendra, MD, Department of Internal Medicine, Respirology and Critical Illness Division, Universitas Indonesia, Dr. Cipto Mangunkusumo General Central National Hospital, Jakarta, Indonesia.

Ersananda Arlisa Putri, MD, Department of Internal Medicine, Respirology and Critical Illness Division, Universitas Indonesia, Dr. Cipto Mangunkusumo General Central National Hospital, Jakarta, Indonesia.
Jordan Sardjan, MD, Department of Internal Medicine, Universitas Indonesia, Dr. Cipto Mangunkusumo General Central National Hospital, Jakarta, Indonesia.
Sidharta Kusuma Manggala, MD, Department of Anesthesiology and Intensive Care, Universitas Indonesia, Dr. Cipto Mangunkusumo General Central National Hospital, Jakarta, Indonesia.

References

1. Chan PS, Tang Y, American Heart Association's Get With the Guidelines®-Resuscitation Investigators (2020) Risk-standardizing rates of return of spontaneous circulation for in-hospital cardiac arrest to facilitate hospital comparisons. J Am Heart Assoc.9(7):e014837
2. Goyal A, Sciammarella JC, Cusick AS, Patel PH. Cardiopulmonary resuscitation. 2023. Dalam: StatPearls [Internet]. In: StatPearls Publ. http://www.ncbi.nlm.nih.gov/books/NBK470402/. Accessed 25 Dec 2023.
3. Al-Alwan A, Ehlenbach WJ, Menon PR, Young MP, Stapleton RD. Cardiopulmonary resuscitation among mechanically ventilated patients. Intensive Care Med. 2014;40:556. https://doi.org/10.1007/s00134-014-3247-2.
4. Jentzer J, Callaway C. Cardiopulmonary resuscitation and critical care after cardiac arrest. Cardiac Intensive Care. 2019;2019:558–579.e6.
5. Teixeira C, Cardoso PRC. How to discuss about do-not-resuscitate in the intensive care unit? Rev Bras Ter Intensiva. 2019;31:386–92.
6. Stapleton RD, Ehlenbach WJ, Deyo RA, Curtis J. Long-term outcomes after in-hospital CPR in older adults with chronic illness. Chest Novemb. 2014;146:1214–25.

4 BALF CD-4 Cell Count in Critical COVID-19

4.1 Case Illustration

A 96-year-old male presented to the hospital with a chief complaint of breathing difficulty for six days before admission. The complaint was accompanied by undulating fever, thick sputum, and decreased appetite. The patient was swabbed before admission for the presence of severe acute respiratory syndrome-coronavirus-2 (SARS-CoV-2) infection, with the results indicating a positive status. A sputum sample was also collected for Gram staining, and the result was positive for the presence of fungus. On the admission day, there was still a complaint of breathing difficulty, and the blood oxygen saturation (SpO_2) was measured at 92–95% in room air using a personal pulse oximeter. A history of controlled hypertension was established, with COVID-19 being contracted from the patient's wife.

The patient underwent comprehensive laboratory (see Table 4.1) and chest X-ray examination (see Fig. 4.1). The chest X-ray imaging revealed massive infiltrations in both lung fields, along with fibrotic lesions on the middle field of the right lung. In addition, signs of emphysema were observed after being assessed. On physical examinations, the patient was conscious, and the airway appeared clear without any obstruction. The vitals were within normal limits (afebrile) but required oxygen supplementation at 3 lpm through a nasal cannula. Based on the initial clinical, laboratory, and radiological findings, a diagnosis of severe COVID-19 was established.

After the examination, the patient was admitted to an isolation ward for COVID-19 patients. The most recent regimen of antiviruses for the disease, along with antibiotics and antifungals, was administered. Supportive treatments were also administered, including intravenous (IV) fluids, anti-inflammatory drugs, vitamins, human albumin, and oxygen supplementation. In addition, anticoagulants were given to reduce the risk of blood coagulation, followed by the insertion of a nasogastric tube (NGT) and urinary catheter.

G. Singh, *Challenging Cases in Respirology and Critical Care*,
https://doi.org/10.1007/978-981-96-5002-6_4

Table 4.1 The patient's initial (first day of admission) laboratory blood test results

Parameters			Results	References	Units
Blood gas analysis	pH		**7.523**	7.350–7.450	
	pCO_2		38.80	35.00–45.00	mmHg
	pO_2		89.80	83.00–108.00	mmHg
	HCO_3		**32.20**	21.00–25.00	mmol/L
Complete peripheral blood	Hemoglobin		**11.7**	13.0–17.0	g/dL
	Hematocrit		**34.0**	40.0–50.0	%
	Erythrocyte		**3.76**	4.50–5.50	$10^6/\mu L$
	Thrombocyte		393	150–410	$10^3/\mu L$
	Leukocyte		**10.09**	4.00–10.00	$10^3/\mu L$
	Differential count	Basophil	0.1	0–2	%
		Eosinophil	**0.0**	1–6	
		Neutrophil	**88.4**	40.0–80.0	
		Lymphocyte	**7.4**	20–40	
		Monocyte	4.1	2–10	
Liver function	AST		**40**	5.00–34.00	U/L
	ALT		35	0.00–55.00	U/L
Kidney function	eGFR		**84.9**	35–81	mL/min/$1.73m^2$
	Creatinine		**0.60**	0.73–1.18	mg/dL
	Urea		32.1	18–55	mg/dL
Glucose	Random glucose test		101	60–140	mg/dL
Proteins	Albumin		**2.7**	2.90–4.50	g/dL
Electrolytes	Natrium		**135**	136–145	mEq/L
	Potassium		**3.1**	3.5–5.1	mEq/L
	Chloride		**96.8**	98.0–107.0	mEq/L
	Magnesium		1.7	1.60–2.60	mg/dL
	Calcium		1.13	1.01–1.31	mmol/L
Coagulation studies	Prothrombin time (PT)		11.0	9.8–12.6	seconds
	Activated partial thromboplastin test (APTT)		**53.9**	31.0–47.0	seconds
	Fibrinogen		371.0	200.0–400.0	mg/dL
	d-dimer		**910**	<440	µg/L
Infection marker	Procalcitonin		**0.09**	<0.05	ng/mL
	C-reactive protein (CRP)		**46.9**	<5.0	mg/L
Covid-19 infection	SARS-CoV-2		**Positive**	Negative	

Bolded numbers indicate out-of-reference values

On the third day after hospitalization, the patient underwent another chest X-ray examination (see Fig. 4.2, box A) and laboratory test (see Table 4.2). Compared to the previous X-ray image, infiltrates on both lungs were reduced, and all the other hallmarks were in status quo. The results also showed that the leukocyte count was elevated ($15.63 \times 10^3/\mu L$) compared to the initial count, as shown in Table 4.1. However, a decrease in percentage (4.7%) was found in the differential blood count for lymphocytes, compared to the initial value of 7.4%, along with a concomitant increase in neutrophil percentage.

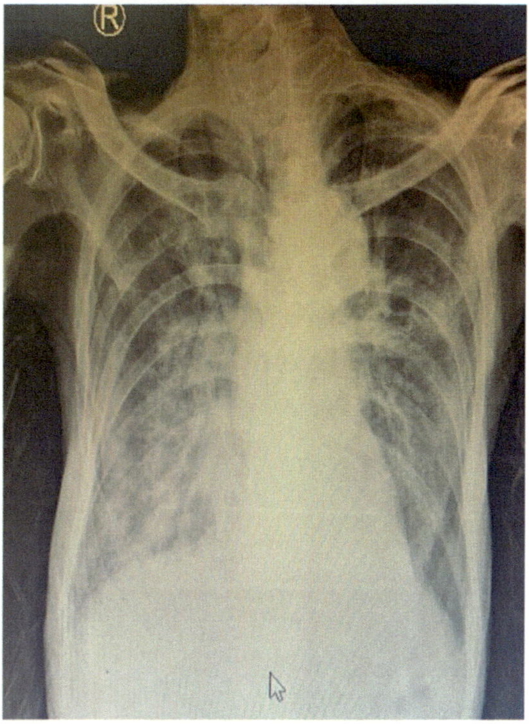

Fig. 4.1 Chest X-ray image on initial hospital admission. Bilateral infiltrates are observed. Fibrosis is in the middle region of the right lung. Both lung fields are emphysematous. (Image Courtesy: Mohamad Yanuar Amal MD)

Around the 6th–7th day of hospitalization, chest X-ray imaging (Fig. 4.2, box B) revealed signs of blunted costophrenic angle and thickened pleural layers, suggesting pleural effusion. Other hallmarks were in status quo compared to the previous third day's examination. The patient was tested for interleukin-6 (IL-6) level, with the results showing a value of 245.5 (reference: 3.12–12.50 pg/mL). The leukocyte count reduced (11.91 × 10^3/μL), but the lymphocyte percentage increased slightly (5.7%). However, the patient complained of strenuous breathing and showed gestures to remove the inserted NGT from the nostril, leading to the increment of oxygen supplementation to 8 lpm. The pleural effusion was sampled and cultured to examine any sign of bacterial growth presence. The result turned negative, including for the presence of mycobacterial infection.

The patient's clinical conditions remained stable over the following days. Follow-up laboratory tests showed a consistent increase in leukocyte count, but the lymphocyte percentage decreased. On the 12th–13th day, the leukocyte count reached 26.40 × 10^3/μ, while the lymphocyte count was suppressed to 2.8%. Subsequently, the serum CD4 (a subset of lymphocytes) absolute count was assessed, and the results yielded 257 (reference: 410–1590 cells/μL). A chest CT scan examination was also performed to monitor the lungs (Fig. 4.3). Consolidations, multifocal ground glass opacity (GGO), and thickening of the interlobular septa were seen on both lungs. Bilateral pleural effusion was observed on the CT imaging, leading to the scheduling of a chest tube insertion procedure to drain the effusions.

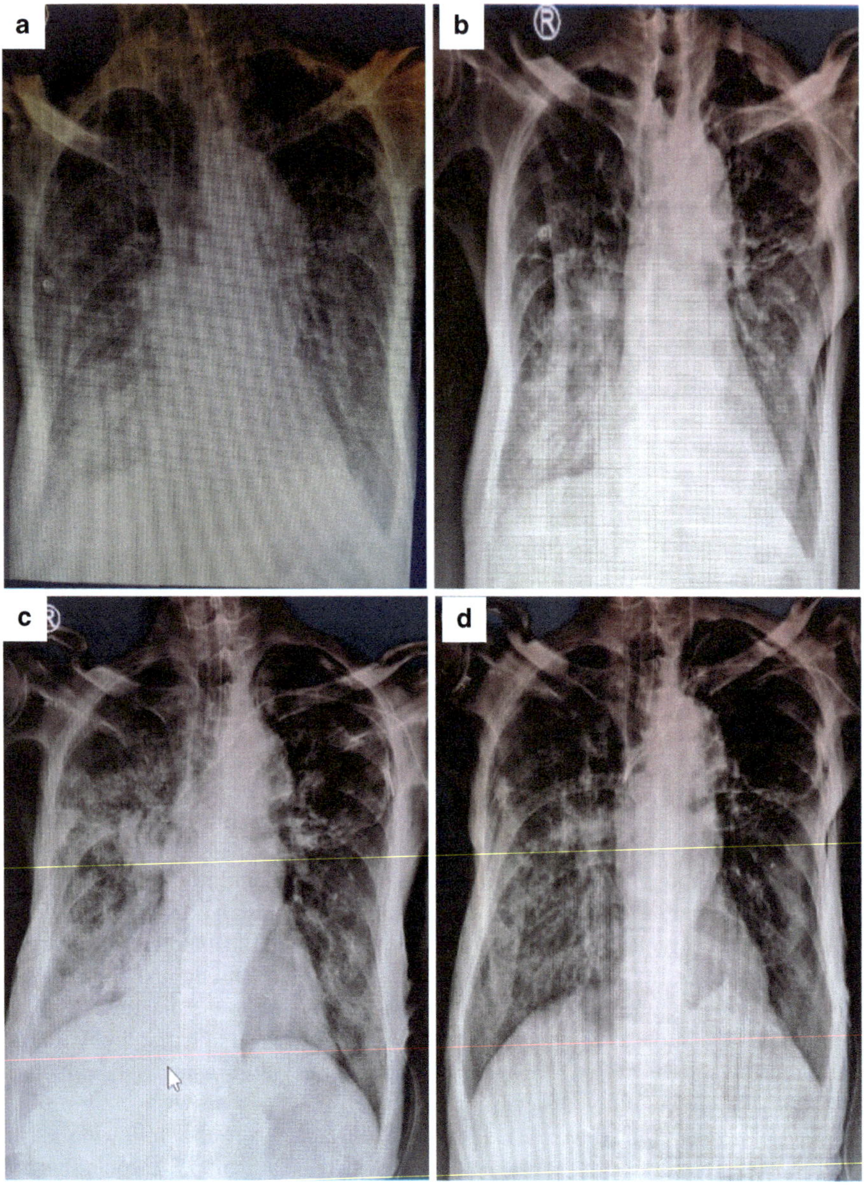

Fig. 4.2 The patient's serial chest X-ray examinations, which were undertaken on the (**A**) 3rd, (**B**) 6th–7th, (**C**) 14th–15th, and (**D**) 18th day. See texts for details. (Image Courtesy: Rahmad Mulyadi MD DM PhD, Sahat Matondang MD DM)

Table 4.2 The patient's serial laboratory test results

Parameters Day since admission		3rd	6th–7th	12th–13th	14th–15th	17th	18th	19th
Leukocytes ($10^3/\mu L$)		15.63	11.91	26.40	31.81	30.34	23.01	19.68
Differential count (%)	Basophil	0.1	0.2	0.2	0.3	0.3	0.2	0.1
	Eosinophil	0	0	0	0.1	0.4	0	0
	Neutrophil	90.7	88.6	90.2	95.1	93.1	88.8	91.0
	Lymphocyte	4.7	5.7	28	0.8	1.1	2.4	2.6
	Monocyte	4.5	5.5	6.8	3.7	5.1	8.6	6.3
Absolute CD4 count (cells/μL)		–	–	257[a]	–	15[b]	–	–
IL-6 (pg/mL)		–	245.5	–	463	–	–	–

IL interleukin, *CD* cluster of differentiation
[a]Obtained from blood serum
[b]Obtained from the bronchoalveolar lavage of the patient's right lung

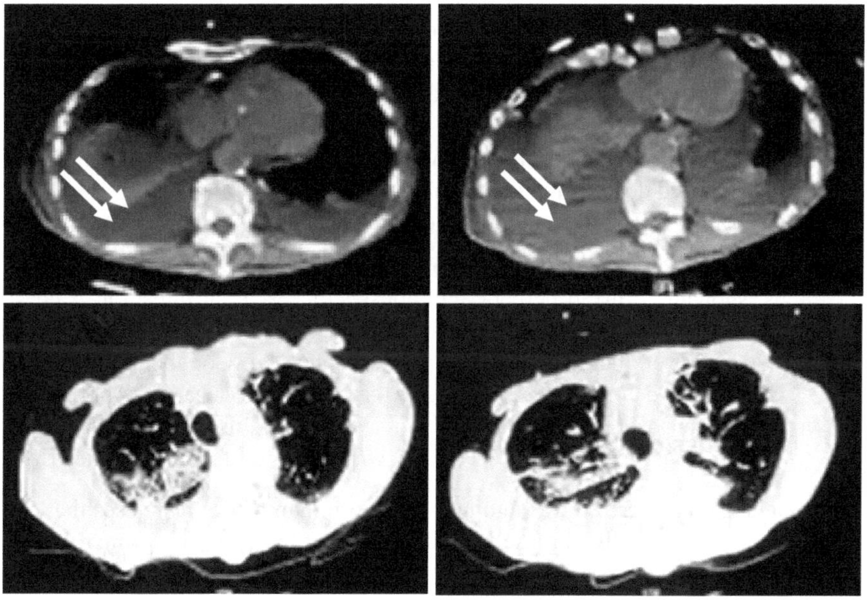

Fig. 4.3 The patient's chest CT scan imaging on the 12th–13th day since hospitalization. Massive effusions had infiltrated most of the patient's lungs, mainly in the right lung. (Image Courtesy: Vally Wulani MD DM)

In the next days (14th–15th day), the procedure was performed and connected to a water-sealed drainage (WSD) system. The post-procedure chest X-ray imaging (Fig. 4.2, box C) showed decreased effusion, but the other hallmarks were unchanged. In addition, subcutaneous emphysema was no longer observed in the patient. Another follow-up laboratory test revealed an IL-6 level of 463 pg/mL (Table 4.2). The leukocyte count was further increased to $31.81 \times 10^3/\mu L$, while the lymphocyte percentage decreased to only 0.8%. The differential blood count shifted to almost consist of only neutrophils (95.1%) (see Table 4.2).

On the 17th day, the patient showed signs of clinical deterioration, with hemodynamics being unstable, leading to the administration of vasopressors. Signs of decreased consciousness (agitation, incomprehensible words) were also observed, and intubation was performed to secure the airway. In addition, a ventilator was installed to support the breathing effort. The results showed that the leukocyte count was slightly decreased to 30.34 × 10^3/μL, and the lymphocyte percentage was also slightly increased to 1.1%. A bronchoalveolar lavage (BAL) procedure was performed. The CD4 absolute cell count from the severely affected right lung was ordered, and a result of 15 cells/μL was obtained.

The next day (18th day), the patient underwent another follow-up chest X-ray examination and laboratory test. Compared to the last imaging, there was a significant decrease in lung opacity (Fig. 4.2, box D). The leukocyte count was also decreased to 23.01 × 10^3/μL, and the lymphocyte percentage was increased to 2.4%. Despite the improvements, hemodynamics were further destabilized, leading to an increase in vasopressor doses to maintain the clinical status. The patient's awareness was under the influence of the given sedation. Subsequently, the family was consulted about the present conditions and decided to taper off the vasopressors and withdraw the ventilator support, with a do-not-resuscitate (DNR) permission granted. The patient's vitals continued to deteriorate after the discontinuation and was finally declared dead on the late 19th day.

The last follow-up laboratory test was ordered on the early 19th day and the leukocyte count had decreased to 19.68 × 10^3/μL, but the lymphocyte count (2.6%; see Table 4.2) was relatively similar to that of the previous day (2.4%). During the treatments, the swab tests for the presence of the SARS-CoV-2 virus were always positive.

4.2 Discussion

Pneumonia is characterized by ongoing localized inflammatory responses that can worsen the severity of the disease by failing to limit the invasion of microbes. A thorough understanding of local inflammation can aid in comprehending the local host's reaction to microbes. According to previous reports, there was a significant increase in the incidence of viral pneumonia cases during the COVID-19 pandemic. Dysregulation of the immune response in COVID-19 can impede viral clearance and hinder healing. A considerable proportion of patients suffering from severe COVID-19 pneumonia encountered acute respiratory failure, leading to their admission to the intensive care unit (ICU), with approximately 80% requiring mechanical ventilation. These individuals exhibit great complexity due to the involvement of multiple organs and the dynamic progression of the condition. In this context, several studies have examined comorbidities, clinical scoring systems, and laboratory profiles as means of assessing disease severity, determining the need for ICU admission, mechanical ventilation, and predicting mortality. However, there is limited data about the local immunopathology responses associated with the increased utilization of the mechanical ventilator. This indicates that enhancing knowledge of the clinical features and immunopathology of bronchoalveolar lavage fluid (BALF) in both severely and less severely afflicted lungs can potentially lead to better outcomes for patients with severe COVID-19 pneumonia. In addition, it is necessary to examine the local inflammatory biomarkers in the lung to assess the extent of damage and identify the factors contributing to death [1].

4.3 Critical Covid-19

Individuals infected with SARS-CoV-2 may exhibit various clinical manifestations, ranging from asymptomatic to severe disease. Adults who have contracted SARS-CoV-2 can typically be classified into different categories based on the severity of their condition. Building on this idea, severe COVID-19 is characterized by respiratory failure, septic shock, and/or multiple organ dysfunction, with a mortality rate among critically ill patients. The integration of IL-6 and D-dimer in the model proved to be highly beneficial in accurately forecasting the mortality rate, demonstrating exceptional performance. In addition, other signs, such as the CD4 cell count, must be assessed. This chapter examines the relationships between CD4 cell count and mortality rate in critical cases of COVID-19 [2].

4.4 Viral Activation of Immunity

The presence of immunity against viral infections is attributed to a range of distinct and non-selective processes. The immune response is influenced by the virus's interaction with host cells, which can be categorized as cytolytic, steady-state, latent, or integrated infections. In addition, the spread of the virus, whether local, primary hematogenous, secondary hematogenous, or through the nervous system, also affects the activation of immune functions and the duration and strength of response. This indicates that viral antigens can be found in several regions, contingent upon the method of transmission and stage of infection. Several studies have shown that infection occurring at surfaces, such as the mucosa, can trigger immune responses that are specific to the affected area, involving both cell-mediated and humoral (IgA) mechanisms. However, these responses may not necessarily confer immunity throughout the entire body. The host possesses several immune defense mechanisms capable of eradicating viruses and/or viral diseases [3].

In line with previous reports, humoral immunity refers to the immune response triggered by viruses or virus-infected cells, which stimulates B lymphocytes to produce antibodies specific to viral antigens. The effectiveness of antibody neutralization is high when the virus is present in abundant liquid areas, such as serum, or on damp surfaces, including the gastrointestinal and respiratory tracts. Antiviral activity has also been demonstrated for IgG, IgM, and IgA. Antibodies can kill viruses through two mechanisms: firstly, by obstructing the contact between the viruses and the host cell, and secondly, by identifying viral antigens on cells that have been infected. This identification can trigger antibody-dependent cytotoxic cells (ADCC) or complement-mediated lysis. IgG antibodies exhibit the primary antiviral function in serum, while IgA plays an essential role in combating viral infections on mucosal surfaces [3].

Cell-mediated immunity comprises the process by which leukocytes recognize and eliminate viruses and virus-infected cells. These cells typically produce various soluble factors known as cytokines when stimulated. Cytotoxic T lymphocytes, natural killer (NK) cells, and antiviral macrophages have been reported to possess the ability to identify and eliminate cells infected by viruses. In this context, helper T cells can identify cells that have been infected by a virus and generate various crucial cytokines. Monocytes, T cells, and NK cells create cytokines known as monokines and lymphokines, which have essential roles in regulating immune activities and creating antiviral immune responses [3].

4.5 Immune Responses in COVID-19

The role of immune cells (innate and adaptive immune) in the anti-SARS-CoV-2 response has increasingly been recognized [4].

4.6 Innate Immune Responses in COVID-19

4.6.1 Monocyte/Macrophage

Macrophages are myeloid immune cells that have a role in both inflammation and tissue repair. Several studies have shown that these cells in the lungs are categorized as either alveolar or interstitial. Alveolar macrophages are mainly located near type I and type II alveolar epithelial cells, whereas interstitial macrophages are primarily situated within the region between the microvascular endothelium and the alveolar epithelium. In this context, activated macrophages operate as the initial defense against infections and other substances that enter the lungs. Several studies have shown that those with a short lifespan can restrict the virus's ability to reproduce. However, when these cells transform into long-lived variants, there is a high probability of becoming infected and remaining in the body [4].

After SARS-CoV-2 infection, macrophages exhibited intensified pro-inflammatory activity, characterized by increased production of inflammatory cytokines such as IL-1β and IL-6, as well as chemokines like CXCL10. The highest levels of IFN-I production were observed in cells located near areas of endothelial cell injury. This IFN-I production may be driven by stimulator of interferon genes (STING)-induced synthesis and the release of mitochondrial DNA (mtDNA) from adjacent endothelial cells. The elevated presence of these pro-inflammatory substances can contribute to the onset of a cytokine storm, a condition linked to poor outcomes in COVID-19 [4].

4.6.2 Dendritic Cell

In severe cases of COVID-19, plasmacytoid dendritic cells (pDCs), which are crucial for antiviral immune response, showed heightened activation of pathways promoting cell death compared to those in moderate cases. This phenomenon is often accompanied by a reduction in the expression of antiviral interferon-stimulated genes (ISGs) and innate immune sensors, such as TLR9, IFNAR, and DHX36. Plasmacytoid dendritic cells (pDCs), which are major producers of IFN-I, may surpass other immune or infected cells in IFN-I production. Furthermore, the infiltration of pDCs, which recognize the presence of SARS-CoV-2, has been positively correlated with increased IFN-I production.

This process contributes to the macrophage-driven cytokine storm in the lungs of COVID-19 patients, potentially exacerbating inflammation. The detection of SARS-CoV-2 by plasmacytoid dendritic cells (pDCs) via TLR7 triggers the production of IFN-α, which induces transcriptional and epigenetic changes in macrophages. These changes heighten the responsiveness of macrophages to environmental stimuli, leading to their hyperactivation. In severe COVID-19 cases, compared to moderate cases, patients exhibited a reduced interferon (IFN) signature and decreased MHC II expression in conventional dendritic cells (cDCs), countering pro-inflammatory pathways. Further investigation revealed that this reduction was linked to lower levels of MHC II regulators, including RFX5, RFXANK, and CIITA, in severe cases. The suppression of antigen presentation by the virus may clarify the worsening of the disease in extreme case and offer new opportunities to enhance the impaired antiviral immune response [4].

4.6.3 Natural Killer Cells

Natural killer (NK) cells from healthy individuals typically exhibit robust antiviral properties, as demonstrated by the reduced levels of SARS-CoV-2 proteins in infected cells co-cultured with these NK cells. Previous studies have shown that NK cells not only exert antiviral effects but also possess antifibrotic activity, reducing the expression of profibrotic genes such as COL1A1 and ACTA2 in lung fibroblasts. However, compared to healthy individuals, COVID-19 patients display NK cells with diminished antiviral efficacy and signs of exhaustion.

COVID-19-related NK cells exhibit a genetic profile that closely resembles those found in the lungs of individuals with pulmonary fibrosis. This is accompanied by a reduced capacity to inhibit the expression of genes that promote fibrosis in lung fibroblasts. IFN-α, a crucial molecule in fighting against viruses, inhibited the generation of IFN-γ by NK cells. However, blocking the effects of IFN-α did not restore their activity [4].

Building on the idea, restoring the diminished antiviral and antifibrotic functions of NK cells in individuals with COVID-19 shows potential as a therapeutic approach against SAR-CoV-2. The initiation of immunity against viral infection mostly occurs through the identification of pattern recognition receptors (PRRs) that are extensively present in various immune and non-immune cells. Activation of PRRs initiates the synthesis of type I/III interferons (IFNs) and pro-inflammatory cytokines, which in turn, stimulate the transcription of interferon-stimulated genes (ISGs) to limit viral infection [4].

4.7 Adaptive Responses to SARS-CoV-2

The primary methods for preserving patients following SARS-CoV-2 infection include the virus-specific cellular and humoral responses. Several studies have shown that the adaptive immune system plays a crucial role in regulating the majority of viral infections. The adaptive immune responses elicited by SARS-CoV-2 are presented below [4].

4.7.1 $CD4^+$ T Cell

Various subsets of CD4+ T cells can have either advantageous or deleterious effects on the advancement of COVID-19. Individuals with severe COVID-19 typically have concurrent presence of highly activated, functional, and functionally exhausted CD4+ T cells. Previous studies showed that 83% of CD4+ T cells in individuals with COVID-19 exhibited reactivity to both the N and C terminus of the S protein. Consequently, there has been a heightened interest in investigating immune responses targeted specifically at the S protein of the virus, including the development of T-cell-responsive COVID-19 vaccines. CD4+ T cells that specifically target SARS-CoV-2 were found to be linked to improved severity of the disease. The development of these SARS-CoV-2-specific CD4+ T cells was also found to be related to a quick reduction in viral load [4].

4.7.1.1 Th1, Th2, and Th17 Cells

The imbalance between T helper type 1 (Th1) and T helper type 2 (Th2) cells has been widely investigated in both COVID-19 patients and high-risk uninfected individuals.

COVID-19 patients, as observed in a study, exhibit a decreased proportion of Th1 and Th17 cells and an increased proportion of activated Th2 cells compared to the control group. In addition, there is a greater percentage of senescent (PD1+/ICOS-) Th2 cells in deceased patients compared to those who survived. Through the assessment of the correlation between Th subsets and mortality, both the overall lymphocyte count and the elevated proportion of senescent Th2 cells are distinct and significant characteristics that contribute to the risk of death. During the recovery stage, the proportion of both Th1 and Th2 cells in patients was lower compared to healthy controls. Therefore, the fluctuating transformation of these cells could serve as a means to track the progression of the disease. Th17 cells have crucial functions in causing tissue damage and excessive inflammation through the release of interleukin-17 (IL-17) and IL-23.

A recent study showed a strong correlation between the expression of IL-17A and the severity of the disease. Other studies have indicated that a systemic neutrophil environment may have a preference for influencing CD4+ T cells toward Th17 and IL-17A promotion, which in turn, worsens inflammation. The findings of another study corroborated this phenomenon, with further experiments revealing that the activation of Th17 cells can be mitigated by inhibitors targeting arginase-1 (Arg-1), nitric oxide synthase (NOS), and reactive oxygen species (ROS), all of which are produced by myeloid cells in response to oxidative stress. Consequently, therapeutic strategies aimed at modulating Th17 activity and inhibiting IL-17 signaling holds promise for managing COVID-19 patients, particularly those experiencing cytokine storm syndrome, to achieve clinical benefits [4].

4.7.1.2 Tfh Cells

Among the various subsets of CD4+ T helper (Th) cells, follicular helper T (Tfh) cells are essential for humoral immunity, facilitating interactions with B cells in germinal centers (GC). These interactions drive the differentiation of B cells into plasma cells capable of producing high-affinity neutralizing antibodies. Studies have reported an absence of GC structures in the thoracic lymph nodes and spleens of COVID-19 patients, along with a marked reduction in Bcl-6+ GC B cells in these organs. The decline in CD4 + CXCR5 + Bcl-6+ GC Tfh cells may explain the loss of germinal centers and the accumulation of activated B cells originating outside these structures. In contrast, SARS-CoV-2 infection has been shown to increase peripheral CD4+ Tfh cells and germinal center responses in rhesus macaques. Additionally, convalescent individuals who experienced severe COVID-19 exhibited elevated levels of peripheral Tfh cells in clinical evaluations. Tfh cells have also been reported to have the potential to expedite the advancement of the disease in some instances, along with their aforementioned preventive functions. Compared to COVID-19 patients who were not hospitalized, severe cases exhibited an increase in the amounts of cytotoxic Tfh cells, which showed an increment in the expression of IFN-γ, IL-2, and TNF-α. An observational study revealed that CCR4+ and CCR6+ Tfh cells had the potential to cause harm to affected individuals [4].

4.7.1.3 Treg Cells

Regulatory T cells (Tregs) are essential for maintaining immunological balance by using several pathways, making their role vital in these processes. Flow cytometric analysis revealed an increased proportion of regulatory T cells (Tregs) within peripheral blood mononuclear cells (PBMCs), accompanied by enhanced FoxP3 expression, which was associated with a poorer prognosis. In this context, COVID-19 patients with acute respiratory distress syndrome (ARDS)—a condition characterized by severe lung inflammation and reduced oxygen levels—exhibited notable alterations in immune cell populations. Specifically, the numbers of CD4+ and CD8+ T cells were diminished, while the proportion of Tregs was elevated in both the lungs and PBMCs [4].

4.7.2 CD8⁺ T Cells

According to several reports, the presence of SARS-CoV-2-specific CD8+ T-cell responses could be linked to the severity of the disease in the early stage, and a lower count of these cells had been detected in severe cases. For instance, a study proposed that inadequate CD8+ T-cell responses, despite elevated antibody levels, could potentially contribute to the development of acute COVID-19. Prior to SARS-CoV-2 infection, the depletion of CD8+ T cells in vaccinated macaques resulted in higher peak viral loads on day 4 in both the upper and lower respiratory tracts. In individuals with COVID-19, CD8+ T cells displayed elevated secretion of IL-2 and IL-17, along with increased expression of the degranulation marker CD107a upon stimulation with anti-CD3/CD28, compared to healthy individuals.

Compared to the previous findings, other studies have indicated that CD8+ T cells from individuals with COVID-19 showed a reduced ability to produce cytokines. Severe COVID-19 patients have been found to have circulating CD8+ T cells exhibiting signs of exhaustion, as indicated by elevated levels of PD-1, TIM-3, LAG-3, CTLA-4, NKG2A, and CD39. Additionally, there is a reverse correlation between the expression of PD-1 and CD38, a marker of T cell activation, in CD8+ T cells. Accumulated evidence shows that PD-1 expression in CD8+ T cells is significantly increased in COVID-19 patients, particularly in those requiring intensive care unit (ICU) admission.

A recent study also found that SARS-CoV-2-specific CD8 + PD-1+ T cells produced higher levels of IFN-γ compared to PD-1-negative populations, independent of the severity of the disease. This suggests that SARS-CoV-2-specific CD8 + PD-1+ T cells are in a functional condition [4].

4.7.3 B Cells

Studies have indicated changes in the subgroups of B cells in individuals with COVID-19, namely in the categories of immature or fully developed cells. In severe and catastrophic cases, there appears to be a modest increase in the frequencies of CD19+ B cells in PBMCs, when compared to healthy individuals. The CD27-IgD- fraction, also known as the double negative (DN) fraction, is a subset of B cells that exhibit notable changes in COVID-19. In addition, the distributions of DN1 (CD21 + CD11c−), DN2 (CD21-CD11c+), and DN3 (CD21− CD11c−) subgroups varied depending on the severity of the disease. Building on this idea, DN1 B cells exhibited a significant decrease in severe and critical patients, while DN2 showed an increase in severe cases compared to mild/moderate and critical cases. The results also revealed that DN3 B cells showed a substantial increase with increasing severity. Furthermore, a significant association was observed between immature, activated naïve B cells and the percentage of DN3 cells with ventilatory parameters, such as respiratory rate, SpO_2, and $PaO2/FiO_2$. A separate study revealed a similar effect involving DN2 B cells in individuals with acute COVID-19 [4].

4.8 BALF CD4 Cell Count as Biomarkers in Critical COVID-19

Biomarkers have been proposed to assist doctors in evaluating the likelihood of mortality and guiding management decisions. The intensity of inflammation in severe cases of COVID-19 is correlated with a decreased count of CD4 T-cells in the bronchoalveolar lavage fluid (BALF). During the process of severe inflammation, CD4 T-cells undergo differentiation into other subsets, such as Tregs. Increased levels of proinflammatory cytokines were detected in both the BALF and plasma of individuals with acute respiratory distress syndrome (ARDS). COVID-19-related ARDS is a characteristic form of ARDS that mostly affects the lungs. The defining characteristic of severe ARDS caused by COVID-19 is a cytokine storm, which occurs due to uncontrolled and imbalanced inflammatory reactions. Meanwhile, the release of proinflammatory substances into the bloodstream can perpetuate and intensify the inflammatory reaction, leading to significant damage to several organs. In this context, endothelial cells play a role in the development of both ARDS and extrapulmonary organ dysfunction, potentially by causing systemic endotheliitis characterized by the presence of inflammatory cells and apoptotic bodies in different tissues and organs. In severe cases of COVID-19, there is widespread inflammation of the endothelial cells lining the blood vessels. This inflammation disrupts the integrity of the artery barrier and promotes a state where blood clots more easily. The condition also contributes to the accumulation of fluid in tissues (edema) and reduced blood flow to organs (ischemia). These effects lead to changes in the structure and function of tissues (histopathologic alterations) and can cause difficulties throughout the body (systemic consequences) [5]. A study conducted by Saris et al. investigated the levels of BALF CD4 T-cells in severe COVID-19 pneumonia patients. The results revealed that non-survivors had lower levels of BALF CD4 T-cells compared to the survivor group [6].

Key Points

Biomarkers have been proposed to evaluate the likelihood of mortality and guiding management decisions. *A low CD4 cell count in bronchoalveolar lavage fluid (BALF) is linked to higher rates of extubation failure and increased mortality in critically ill COVID-19 patients.*

Questions

1. Criteria of critical COVID-19:
   (a) Respiratory failure, septic shock, and/or multiple organ dysfunction
   (b) Respiratory failure, septic shock, without multiple organ dysfunction
   (c) ARDS, septic shock, prolonged fever, without multiple organ dysfunction
   (d) ARDS, septic shock, without multiple organ dysfunction
   (e) ARDS, septic shock, and/or multiple organ dysfunction

2. The following is a mortality prediction factor in COVID-19:
   (a) Th1
   (b) Th2
   (c) IFN 1
   (d) IL-17
   (e) D-Dimer
3. The following are the adaptive responses of SARS-COV-2, except:
   (a) $CD8^+$ T cells
   (b) $CD4^+$ T cells
   (c) B Cells
   (d) Treg Cells
   (e) Dendritic Cells
4. What local inflammatory biomarker of the lung is required to measure the severity and mortality of lung injury?
   (a) IFN-α
   (b) IL16
   (c) D-Dimer
   (d) PD-1
   (e) $CD4^+$ Cell Count
5. In Covid-19 patients, which $CD8^+$ T cells exhibit enhanced production?
   (a) IL-6 and D-Dimer
   (b) IFN-γ, IL-2, and TNF-α
   (c) IL-2, IL-17, and the expression of degranulation marker CD107
   (d) DN1 ($CD21^+CD11c^-$), DN2 ($CD21^-CD11c^+$), and DN3 ($CD21^-CD11c^-$)
   (e) PD-1, TIM-3, LAG-3, CTLA-4, NKG2A, and CD39

Answer Keys

1. A
2. E
3. E
4. E
5. C

Acknowledgments Cipta Mahendra, MD, Department of Internal Medicine, Respirology and Critical Illness Division, Universitas Indonesia, Dr. Cipto Mangunkusumo General Central National Hospital, Jakarta, Indonesia.

Ersananda Arlisa, Putri MD, Department of Internal Medicine, Respirology and Critical Illness Division, Universitas Indonesia, Dr. Cipto Mangunkusumo General Central National Hospital, Jakarta, Indonesia.

Dita Aditianingsih, MD, PhD, Department of Anesthesiology, Universitas Indonesia, Dr. Cipto Mangunkusumo General Central National Hospital, Jakarta, Indonesia.

Adhrie Sugiarto, MD, PhD, Department of Anesthesiology, Universitas Indonesia, Dr. Cipto Mangunkusumo General Central National Hospital, Jakarta, Indonesia.

Sidharta Kusuma Manggala MD, Department of Anesthesiology, Universitas Indonesia, Dr. Cipto Mangunkusumo General Central National Hospital, Jakarta, Indonesia.

References

1. Singh G, Martin Rumende C, Sharma SK, Rengganis I, Amin Z, Loho T, Hermiyanti E, Harimurti K, Low WH, B.A.L.F. CD4 T cells count is associated with extubation failure and mortality in critically ill covid-19 pneumonia. Ann Med Dec. 2022;54:1894–905.
2. Riou C, Bruyn E, Stek C, et al. HIATUS consortium. Relationship of SARS-CoV-2-specific CD4 response to COVID-19 severity and impact of HIV-1 and tuberculosis coinfection. J Clin Invest. 2021;15(131):e149125.
3. Klimpel GR. Immune defenses. In: Medical microbiology. Galveston: University of Texas Medical Branch at Galveston; 1996.
4. Zhu Q, Xu Y, Wang T, Xie F. Innate and adaptive immune response in SARS-CoV-2 infection-current perspectives. Front Immunol. 2022;13:1053437. https://www.frontiersin.org/articles/10.3389/fimmu.2022.1053437
5. Ning Q, Wu D, Wang X, Xi D, Chen T, Chen G. The mechanism underlying extrapulmonary complications of the coronavirus disease 2019 and its therapeutic implication. Signal Transduct Target Ther. 2022;7:57.
6. Saris A, Reijnders TDY, Nossent EJ, Schuurman AR, Verhoeff J, van Asten S. Distinct cellular immune profiles in the airways and blood of critically ill patients with COVID-19. Thorax Oct. 2021;76:1010–9.

Infective Endocarditis in COVID-19

5

5.1 Case Illustration

A 67-year-old male patient was presented to the hospital with shortness of breath. Around 4–5 days before the hospital admission, body aches and fever were experienced, with blood oxygen saturation decreasing to 92% when measured at home. A chest CT scan (Fig. 5.1) and a swab test confirmed a positive result for severe acute respiratory syndrome coronavirus 2 (SARS-CoV-2). Subsequently, the patient was managed in a COVID-19 isolation ward, receiving standard treatments for 7 days. Before discharge, additional antivirals and antibiotics were administered to further clear the infection. The patient felt better, and the lungs were also improved (Fig. 5.1).

A week after completing the prescribed medication, the patient started experiencing night chills and vomiting. A blood test showed positive results for enterococcal and pseudomonal infection, which was contracted during the hospitalization period. Subsequently, the patient was treated at home with antibiotics to eradicate the bacterial infections by taking the medication for 2 weeks. After consuming all the antibiotics, another blood test returned negative for the infection, and there was no complaint of night chills and vomiting. Approximately a week after, the same symptoms were experienced with decreased appetite and swollen joints (Fig. 5.2), described by the patient as migrating. Although hospitalization and further investigations were suggested, the patient refused and opted for home medication treatment.

The patient endured this "free-and-relapse" cycle for approximately 2.5 months before finally returning to the hospital. The hemoglobin (Hb) level had plummeted to 6.6 g/dL, and N-terminal-prohormone BNP (NT-proBNP) reached 28.000 pg/mL. Subsequently, the patient was admitted to manage the symptoms and investigate for the possible causes of decreased Hb and increased NT-proBNP. Antibiotics and blood transfusions were administered for two weeks before an echocardiography evaluation.

G. Singh, *Challenging Cases in Respirology and Critical Care*,
https://doi.org/10.1007/978-981-96-5002-6_5

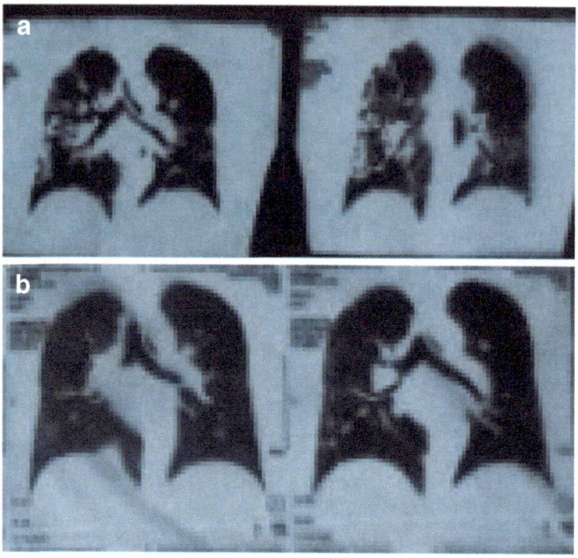

Fig. 5.1 The patient's chest CT scan, at initial hospital admission (**a**) and the discharge (**b**). Compared to box **b**, the lungs' appearance in box **a** was more fibrotic and patchier. This suggests that the lungs had improved after the COVID-19 treatment. (Image Courtesy: Dewi Tantra MD)

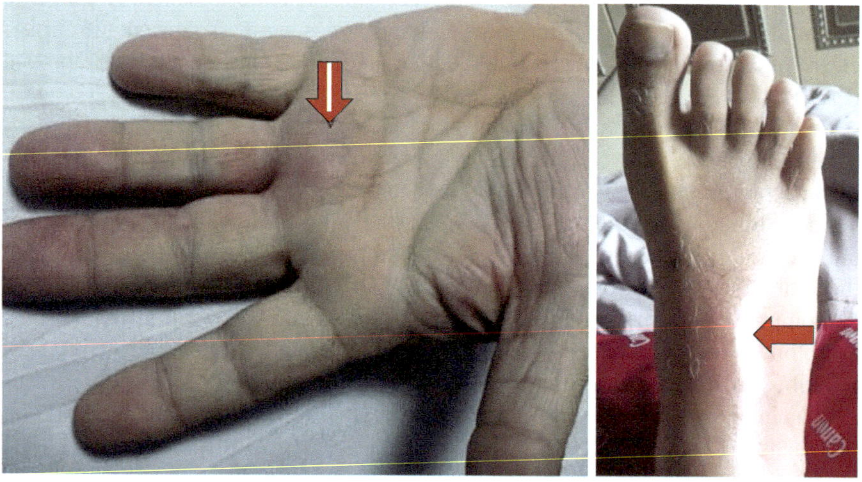

Fig. 5.2 The locations and appearance of the complained swollen joints (pointed by the arrows). The patient claimed that at times, the swollen joints were migrating to other sites of his body

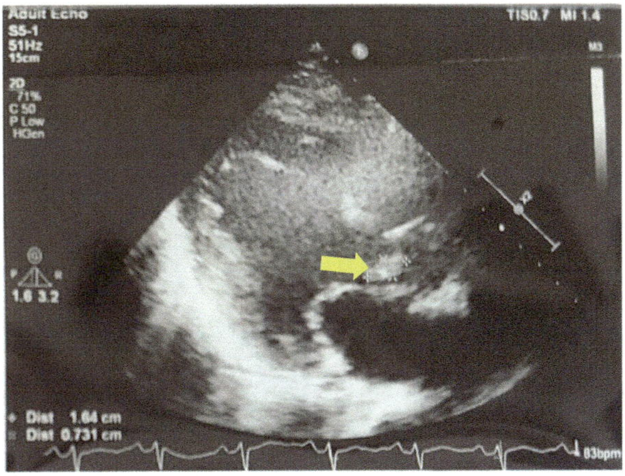

Fig. 5.3 Initial echocardiography imaging, showing moving vegetation infested on the aortic valve (pointed by yellow arrow). (Image Courtesy: Denio Adrianus Ridjab MD)

The initial echocardiography test showed a suspected moving vegetation sitting on the aortic valve (Fig. 5.3), suggesting the potential cause of the symptoms, Hb, and NT-proBNP level abnormality. The patient was subjected to a transesophageal echocardiography (TEE) procedure, and the presence of the vegetation was finally confirmed (Fig. 5.4), leading to a diagnosis of IE.

A week after the definitive diagnosis, the treatment received managed to reduce the NT-proBNP level of the patient to 10.000 pg/mL. The Hb level was also increased, but only to a suboptimal level (~9 to 10 g/dL). A final echocardiography imaging was performed, suggesting valve replacement surgery. Moreover, the replacement was successfully carried out, and the patient was delayed for a month after receiving additional antibiotic treatment. After being discharged from the hospital, there were no significant issues. Three months following the discharge, the Hb level finally reached a normal value (>12 g/dL), alongside the NT-proBNP level, which was found in a normal range.

The removed heart valve was examined microscopically and showed signs of chronic nonspecific inflammation in the valve tissues (Fig. 5.5, box b). However, there was no microbiological examination to determine the microorganism infecting the valve.

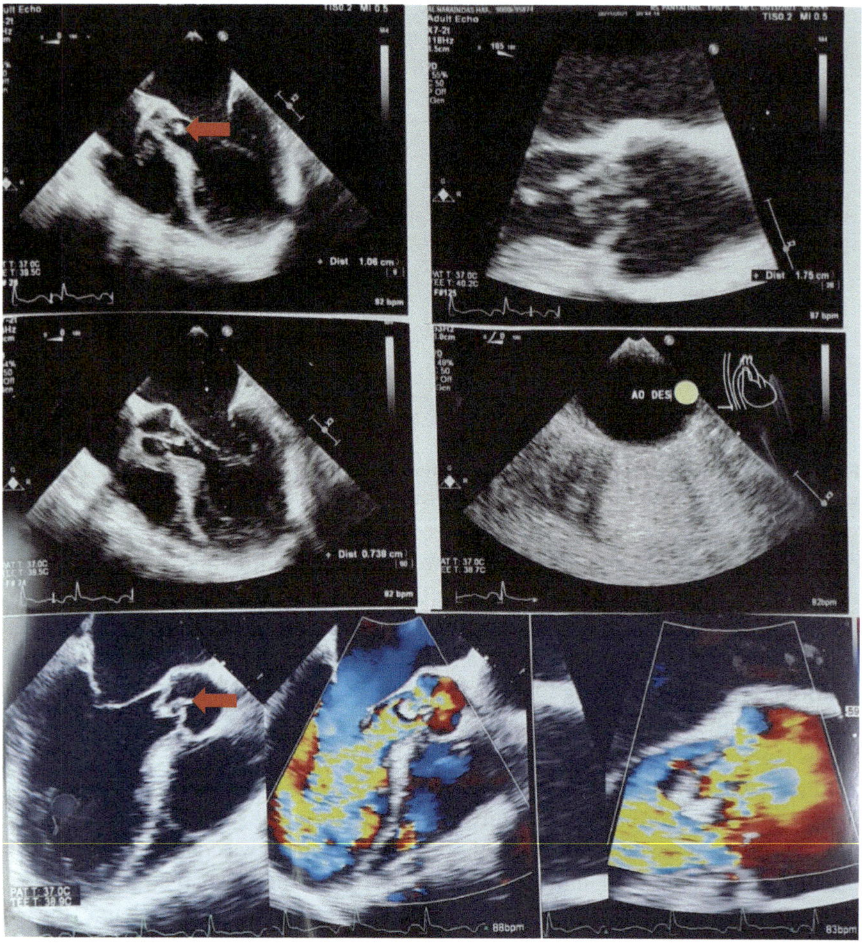

Fig. 5.4 Transesophageal echocardiography (TEE) imaging, revealing the presence of the vegetation as indicated by the arrows. The measured size of the vegetation was approximately 2 cm. (Image Courtesy: Denio Adrianus Ridjab MD)

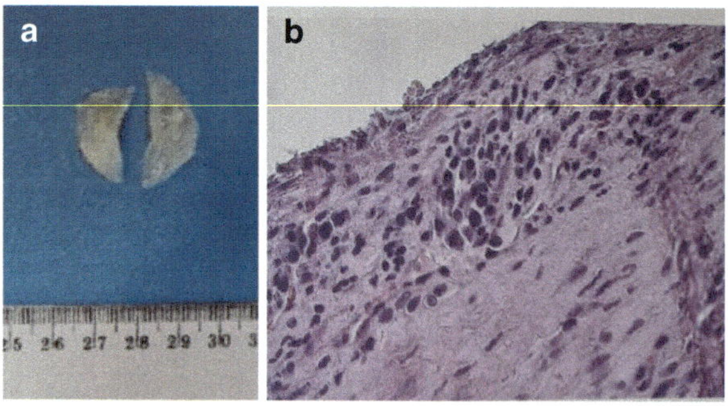

Fig. 5.5 (a) Macroscopic appearance of the removed heart valve. (b) Signs of chronic nonspecific inflammatory reactions were microscopically seen on the valve. (Image Courtesy: Stella Marleen MD)

5.2 What Is the Patient's Problem?

The patient was admitted to the hospital with a diagnosis of COVID-19. After hospitalization, antibiotics were prescribed as take-home medication. However, there was the experience of night chills and vomiting a week after completing all prescribed antibiotics. These symptoms were addressed by administering antibiotics but reoccurred when the medication had finished. Moreover, there were additional signs and symptoms, which included swollen joints, loss of appetite, increased NT-proBNP level, and decreased Hb refractory to blood transfusion. Echocardiography examinations showed infective endocarditis (IE), and valve replacement surgery was conducted. The results showed no relapse or additional complaint ever since the replacement procedure.

5.3 Discussion

Infective Endocarditis (IE) poses a significant public health concern, with an anticipated 13.8 occurrences per 100,000 individuals per year in 2019, resulting in a total of 66,300 deaths globally. Due to the high morbidity and mortality rates, there were 1723.59 disability-adjusted life years and 0.87 death cases per 100,000 individuals. Moreover, IE is a bacterial, viral, or fungal infection that affects the inner lining of the heart, particularly the surfaces of one or more cardiac valves. It also affects the inner lining of the heart muscle or a septal defect, although to a lower extent. The significant effects include serious valve leakage, uncontrollable heart failure, abscesses in the heart muscle, infected and non-infected blood clots, as well as various immune system reactions. Since 2008, there has been a significant increase in the occurrence, severity, and death rate due to IE [1].

Resistant to several recognized antimicrobial treatments are increasingly becoming widespread recently. Another problem is the management of "novel" viruses that occur from foreign sources or due to the growing population of immunocompromised patients. Additionally, the prevalence of intravascular infections has increased due to the high demand for intravascular lines caused by the successive waves of COVID-19 [2].

5.4 Epidemiology

The epidemiological composition of Infective Endocarditis (IE) has experienced substantial modification. Recently, Staphylococcus aureus has become the predominant bacterium causing infections in the developed world, even when the total incidence of IE has remained constant. An influential aspect in the increase of staphylococcus aureus IE is the increasing importance of healthcare contact as a key source of infection risk. Additionally, there has been an increase in the average age of patients with IE, a rise in the proportion of prosthetic valves and other cardiac devices, as well as a decreased percentage of cases related to rheumatic heart disease. The proportion of patients with IE who have surgery has also increased to over 50% [3].

The incidence rate of IE in the western population is 10 cases per 100,000 population years. Extensive population-based investigations have shown that the proportion of individuals with newly diagnosed IE is unchanged compared to the previous two decades. However, staphylococcus aureus IE has been misdiagnosed as Multisystem Inflammatory Response Syndrome. Both conditions show comparable symptoms, chest x-ray findings, vital signs, and screening laboratory testing. To effectively address these circumstances, there is a need to implement a strategic approach (SA) that includes a COVID-19 test alongside an initial evaluation screening. Cardiac infection may occur several months after a COVID-19 infection in individuals who do not have any preexisting risk factors. It can manifest as non-bacterial thrombotic endocarditis, bacterial infective endocarditis, or myocarditis with the virus persisting in the myocardium. Both conditions are caused by the viral infection, along with a severe systemic inflammatory and thrombotic response. COVID-19 infection can lead to visceral thrombosis, resulting in the development of IE. These occurrences may take place before receiving treatment in the community or various medical facilities. The primary cause is the presence of several intravascular lines, leading to a temporary bloodstream infection. The early fever generated by COVID-19 is mostly attributed to the virus, including the thrombotic and inflammatory processes. After seven days, there is a need to eliminate the possibility of bacterial or fungal infections, alongside thorough reassessment for IE using echocardiography [4, 5].

5.5 Clinical Signs and Symptoms

Medically, infective endocarditis (IE) can manifest with a wide range of signs and symptoms. Therefore, doctors should consider this potential diagnosis when evaluating patients with risk factors showing fever or sepsis of uncertain cause. Patients frequently report the gradual onset of fever, chills, malaise, and weariness, which typically leads to medical assessment within the initial month. In a comprehensive multinational prospective cohort study, fever, commonly defined as a temperature over 38.0 °C (100.4 °F), was observed in more than 95% of all patients. However, the presence and occurrence rate may be hindered by several factors such as immunosuppression, advanced age, the use of antipyretic medications, or prior administration of antibiotics. Additional non-specific symptoms that can indicate a systemic illness include loss of appetite, headache, and overall weakness. Less frequently observed symptoms, such as chest pain, dyspnea, reduced exercise capacity, orthopnea, and paroxysmal nocturnal dyspnea, also facilitate the identification of the specific inclusion of the cardiopulmonary system. These symptoms should be considered potential indicators of underlying aortic or mitral valve insufficiency. When a patient experiences acute valvular incompetence, there can be an appearance of a critical condition with a sudden onset of heart failure symptoms [6].

5.6 Pathophysiology

The undamaged and healthy inside tissue of the heart, known as the endocardium, usually has a natural resistance to the colonization of bacteria. However, the occurrence of Infective Endocarditis (IE) requires initial damage to the endocardium, followed by a phase of bacteria. The initial rupture of the endocardium can occur due to turbulent flow around valves that are affected by illness or direct mechanical injury produced by the insertion of a catheter or electrode. Regarding intravenous drug usage, repeated obstruction of the valves by co-injected particles causes the required damage. The presence of vegetations on the ventricular surface of the aortic valve and the atrial surface of the mitral valve shows that hemodynamics is a significant factor in the development of IE. The presence of vegetation is observed in the areas directly following the backward flow of blood. This suggested that reduced blood flow to the inner layer of the heart can make the regions more susceptible to damage. Additionally, IE is more prevalent in cases of high turbulence lesions, such as a tiny ventricular septal defect with a jet lesion or stenotic valves. Based on the previous assumption, the high-pressure flow causes greater local damage compared to defects with larger surface areas or low flow. The injured inner lining of the heart (endocardium) acts as a site for blood platelets to accumulate and trigger the process of blood clotting. This process leads to the development of a non-infectious blood clot (thrombus) on the heart valve, which is known as thrombotic vegetation [6].

After the occurrence of bacteremia, the colonization of the vegetation takes place. Bacteremia can occur due to an existing illness in a distant part of the body or occasional introduction of oral bacteria into the bloodstream during dental or gum procedures. The lowest bacterial load required to cause IE is currently undetermined. However, animal models have successfully induced instances of IE by administering gradual infusions of 1 mL containing 106 colony-forming units of bacteria. Pathogenesis in the context of endocardial damage and bacteremia requires the presence of a highly pathogenic organism that can effectively bind to and promote the formation of platelet-fibrin deposits. Moreover, three proteins from the Staphylococcus aureus bacterium, including clumping factors A, B, and serine-aspartate repeat protein, have been discovered to individually facilitate the process of platelet aggregation. Theoretically, the expansion of the initially sterile platelet-fibrin deposits protects pathogens against the immunological response of the host, facilitating vegetation growth [6].

5.7 Workup

5.7.1 Blood Culture-Positive Infective Endocarditis

Blood cultures that produce positive results are essential for diagnosing Infective Endocarditis (IE), offering viable bacteria for both identification and susceptibility testing. Before initiating antibiotic medication, there is a need to collect a minimum of three sets of blood cultures at 30-min intervals. Each set should consist of 10 mL of blood, cultured in both aerobic and anaerobic environments. Samples should also be obtained from a peripheral vein using a careful and clean procedure instead of a central venous catheter due to the potential for contamination and misinterpretation. Without prior use of antimicrobial treatment, this method is effective in identifying the typical microorganisms responsible and requires the establishment of a culture before administering antibiotics. In Internet Explorer, the occurrence of bacteremia is consistently present and has two important consequences. These include (i) the absence of a logical need to postpone blood collecting to correlate with periods of high temperature and (ii) all blood cultures yield positive results during bacteremia. Therefore, there is a need to exercise caution when using a single positive blood culture to establish a diagnosis of IE. The microbiology laboratory must be aware of clinical suspicion of IE. Automated equipment conducts ongoing surveillance of bacterial proliferation, ensuring prompt delivery of reports to specialists.

Gram staining is also used for presumptive identification when a positive blood culture is detected. The practitioners are promptly provided with this information to modify the empirical antibiotics treatment. Current methods, such as matrix-assisted laser desorption ionization time-of-flight mass spectrometry (MALDI-TOF MS), can typically achieve complete identification within one or two days. However, for more delicate or unusual species, the process can be prolonged to enhance accuracy. Due to the significant time gap between collecting blood samples for culture and accurately identifying the specific organism causing the bloodstream infection and testing its susceptibility to antibiotics, various enhancements have been suggested to facilitate the process. A cutting-edge method for quickly identifying bacteria is dependent on peptide spectra acquired by MALDI-TOF MS. Despite advancements in technology and the move towards quick susceptibility testing using MALDI-TOF MS, the most reliable method is still the measurement of minimal inhibitory concentrations (MICs). This is crucial for selecting the appropriate antibiotic treatment and must be carried out using validated and standardized procedures [2].

5.7.2 Blood Culture-Negative Infective Endocarditis

Blood culture-negative infective endocarditis (BCNIE) is a condition characterized by the absence of detectable bacteria using standard blood culture methods, despite the presence of infective endocarditis (IE). The incidence of BCNIE as the etiology of IE shows significant variability and frequently presents substantial challenges in terms of diagnosis and treatment decisions. BCNIE often occurs due to earlier antibiotic usage, showing the significance of conducting blood cultures before starting antibiotic treatment. This is particularly important for patients who have recognized risk factors for IE. In stable patients with subacute symptoms, no evidence of local or distant problems, and receiving a relatively short course of antibiotics, it may be necessary to withdraw the medication and recheck blood cultures. Fungal or fastidious bacteria, particularly obligatory intracellular bacteria, can also induce IE with negative blood culture results. The isolation of these bacteria shows the need for their cultivation on specialist media, although the growth rate is very slow. Based on the local epidemiology, it is recommended to conduct systematic serological testing for Coxiella burnetii, Bartonella spp., Aspergillus spp., Mycoplasma pneumoniae, Brucella spp., and Legionella pneumophila. This should be followed by specific polymerase chain reaction (PCR) assays for Tropheryma whipplei, Bartonella spp., and fungi (Candida spp., Aspergillus spp.) from blood and tissue samples [2].

Testing for antinuclear antibodies and antiphospholipid syndrome (APLs), specifically anticardiolipin antibodies (immunoglobulin (Ig)G) and anti-β2-glycoprotein 1 antibodies (IgG and IgM), should be conducted. Moreover, these antibodies can be found in individuals with confirmed IE. Performing a pathological examination of surgically removed tissue or embolized fragments remains the most reliable method for diagnosing IE. All tissue samples removed during surgical valve debridement/resection should be collected in a sterile container, without fixative or culture medium. These samples are sent to the pathology department and the microbiology laboratory for microorganism identification. The histological analysis of removed valve tissue shows varying patterns and degrees of inflammation, which are contingent upon the infecting organism. Staining methods can be used to identify bacteria, mycobacteria, and fungi, while immunohistochemistry stains specific to each organism play a significant role in the definitive diagnosis. Histopathological investigation is also crucial in aiding the diagnosis of non-infectious causes of endocarditis, including neoplastic and autoimmune origins [2].

5.8 Echocardiography

Echocardiography has become the preferred indirect diagnostic method, particularly in individuals who show clinical symptoms of Infective Endocarditis (IE) but yield inconclusive results from blood culture tests (e.g., certain cases of fungal endocarditis). However, the exclusion of IE cannot be definitively determined based on negative findings from transthoracic echocardiography (TTE) or transesophageal echocardiography (TEE) [7].

The American Heart Association (AHA) guideline on cardiac implantable electronic device (CIED) infections recommends the use of TEE to assess the left-sided heart valves in all adults suspected of having CIED-related endocarditis, without considering the adherence of detected TTE. When the TTE images are satisfactory, the result might be adequate for pediatric patients. However, patients who have tested positive for blood culture or negative after receiving recent antimicrobial medication should receive TEE to assess for infection CIED or valvular endocarditis [7].

The presence of observable vegetation shows a more unfavorable prognosis. Both TTE and TEE have a high degree of specificity in detecting valvular vegetation, but their sensitivity levels vary. Cardiac Doppler ultrasonography scanning in two dimensions represents a significant progression in the diagnosis and assessment of IE. It offers data regarding the existence and dimensions of vegetation, aiding in diagnosis and forecasting embolization to a certain extent. TEE is highly effective in identifying anterior myocardial abscesses and accurately measuring the severity of valvular dysfunction [7].

The Doppler method is capable of identifying aberrant blood flow and specific heart abnormalities that are not observable with conventional echocardiography. It is also beneficial for visualizing jet lesions and distinguishing cusp perforation from valvular insufficiency. The use of TEE and color Doppler imaging is highly effective in the identification of intracardiac fistulas. The real-time resolution of both TEE and TTE is approximately 2 mm. Factors that contribute to the identification of valvular thrombi include the poor visibility of right-sided structures, particularly with TEE, disease duration beyond two weeks, presence of valve or myocardial abscesses, and sinus of Valsalva aneurysms [7].

5.9 Radiography

5.9.1 Computed Tomography

The indications for computed tomography (CT) in patients with suspected or diagnosed IE include:

(i) Diagnosis of IE and associated cardiac problems. Cardiac CT is a superior method compared to transesophageal echo (TOE) for accurately diagnosing complications related to perivalvular and periprosthetic infections, such as abscesses, pseudoaneurysms, and fistulae. It is recommended to use cardiac CT in cases of both native valve endocarditis (NVE) and prosthetic valve endocarditis (PVE) when TOE results are inconclusive or not possible. Furthermore, cardiac CT has the potential to significantly impact subsequent surgical decision-making. Echocardiography remains the preferred method for identifying valve abnormalities, particularly tiny vegetations measuring less than 10 mm, which are often undetected by CT scans. Additionally, echocardiography is effective in detecting leaflet perforations and fistulae. Cardiac CT should be obtained in accordance with the standard criteria to ensure a high level of diagnostic accuracy. It can be performed alone or in conjunction with Positron Emission Tomography (PET) [1].

(ii) Detecting remote lesions and sources of bacteremia. Whole-body and brain CT scans are valuable for evaluating systemic consequences of IE, including septic emboli. Identifying distant lesions is a minor diagnostic factor that contributes to a more definitive diagnosis of confirmed or ruled-out IE, playing a significant role in making decisions. CT angiography is capable of identifying mycotic artery aneurysms that occur as a complication of infective endocarditis in several locations throughout the vascular system, including the central nervous system (CNS). Although MRI is more effective in diagnosing neurological complications, CT is practically used in emergency situations as a viable alternative. CT has a sensitivity of 90% and specificity of 86% in identifying ischemic and hemorrhagic lesions. It can also identify sources of bacteria outside the heart, such as early cancerous growths. This information is crucial for managing the patient and should preferably be addressed before heart valve surgery. However, CT scanning is not a substitute for the specific test recommended for diagnosing the source of bacterial infection outside the heart, such as colonoscopy for colon tumors [1].

(iii) Evaluation before surgery. Heart CT is a useful substitute for non-invasive evaluation of coronary artery disease (CAD) before heart surgery in patients with IE [1].
(iv) Alternative medical assessment in cases where IE has been ruled out, or in patients with uncertain diagnosis of IE, whole-body CT can be used to identify other probable sources of infection. However, [18] FDG positron emission tomography/computed tomography (PET/CT) is the favored imaging method [1].

5.9.2 Magnetic Resonance Imaging

The roles of MRI in the diagnostic workup of Infective Endocarditis (IE) include:

(i) Diagnosis of IE and associated cardiac problems. The diagnostic capabilities of cardiac MRI in identifying IE are restricted due to inferior spatial resolution when compared to cardiac CT. Additionally, the presence of some prostheses might create signal voids, which hinder the accurate evaluation of prosthetic valve architecture and function [1].
(ii) Neurological problems associated with IE diagnosis. MRI shows more sensitivity than CT in diagnosing neurological abnormalities. This enhances the probability of identifying neurological problems in patients with IE, showing central nervous system (CNS) lesions. The presence of CNS lesions might be included as an additional diagnostic criterion for patients without neurological symptoms and an inconclusive diagnosis. Brain magnetic resonance imaging (MRI) has the ability to reclassify 25% of patients who initially had an equivocal diagnosis for IE to a more definitive diagnosis, resulting in an earlier identification of the condition. Cerebral microbleeds, which are present in 50–60% of patients with IE, can be identified using gradient echo T2* sequences. However, cerebral microbleeds should not be considered a minor criterion due to the lack of agreement with ischemic lesions [1].
(iii) Spine lesion diagnosis. MRI is the preferred diagnosis method for spondylodiscitis and spinal osteomyelitis, with an accuracy ranging from 89% to 94%. The results of the MRI show the presence of swelling in the vertebrae and discs, inflammation or abscess in the surrounding area, and erosion of the bones, as well as enhanced visibility of the vertebrae and discs due to the use of gadolinium. Moreover, there is a need to recognize that early MRI can lead to a higher occurrence of false-negative results [1].

5.10 Diagnostic Criteria

The modified Duke criteria, implemented since 2000, have successfully included clinical, microbiological, and imaging data to diagnose Infective Endocarditis (IE) with an impressive overall sensitivity of 80%. However, the manifestation of IE in a clinical setting can show significant variability. Several significant drawbacks of the modified Duke criteria have also become evident, particularly in cases including prosthetic materials such as PVE, aortic grafts, cardiac devices, and CHD. Under these circumstances, echocardiography can appear normal or inconclusive in approximately 30% of patients, even when IE is present. Therefore, the 2015 ESC diagnostic criteria implemented a multimodality imaging strategy including echocardiography, cardiac/whole-body CT, cerebral MRI, [18F]FDG-PET/CT, and WBC SPECT/CT to enhance the accuracy of diagnosis. This novel method has shown its superiority over the conventional diagnostic criteria (Table 5.1) [1, 8].

Table 5.1 Definitions of the 2023 European Society of Cardiology modified diagnostic criteria of infective endocarditis

Major Criteria
I. Blood Cultures positive for IE:
(a) Typical microorganisme consistent with IE from two seperate blood cultures: oral streptococci, streptococcus gallayticus (formerly S. Bovis), HACEK group, S. aureus, E faecalis
(b) Microorganisms consistent with IE from continuosly positive blood cultures: ≥2 positives blood cultures of blood samples drawn >12 h apart
All of 3 or a majority of ≥4 separate cultures of blood (with first and last samples drawn ≥1 h apart
(c) Single positive blood culture for C.burnetii or phase I IgG antibody titre > 1:800
II. Imaging positive for IE:
Valvular, perivalvular/periprosthetic and foreign material anatomic and metabolic lesions characteristic of IE detected by any of the following imaging techniques:
Enchocardiography (TTE and TOE)
Cardiac CT
[18F]-FDG-PET/CT(A)
WBC SPECT/CT
Minor Criteria
I. Predisposing conditions
II. Fever defined as temperature >38 °C
III. Embolic vascular dissemination
IV. Immunological phenomena
V. Microbiological Evidence
IE Classification (at admission and during follow-up)
Definite:
2 major criteria
1 major criterion and at least 3 minor criteria
5 minor criteria
Possible:
1 major criterion and 1 or 2 minor criteria
3–4 minor criteria
Rejected:
Does not meet criteria for definitie or possible at admission with or without a firm alternative diagnosis

Source: ESC Guideline, Ref. [1]

[18F]-FDG-PET/CT, ^{18}F-fluorodeoxyglucose positron emission tomography; CT(A), computed tomography (angiography); HACEK, *Haemophilus*, *Aggregatibacter*, *Cardiobacterium*, *Eikenella*, and *Kingella*; IE, infective endocarditis; Ig, immunoglobulin; PWID, individuals who inject drugs; TOE, transoesophageal echocardiography; TTE, transthoracic echocardiography; WBC SPECT/CT, white blood cell single photon emission tomography/computed tomography

5.11 Management and Prognosis

Typically, the treatment of Infective Endocarditis (IE) should focus on administering antibiotics that specifically target the microorganism identified in blood cultures. The therapeutic duration should be determined starting from the initial day of negative blood cultures [1].

5.12 Antibiotic therapy

Indications—In cases where patients are suspected of having Infective Endocarditis (IE) but do not show immediate symptoms, it is not always necessary to start treatment based on assumptions. However, treatment can be postponed until the results of blood culture tests are obtained. This is particularly important because a precise diagnosis of the specific microorganism causing the infection is crucial in determining the most effective treatment method. Empiric treatment can be indicated for acutely unwell patients showing clear signs and symptoms highly indicative of IE. This treatment should only be given after obtaining at least two (preferably three) sets of blood cultures from independent venipunctures, within an ideal space of 30 to 60 min [1].

Selection—When selecting empiric treatment, it is important to consider the most probable infections. This treatment should typically include staphylococci such as methicillin-susceptible and methicillin-resistant strains, streptococci, and enterococci [1].

The effective management of IE depends on the complete elimination of microorganisms through the use of antimicrobial medications, with surgery contributing by removing infected material. Treatment regimens that kill bacteria are more successful compared to growth inhibition. Aminoglycosides show synergistic effects with cell wall inhibitors such as beta-lactams and glycopeptides, resulting in bactericidal activity. These antibiotics are valuable in reducing the length of treatment, particularly for oral streptococci, and eliminating troublesome organisms. However, there is a need to consider the potential adverse effects of aminoglycosides. The combination of ampicillin with ceftriaxone has proven to be effective in treating IE caused by E. faecalis, regardless of the presence of high-level aminoglycoside resistance (HLAR). This combination also helps to minimize the risk of kidney damage (nephrotoxicity). Bacterial antibiotic resistance is a significant obstacle to drug-induced killing. Although tolerant microorganisms are not immune to the drug's growth inhibitory effects, they are capable of evading drug-induced death and continue growing after treatment cessation.

Microbes that grow slowly and are inactive show phenotypic tolerance to most antimicrobials, except rifampin to a certain degree. Bacteria are found in plants and biofilms, which are intricate communities living inside a matrix of exopolysaccharides and attached to surfaces, such as in PVE. This shows the need for extended treatment to eliminate infections in heart valves. Certain bacteria possess mutations that are resistant to adverse conditions, such as both active growth and dormant stages. Combining bactericidal drugs is more favorable than using a single antibiotic when dealing with tolerant organisms. For instance, in cases of infective endocarditis caused by E. faecalis, the combination of ampicillin and ceftriaxone is favored. The duration of drug treatment for PVE should be extended to a minimum of 6 weeks, while native valve endocarditis (NVE) often ranges from 2 to 6 weeks. Except for differences in duration, the treatment methods for both types of endocarditis are generally comparable. In cases of staphylococcal PVE, the treatment plan should incorporate rifampin when the strain is susceptible, despite recent evidence showing no significant differences in outcomes between patients treated with and without rifampin. In patients with NVE who require valve replacement with a prosthesis when receiving antibiotics, the post-operative antibiotic regimen is often recommended. For both NVE and PVE, the length of treatment is determined by the start of effective antibiotic therapy (when the blood culture becomes negative after initially testing positive), rather than the day of surgery. Commencement of a fresh comprehensive treatment regimen should only occur when valve cultures yield positive results (Fig. 5.6) [1].

When a new complication of IE is suspected, it is recommended to perform a repeat echocardiogram (either TTE or TEE) during antibiotic treatment. Repeat echocardiography, either transthoracic echocardiography (TTE) or transesophageal echocardiography (TEE), is clinically indicated in cases of a

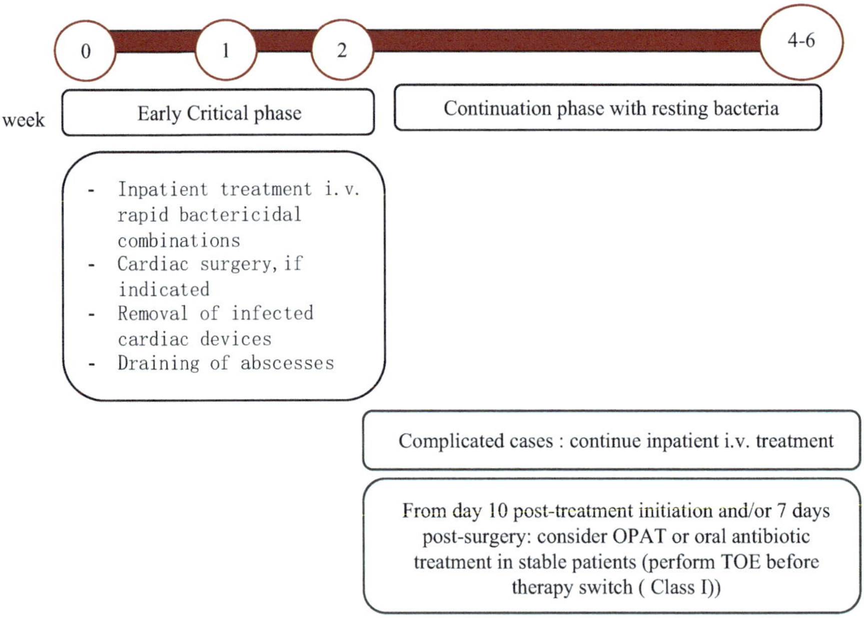

Fig. 5.6 Antibiotic Phase of Infective Endocarditis; OPAT, outpatient parenteral antibiotic treatment; TOE, transoesophageal echocardiography. *A Criteria for switching to OPAT or partial oral treatment of endocarditis (Adapted: ESC Guideline). [1]

newly detected murmur, embolic complications, worsening heart failure, and the occurrence of atrioventricular block. Furthermore, those experiencing prolonged fever or bacteremia lasting more than five to seven days should receive another echocardiography examination to assess the presence of an abscess. When contemplating a transition from a parenteral to an oral antibiotic regimen to finish a therapeutic course, it is recommended to conduct a repeat echocardiogram to exclude the presence of an abscess or any other justification for surgery. However, repeat echocardiography is not necessary to assess the extent of vegetation, and the method of repeating the echocardiogram remains the same regardless of the pathogen [1].

5.13 Role of Valve Surgery

Patients with Infective Endocarditis (IE) who receive antibiotic treatment may experience several consequences that have a negative impact on their prognosis. These issues may require early surgical intervention before the completion of antimicrobial treatment. Early surgery should be promptly performed unless there are significant cerebrovascular complications such as hemorrhagic stroke, high risk for surgery, or poor long-term prognosis due to other medical issues. Patients who suffer from embolic events in the CNS, without any bleeding or significant neurological damage, can still be subjected to cardiac surgery with an acceptable level of risk. However, those who have experienced a hemorrhagic stroke should wait for a minimum of 4 weeks before surgery [9].

5.14 For Native Valve IE

For left-sided native valve IE—Left-sided native valve endocarditis (NVE) patients often require prompt valve surgery due to several problems. These include valve dysfunction associated with infective endocarditis (IE) worsened by heart failure, intracardiac abscess, challenging-to-treat pathogens, and chronic infection [9].

For right-sided native valve IE—Surgical intervention is warranted in cases of right-sided NVE when there is exceptionally large vegetation, measuring 20 mm or more in diameter. Other conditions include recurrent septic pulmonary emboli, extremely resistant pathogens, and chronic bacteremia. Severe tricuspid valve regurgitation is better tolerated from a hemodynamic perspective than severe left-sided regurgitation in right-sided NVE. Therefore, early surgery is not commonly recommended for heart failure (HF) in these cases. Severe tricuspid regurgitation, which leads to right heart failure and does not respond well to conventional treatment, is not a major factor for surgery. Valve repair is typically favored over replacement in similar cases, particularly among individuals who take injectable drugs [9].

5.15 Prognosis

The prognosis can significantly differ based on factors such as the strength of the infectious pathogen, the development of further complications, coexisting medical conditions, and whether the valve affected is natural or artificial. The death rate within the hospital remains at approximately 18%, while the mortality rate within one year is approximately 40%. Typically, instances of prosthetic valve endocarditis (PVE) that occur within the initial 60 days after surgery have the most elevated mortality rate of approximately 30% during the patient's hospital stay. A comprehensive study conducted in Japan showed that staphylococcal infection and heart failure were identified as the most significant factors in predicting fatality rates after hospitalization. Although surgical intervention is performed in approximately 50% of IE cases, it does not seem to increase the risk of in-hospital mortality rate [6].

Key Point

Cardiac infection may occur several months after a COVID-19 infection in individuals who do not have any preexisting risk factors. COVID-19 infection can lead to visceral thrombosis, resulting in the development of Infective Endocarditis.

Questions

1. What is the most common bacterial cause of infective endocarditis?
   (a) Staphylococcus Aureus
   (b) Brucella spp.
   (c) T. whipplei
   (d) Mycoplasma spp.
   (e) C. burnetti
2. What is the main role of COVID-19 as a pathogenic cause of infective endocarditis?
   (a) Triggered Myocarditis infection
   (b) Triggered visceral thrombosis
   (c) Triggered system inflammatory response syndrome
   (d) Triggered atrioventricular block
   (e) Aneurysms of the sinus of Valsalva
3. In infective endocarditis blood culture, a negative result may be caused by:
   (a) Viral
   (b) Fungi
   (c) S. Aureus
   (d) COVID-19
   (e) Obligatory extracellular bacteria
4. Below are the minor criteria of infective endocarditis according to the European Society of Cardiology, except:
   (a) Fever defined as temperature > 38 °C
   (b) Glomerulonephritis

   (c) Janeway's lesson
   (d) Single positive blood culture for C. Brunetti
   (e) Serological evidence of active infection with organism consistent with IE
5. The following are clinical indications for repeating TTE and/or TEE, except
   (a) New murmur
   (b) Embolic complications
   (c) New or progressive heart failure
   (d) Development of atrioventricular block
   (e) Acute myocarditis

Answer Keys
1. A
2. B
3. B
4. D
5. E

Acknowledgment Cipta Mahendra, MD, Department of Internal Medicine, Respirology and Critical Illness Division, Universitas Indonesia, Dr. Cipto Mangunkusumo General Central National Hospital, Jakarta, Indonesia.
Ersananda Arlisa Putri, MD, Department of Internal Medicine, Respirology and Critical Illness Division, Universitas Indonesia, Dr. Cipto Mangunkusumo General Central National Hospital, Jakarta, Indonesia.
Denio Adrianus Ridjab, MD, Department of Cardiovascular, Pantai Indah Kapuk Hospital, Jakarta, Indonesia.
Rajesh Kalwani, MD DM, Department of Internal Medicine, Medical Hematology and Oncology Division, Pantai Indah Kapuk Hospital, Jakarta, Indonesia.

References

1. Delgado V, Ajmone Marsan N, Waha S, Bonaros N, Brida M, Burri H. 2023 ESC Guidelines for the management of endocarditis. Eur Heart J. 2023;14(44):3948–4042.
2. Brusch JL. Infective endocarditis and it's mimics in the critical care unit. In: Infectious diseases in critical care medicine. 4th ed. New York: CRC Press; 2020. p. 255–63.
3. Barahimi E, Defaee S, Shokraei R, Sheybani-Arani M, Salimi Asl A, Ghaem HM. Bacterial endocarditis following COVID-19 infection: two case reports. J Med Case Rep. 2023;17(1):274.
4. Quintero-Martinez JA, Hindy J, Mahmood M, Gerberi D, DeSimone D, Baddour L. A clinical profile of infective endocarditis in patients with recent COVID-19: a systematic review. Am J Med Sci. 2022;364(1):16–22.
5. George A, Alampoondi Venkataramanan SV, John KJ, Mishra AK. Infective endocarditis and COVID-19 coinfection: an updated review. Acta Biomed. 2022; https://doi.org/10.23750/abm.v93i1.10982.
6. Yallowitz AW, Decker LC Infectious Endocarditis.
7. Ten Hove D, Slart R, Sinha B, Glaudemans A, Budde B. 18F-FDG PET/CT in infective endocarditis: indications and approaches for standardization. Curr Cardiol Rep. 2021;23

8. Durack DT, Lukes AS, Bright DK. New criteria for diagnosis of infective endocarditis: utilization of specific echocardiographic findings. Duke Endocarditis Service. Am J Med. 1994;96:200–9.
9. Overview of management of infective endocarditis in adults – UpToDate. Internet. https://www.uptodate.com/contents/overview-of-management-of-infective-endocarditis-in-adults/print. Accessed 26 Dec 2023

Carotid Doppler Ultrasonography in Diabetic Mellitus

6

6.1 Case Illustration

A 62-year-old female patient came to the hospital with a major complaint of breathing difficulty and fever for 2–3 weeks before admission. The patient was referred after receiving prior treatments for pneumonia at another hospital due to recurrent symptoms. The medical history included type 2 diabetes mellitus (T2DM), hypertension, and chronic kidney disease (CKD), but there was no allergy. The patient admitted being noncompliant, with infrequent visits to a doctor for regular check-ups, particularly to control the blood glucose level (BGL).

Physical examinations showed rhonchi in the right lung and pitting edema in both lower extremities. The patient was fully conscious, and most vital signs were in the abnormal range, including blood pressure (BP) of 151/69, heart rate (HR) of 104 times/min, respiratory rate (RR) of 26 times/min, and body temperature of 36.6 °C. A urinary catheter was found inserted into the patient's urethra. Blood tests showed hyperuricemia and hypoalbuminemia, with slightly elevated liver enzyme levels. An initial ultrasonography (USG) examination showed minimal pleural effusion in both lungs but no ascites. Heart examination showed a 75% ejection fraction (classified as heart failure with preserved ejection fraction (HFpEF)) on echocardiography, as well as sinus arrhythmia and Q-wave infarctions (multiple leads) on electrocardiography (ECG). Based on the previous histories and examination results, the patient was diagnosed with T2DM, HFpEF, hypertension, and CKD, with a suspicion of pneumonia.

The patient was given appropriate treatment to alleviate symptoms and problems related to diagnosis. Oxygen supplementation, antihypertensive, and antidiabetic medications were administered. Regarding the T2DM, hypertension, and CKD status, restriction of calorie and fluid intake was also initiated. Antidiuretics were given to decrease the pleural effusion and alleviate the edema in the extremities. By the end of the 2nd to 3rd day of admission, breathing effort was improved, alongside a reduction in severity of the edema. A repeat USG examination showed decreased pleural effusion compared to the initial USG finding.

G. Singh, *Challenging Cases in Respirology and Critical Care*,
https://doi.org/10.1007/978-981-96-5002-6_6

In the following days, the patient complained of itchiness and tenderness of the genitals. A smear and blood test were obtained and examined for the presence of infections, showing a mixed herpetic and nonspecific bacterial infection. A chest X-ray imaging was also obtained, showing multiple fibrotic lesions suggestive of pneumonia. However, there was no heart contour abnormality on the imaging. The patient was swabbed for SARS-CoV-2, and the result was negative. Appropriate antibiotics, antifungals, and antivirals (acyclovir) were administered to address and manage the findings. A new urinary catheter was also inserted, and another USG examination found no abnormality observed on the patient's urinary tracts.

Around the middle days during the hospitalization period, a repeat chest X-ray procedure was performed. The imaging showed relatively unchanged findings with multiple fibrotic lesions compared to the previous imaging. Additionally, bladder training was initiated, leading to spontaneous urination several days after the training.

One to two days before the discharge from the hospital, the patient was relieved from the genital infection and the edema in the extremities. A slight breathing difficulty was complained of, but the symptom significantly improved compared to the initial admission. Laboratory examination found no significant abnormality except for the glucose level. During the whole hospitalization period (15 days since admission), the patient's BGL was fluctuating (Table 6.1), with results ranging from <100 to >200 mg/dL. Besides the glucose, the blood pressure readings were also fluctuating but not <130 for the systolic pressure, except on the 8th day (Table 6.1).

The patient was shortly discharged based on request, and take-home medications for the continuing T2DM, HfpEF, hypertension, and CKD management were prescribed. Subsequently, the patient was informed to visit the hospital the following week. Hypoglycemia was observed upon arrival, with symptoms of weakness, lack of appetite, and occasional fever. Although a recommendation was made for hospitalization, the patient opted for home treatment.

The next day, the patient came back to the hospital with the same complaint as the initial hospitalization, which was breathing difficulty and fever. Pneumonia that did not clear thoroughly on the previous admission was suspected and treated for a lung infection. After 4 days of treatment, the patient suddenly appeared very weak and unresponsive to instruction, unable to move or lift extremities, particularly on the right side. Subsequently, the patient was suspected of stroke and transported to the intensive care unit (ICU).

Regarding the recurrent hospital admission, lumbar puncture was performed to determine the possibility of central nervous system (CNS) infection. The result was negative, showing no infection, including tuberculosis. A head CT scan was conducted to examine the brain, and the imaging showed no abnormality, resulting in a negative for the suspected stroke.

Head magnetic resonance angiography (MRA) was carried out to clarify whether the brain was eventually cleared from any stroke. The MRA imaging showed abnormalities in two lobes of the brain, including acute infarcts on the left parietal lobe and subacute infarcts on the left frontal lobe (Fig. 6.1). However, there was no sign of stenosis, arteriovenous malformation (AVM), or aneurysm observed in the imaging.

Table 6.1 The patient's blood glucose levels (BGL) and blood pressure (BP) readings during hospitalization

Day since admission	2nd	3rd	4th	5th	6th	7th	8th	9th	10th	11th	12th	13th	14th	15th
BGL	234	157	147	296	*	205	256	160	117	247	73	148	90	219
BP	150/89	164/98	171/102	160/82	166/82	137/74	120/84	138/76	160/88	146/72	160/86	154/87	150/80	*

*No measurement was performed on the indicated day

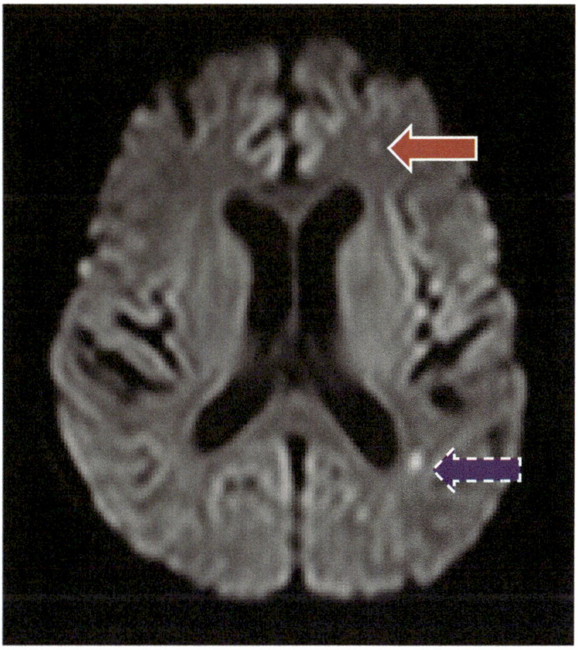

Fig. 6.1 The patient's head magnetic resonance angiography (MRA) imaging. Hyperintense lesion on fluid-attenuated inversion recovery (FLAIR) method, and restricted diffusion on diffusion-weighted imaging (DWI) method were found on the left parietal lobe of the brain (dashed-line arrow). Meanwhile, the same hyperintense lesion on FLAIR was found on the left frontal lobe (solid-line arrow). The patient was diagnosed with an ischemic stroke. (Image Courtesy: Dewi Tantra MD)

In addition to MRA, carotid USG imaging was also performed, showing the narrowing of both carotid sinuses caused by the plaques. The discovered plaques resulted in 30% stenosis of both carotid sinuses (Fig. 6.2), without signs of thrombus and obstructed carotid flows.

Despite the aggressive treatments administered in response to the radiological findings, the clinical condition did not improve. The patient's family was informed regarding the clinical deterioration and prognosis. A decision was made against resuscitation (do not resuscitate (DNR) and intubate), opting for supportive treatments. A week after the ICU admittance, the patient was finally declared dead.

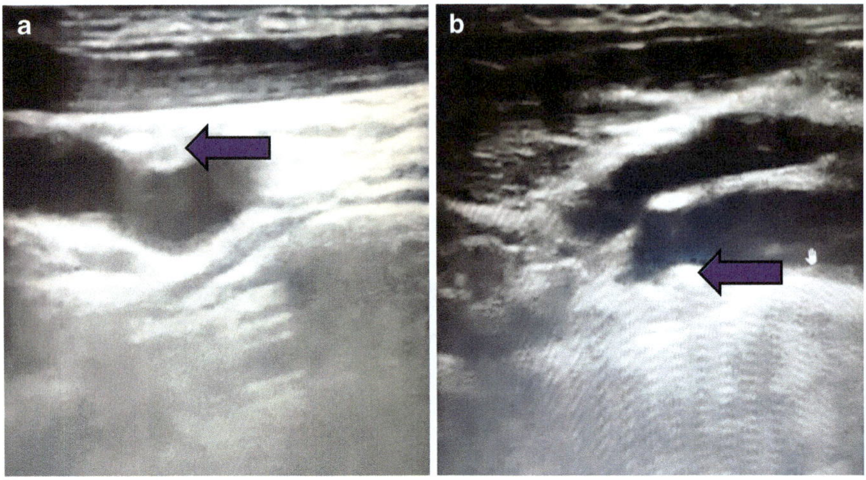

Fig. 6.2 The patient's carotid ultrasonography (USG) imaging. Both the left (box **a**) and right (box **b**) carotid sinuses were obstructed with plaque as shown by the arrows, which caused 30% stenosis in each carotid sinus. (Image Courtesy: Arif Sejati MD)

6.2 What Is the Patient's Problem?

The patient initially came to the hospital with a major complaint of breathing difficulty and fever. A chest X-ray examination suggested the presence of pneumonia, with multiple comorbidities including hypertension, heart failure, type 2 diabetes mellitus (T2DM), and chronic kidney disease (CKD). Subsequently, treatment was administered for both pneumonia and the comorbidities during hospitalization, without carotid USG imaging.

After discharge, the patient was readmitted to the hospital with the same complaint as the first initial admission. Several days after the readmission, an ischemic stroke occurred, confirmed by the MRA imaging. Carotid USG imaging was also performed, showing plaques in both carotid sinuses. A week later, the patient was declared dead due to the acquired stroke. Moreover, there was relative noncompliance with treatments before the hospital admissions.

6.3 Discussion

Diabetes mellitus (DM) is associated with increased illness, and death rates, as well as various acute and predominantly chronic issues arising from both functional and structural damage to the blood vessels. Specifically, diabetic vasculopathy primarily entails alterations to the vascular wall, resulting in impaired function of both endothelial and smooth muscle cells. Multiple clinical studies have analyzed the relationship between specific sonographic characteristics of the carotid arteries and the immediate clinical results of individuals with carotid atherosclerosis in diabetes [1].

Type 2 diabetes is regarded as a component of metabolic syndrome, leading to both small and large blood vessel issues. Diabetes is a contributing factor in the progression of atherosclerosis and carotid artery disease, including a cerebrovascular accident. The most prevalent imaging method for diagnosing carotid disease is Doppler ultrasonography [2]. Stenosis of more than 50% in the extracranial internal carotid arteries is associated with approximately 8–15% of ischemic strokes. Diabetics with unstable and vulnerable plaques were discovered to have carotid artery disease, which could lead to thromboembolism. The development of carotid artery disease in individuals with type 2 diabetes is influenced by a group of metabolic factors, including insulin resistance, hyperlipidemia, obesity, and arterial hypertension [3].

Generally, DM is a long-term metabolic condition defined by consistently high levels of glucose in the blood. The cause is attributed to compromised insulin secretion, resistance to insulin's peripheral effects, or a combination of both. DM is categorized into three main kinds based on its cause and clinical manifestation, including type 1, type 2, and gestational diabetes mellitus (GDM). Type 2 diabetes mellitus (T2DM) comprises approximately 90% of the total number of cases, characterized by reduced sensitivity to insulin, namely insulin resistance. Uncontrolled DM can lead to various consequences, both immediate and long-term, due to consistently high blood sugar levels. This medical condition is a prominent contributor to the development of cardiovascular disease (CVD), vision loss, renal failure, and lower limb amputation. Acute consequences of DM include hypoglycemia, diabetic ketoacidosis, hyperglycemic hyperosmolar condition, and hyperglycemic diabetic coma. The chronic microvascular problems include nephropathy, neuropathy, and retinopathy. Meanwhile, chronic macrovascular complications consist of coronary artery disease (CAD), peripheral artery disease (PAD), and cerebrovascular disease. Annually, a CVD incident occurs in approximately 1.4 to 4.7% of middle-aged DM patients. These patients have a threefold higher risk of developing CVD, including conditions such as coronary and carotid artery disorders, as well as stroke, compared to those without DM. The carotid bifurcation, commonly impacted by atherosclerosis and serving as a potential origin for both transient ischemic episodes and strokes, is a crucial area for examination. Doppler ultrasonography (DU) is a precise and widely accepted method that does not require any invasive procedures to assess carotid artery disease [4].

Carotid DU is a widely used method for assessing the presence of atherosclerosis in the carotid artery. The two-dimensional grayscale of the image can be used to measure the intima-media thickness, serving as an excellent biomarker for atherosclerosis and can assist in characterizing plaques. The appearance of the plaque is associated with the possibility of experiencing stroke [5].

6.4 Carotid Artery Anatomy

The right carotid artery originates from the right brachiocephalic artery. Ultrasonography (USG) can visualize the closest section of the common carotid artery. The left common carotid artery originates from the aortic arch. However, USG is unable to visualize the proximal portion of the left common carotid artery.

The examiner must possess the ability to distinguish between the internal carotid artery (ICA) and the external carotid artery (ECA). The ICA is situated in a posterior, laterally positioned relative to the ECA, and is marginally larger. Moreover, the ECA possesses branches, such as the lingual artery, while the ICA does not have branches [5].

6.5 Intima Media Thickness

The intima-media thickness (IMT) is commonly used as a measure for assessing atherosclerosis and is quantified using a two-dimensional (2D) grayscale picture. The ideal monochromatic image of the longitudinal scan of the carotid artery, which traverses through the middle of the carotid artery, shows two luminous boundaries along the arterial wall. The upper bright line in the far wall represents the boundary between the blood and intima. Meanwhile, the lower bright line represents the boundary between the media layer and the adventitia layer. The boundary between the intima and media layers does not generate any interface. The disparity between the upper and lower luminous boundaries signifies the magnitude of the intima and media layer's thickness. For more accurate results, the carotid artery should be arranged parallel to the surface of the probe. This will help reduce any potential overestimation of the IMT that may occur when measuring diagonally. The IMT is often assessed on the far wall of the distal common carotid artery. This option is made because the common carotid artery is more easily visualized and shows less variability compared to the Internal Carotid Artery (ICA), primarily due to the angle of the ultrasonography beam or the depth of the vessel [5].

6.6 Plaque Morphology

Plaque morphology, such as echogenicity, surface, and ulceration, as well as the presence of plaque and stenosis, is important for predicting future cardiovascular events. A description of the plaque morphology from a gray-scale image is highly recommended during carotid Doppler ultrasonography (DU). This description should include the echogenicity, surface, and the presence of ulceration. The echogenicity of the plaque could be described as echogenic, isoechoic, echolucent, or heterogeneous. Isoechoic plaque shows that the echogenicity is the same as the intima-media complex. The surface can be described as smooth, irregular, or ulcerated, while plaque ulceration is associated with an increased risk of stroke. However, detecting plaque ulceration through USG examination is very challenging and highly operator-dependent. The sensitivity of detecting carotid plaque ulceration ranges from <30% to >80% compared to pathological specimens. The effort to detect ulceration should be applied to increase the accuracy of risk assessment of the patient with carotid plaque. Another problem is the inability to correlate with symptoms and detect without careful gray-scale examination. The depression of the plaque surface by more than 2 mm is thought to indicate ulceration, showing various patterns, including cystic, bridge-shaped, sponge-shaped, or a simple depression [5, 6].

Regarding echogenicity, it has been observed that symptomatic lesions are commonly correlated with plaques that are primarily or mostly hypoechoic. An effort has been made to quantitatively evaluate the echogenicity of plaque using longitudinal images of the plaque and vessel wall to quantify the gray-scale median (GSM). Based on categorization, the GSM of the blood pool ranged from 0 to 5, while the adventitia of the wall varied between 185 and 195. Moreover, it was discovered that the possibility of having a stroke during carotid stenting procedures was influenced by the GSM (GigaHertz Square) value of the plaque. GSM values of 25 or lower showed a stroke risk of 7.1%, while plaque with values over 25 had a stroke risk of only 1.5%. Consequently, echolucent plaque has a higher susceptibility to damage [5].

6.7 Management

Platelet inhibition and anticoagulation are essential in diabetic patients with CAD. These interventions reduced the overall risk of vascular mortality, myocardial infarction (MI), and stroke by 19% in patients with diabetes. Low molecular weight heparin provides a similar reduction in events for patients with diabetes, as it does for those without diabetes in cases of unstable angina. The inclusion of tirofiban alongside heparin resulted in a greater reduction in mortality and myocardial infarction rates among patients with diabetes compared to those without diabetes [7].

6.8 Coronary Revascularization

Both diabetes and nondiabetes patients have comparable percentages of initial success following percutaneous coronary revascularization. Shortly after patients with diabetes depart from the catheterization laboratory, there are clinical occurrences at elevated frequencies compared to nondiabetic patients. Moreover, patients diagnosed with diabetes often show a distinct pattern of elevated incidence of in-stent thrombosis. Multiple studies have shown an increased long-term risk of restenosis following balloon angioplasty [7].

6.9 Cerebrovascular Disease

Patients with diabetes and cerebrovascular atherosclerosis should additionally be prescribed platelet antagonists, statins, and ACE inhibitors. The implementation of surgical revascularization in cases of hemodynamically severe internal carotid artery atherosclerosis led to a reduced incidence of strokes compared to relying solely on medicinal therapy [7].

Question

1. Below are acute complications of diabetes mellitus, except?
   (a) Hypoglycemia
   (b) Diabetic ketoacidosis
   (c) Hyperglycemic hyperosmolar state
   (d) Hyperglycemic diabetic coma
   (e) Cerebrovascular Disease
2. The most common imaging technique for the diagnosis of carotid disease is?
   (a) MRI
   (b) CT Scan
   (c) Rontgen
   (d) PET Scan
   (e) Doppler Ultrasonography
3. What is a good biomarker for atherosclerosis and can aid in plaque characterization?
   (a) Measuring the intima-media thickness
   (b) Measuring the tunica adventitia thickness
   (c) Identify the plaque morphology
   (d) Carotid bifurcation
   (e) The plaque ulceration
4. How to measure the intima-media thickness using Doppler ultrasonography?
   (a) Measure the distance between the upper and lower bright lines
   (b) Measure the distance between the upper and lower depth lines
   (c) Estimation of the IMT from the vertical measurement
   (d) Shows two bright interfaces along the vein wall
   (e) Shows upper bright lines along the artery wall
5. Treatment given to diabetic patients with CAD:
   (a) Fibrinolytic
   (b) Platelet Inhibition
   (c) Anticoagulant
   (d) Anticoagulant and Platelet inhibition
   (e) Fibrinolytic, Platelet Inhibition, and Anticoagulants

Answer Keys

1. E
2. E
3. A
4. A
5. D

Acknowledgment Cipta Mahendra, MD, Department of Internal Medicine, Respirology and Critical Illness Division, Universitas Indonesia, Dr. Cipto Mangunkusumo General Central National Hospital, Jakarta, Indonesia.

Key Point
Diabetes Mellitus is a contributing factor in the progression of atherosclerosis and similarly carotid artery disease, including a cerebrovascular accident. Carotid Doppler Ultrasonography is a widely used method for assessing the presence of atherosclerosis in the carotid artery.

Ersananda Arlisa Putri, MD, Department of Internal Medicine, Respirology and Critical Illness Division, Universitas Indonesia, Dr. Cipto Mangunkusumo General Central National Hospital, Jakarta, Indonesia.
Arif Sejati, MD DM, Department of Internal Medicine, Cardiovascular Division, Universitas Katolik Indonesia Atma Jaya, Mochtar Riady Comprehensive Cancer Center (MRCCC) Siloam Hospital, Jakarta, Indonesia.
Anne Dinna Subroto, MD, PhD, Department of Neurology, Mochtar Riady Comprehensive Cancer Center (MRCCC), Siloam Hospital, Jakarta, Indonesia.

References

1. Hoke M, Schillinger M, Minar E, Goliasch G, Binder CJ, Mayer FJ. Carotid ultrasound investigation as a prognostic tool for patients with diabetes mellitus. Cardiovasc Diabetol. 2019;12(18):90.
2. Sultana N, Islam MR. Doppler evaluation of carotid vessels in type 2 diabetes. Mymensingh Med J. 2020;29:572–8.
3. Areej H, Farooq SMY, Asad N, Fatima M, Mahmood A, Attique UKA, Tahir MU, Khan HN. Carotid artery disease assessed by color Doppler flow imaging: comparison between diabetic and non-diabetic patients. Adv Life Sci. 2023;10:66–71.
4. Goyal R, Singhal M, Jialal I. Type 2 diabetes. StatPearls Publ; 2023. https://www.ncbi.nlm.nih.gov/books/NBK513253/
5. Lee W. General principles of carotid Doppler ultrasonography. Ultrasonography. 2014;33:11–7.
6. Rafailidis V, Chryssogonidis I, Tegos T, Kouskouras K, Charitanti-Kouridou A. Imaging of the ulcerated carotid atherosclerotic plaque: a review of the literature. Insights Imaging. 2017;8:213–25.
7. Beckman JA, Creager MA, Libby P. Diabetes and atherosclerosis. JAMA. 2002; https://doi.org/10.1001/jama.287.19.2570.

Cytomegalovirus Pneumonia in Critically Ill Patient

7

7.1 Case Illustration

A 68-year-old male patient was presented to the emergency ward with the chief complaint of awareness impairment. According to family members, the impairment occurred suddenly with no preceding events, and a history of head injury, headache, vomiting, double vision, hearing disturbance, slurred speech, and pouting mouth was denied. However, the patient had a history of hypertension and diabetes and was relatively noncompliant with regular visits to the doctor.

Approximately 6 days before admission, an episode of convulsion was experienced for 15 minutes, with continuous jerking of the left hand. The patient was unconscious during and after the convulsion and was then brought to the nearest hospital. A head CT scan was performed, leading to a diagnosis of stroke after the imaging procedure. Subsequently, healthcare management was performed in a high-care unit (HCU) ward, where another episode of convulsion occurred during the treatment period. The patient was then discharged and treated as an outpatient, but the level of awareness started declining again. This led to a return to the hospital and eventual transfer to the current facility.

On physical examination, the patient was apathetic in appearance, and vital signs were within normal range except for the blood pressure (185/105 mmHg). Neurological examination revealed relative weakness on the left side of the body compared to the right side, with decreased motoric powers and no pathological reflexes. In addition, chest auscultation showed minimal rhonchi and stridor at the base of the lungs. All other body systems and organs were within normal findings and limits. Subsequently, the patient underwent an initial chest X-ray, with the results showing reticular opacities of the left lung's basal field. Laboratory examinations revealed numerous abnormalities in fibrinogen (900 mg/dL; normal: 200–400), D-dimer (4820 μg/L; normal: <440), creatinine (2.8 mg/dL), blood urea (122 mg/dL), eGFR (22.2 mL/min/1.73 m^2), blood glucose (255 mg/dL), procalcitonin (1.08 ng/mL), and C-reactive protein (226 mg/L; normal: 5 mg/L). The lipid profile was also relatively anomalous, with

G. Singh, *Challenging Cases in Respirology and Critical Care*, https://doi.org/10.1007/978-981-96-5002-6_7

elevated triglyceride and decreased HDL cholesterol values. The blood urate levels were increased, and SARS-CoV-2 infection was found negative.

Based on the history and initial examination findings, the patient was diagnosed with nonconvulsive status epilepticus (NCSE) caused by ischemic stroke, with multiple comorbidities. These included hospital-acquired pneumonia (HAP), hypertension, acute kidney injury (AKI), and type 2 diabetes mellitus (T2DM). The patient was then given the appropriate drugs according to the diagnosed conditions, including topiramate, lamotrigine, heparin, candesartan, amlodipine, simvastatin, insulin, allopurinol, and levofloxacin. Intravenous (IV) fluids and supporting supplementations (oxygen, vitamin B) were also administered.

During the first week after admission, the patient's awareness level fluctuated, with no sign or event of seizure or convulsion. However, slimes were found obstructing the airway and necessitating a suction procedure for evacuation. The patient also underwent blood drawing and culture to detect the presence of any bloodstream infection, with the results being negative (sterile). In the following week, another chest X-ray was obtained, showing increased infiltrates and opacities on both lung fields, with pleural effusion on the left lung. Examination also revealed that the awareness level continued to fluctuate. Considering the elevation of the blood urea level, an additional diagnosis of uremic encephalopathy was established, leading to a hemodialysis schedule.

At the beginning of the third week after admission, the patients exhibited a marked increase in work of breathing and a reduction in blood pressure. Sputum samples were collected and subjected to Gram staining and culture, which revealed the presence of Gram-negative bacteria, specifically *Escherichia coli* (*E. coli*). Testing for SARS-CoV-2 infection was still negative, and hypernatremia was also found on blood electrolyte analysis. Subsequently, an endotracheal tube (ETT) was inserted to secure the airway, and a ventilator was used to support breathing. The patient was transferred to the HCU ward due to the condition, where additional antibiotics and antifungals were given to prevent further nosocomial infections. Vasopressors were also administered to support and stabilize the blood pressure.

Further analysis showed that *Mycobacterium tuberculosis* bacteria were not found on the sputum samples. Bronchial washing (BW) was then performed and sent to the laboratory for examination, confirming the absence of tuberculosis infection (by GeneXpert MTB/RIF). However, cytomegalovirus (CMV) infection was detected, prompting the quantification of viral load. Based on the findings obtained, the patient was suspected of CMV pneumonitis.

In the late third week, the patient underwent the first hemodialysis session. The hemoglobin (Hb) level was found to decrease to 8.7 g/dL, necessitating blood transfusion to restore the Hb level. In addition, an electroencephalography (EEG) test was performed, which revealed patterns of brief potentially ictal rhythmic discharges (BIRDs). The BW analysis revealed the presence of another infection by Gram-positive cocci alongside CMV. Another blood culture was then performed, showing the presence of *Staphylococcus epidermidis* (*S. epidermidis*) bacteria. A Galactomannan (GM) antigen test was ordered to assess the presence of aspergillosis.

During the fourth week, the patient's clinical conditions were relatively stable, with no convulsion or seizure occurring. Wet crackles were heard on lung auscultation, predominantly on the right side. An echocardiography examination showed a dilated left atrium, global hypokinesis, and signs of reduced ejection fraction on the imaging. This led to a new diagnosis of heart failure with reduced ejection fraction (HFrEF). Despite insulin injections, blood glucose control was still suboptimal. Another chest X-ray image was carried out, which showed no change in the patient's lung fields compared to the previous imaging.

The GM antigen test result was positive (3.56; cut-off value: <1.8), leading to a diagnosis of lung aspergillosis. The ventilator remained connected to the patient's ETT to support the breathing. A tracheostomy was then scheduled after considering the length of stay in the hospital and the current clinical status, and the procedure was finally performed at the end of the week. While waiting for the CMV viral load result, ganciclovir antiviral treatment was planned based on the presence of CMV on the BW analysis. In addition, a urinalysis was carried out, which showed the presence of albumin and blood in the urine.

The CMV viral load test result was issued the following week, revealing the presence of 250 cells/mL of CMV particles. An internal multidisciplinary meeting was held, and the decision was to withhold the antiviral treatment as the viral load was deemed too low. The patient's condition began to deteriorate, and elevation of liver transaminases was found, leading to the postponement of simvastatin treatment. Another BW fluid was sampled and analyzed, showing the presence of *Acinetobacter* bacteria. Gram-positive cocci were still positive on the fluid, and the patient's Hb level did not return to normal range despite several blood transfusions since the third week of hospitalization. Blood pressure also started to drop consistently despite the administration and increased dose of vasopressors. At the end of the week, the patient was observed to be asystolic. The family was informed of the clinical conditions and approved the do-not-resuscitate initiative. Consequently, resuscitation was not performed, and the patient was declared dead. During the five-week hospital stay, there was no episode of seizure or convulsion, and the presence of SARS-CoV-2 remained negative.

7.2 What Is the Patient's Problem Focus?

A 68-year-old male presented to the hospital with the chief complaint of awareness impairment after previously experiencing a 15-minute convulsion 6 days before admission. The patient was diagnosed with NCSE caused by ischemic stroke, accompanied by multiple comorbidities (HAP, AKI, T2DM, hypertension, HFrEF). During treatments, bacterial and fungal infections were contracted, including *E. coli, S. epidermidis, Aspergillus,* and *Acinetobacter*. In addition, examination also showed the presence of cytomegalovirus (CMV) viral infection. All these infections were suspected to contribute to the patient's pneumonic condition, particularly CMV (based on the BW analysis). Several laboratory parameters were also out of range in values, such as decreased Hb, increased blood urea, and elevated glucose level. Antibiotics and antifungals were then given to treat the conditions. However, the ganciclovir antiviral was not approved to be administered because the patient's CMV viral load was too low. During the hospitalization weeks, the patient never experienced any seizure or convulsion.

7.3 Discussion

Cytomegalovirus (CMV) is a prominent member of the beta herpes virus family and a significant human pathogen. Several studies have shown that it has a high infection rate, with the prevalence of antibodies increasing from 65% in individuals aged 40–49, to 91% in those aged ≥80 years. After the first infection, CMV, in similarity to other beta herpes viruses, enters a state of long-term latency. Individuals with a robust immune system may exhibit asymptomatic viral shedding, which can be identified in their saliva or urine. However, the cell-mediated responses of the immune system hinder the manifestation of overt CMV infection [1].

7.4 Definition

Primary cytomegalovirus (CMV) infection typically occurs in infancy and early adolescence. In individuals with a healthy immune system, it is often asymptomatic or causes moderate and self-limiting symptoms. After the resolution of an acute infection, CMV enters a latent phase within leukocytes, specifically mononuclear cells. This stage is identified by a positive anti-CMV IgG serology (indicating seropositivity) and is characterized by the presence of the viral genome without the production of active infectious virions. However, the viral genome retains the ability to reactivate under specific conditions. Several studies have shown that immunocompetent individuals who are critically ill can develop the infection. CMV infection has been widely documented in severely ill immunocompetent patients undergoing surgery or experiencing sepsis, burns, or trauma [2].

7.5 Epidemiology

Several epidemiological studies have investigated the prevalence of cytomegalovirus (CMV) infection in individuals who are severely ill. These studies vary in their inclusion criteria, with some only considering individuals who tested positive for CMV antibodies. Therefore, only the frequency of the virus's reactivation was investigated, rather than the overall frequency of the infection, which could be significantly greater if seronegative patients who acquire new infections were also considered. The studies also differ in terms of the populations examined, comprising all patients in intensive care units to specific subgroups, such as those with sepsis, undergoing surgery, experiencing burns, or recovering from cardiac surgery. These subgroups could possess distinct susceptibilities to acquiring CMV infection [2].

7.6 Clinical Manifestation

Diagnosing cytomegalovirus (CMV) illness in individuals with a robust immune system is challenging due to its non-specific symptoms, involvement of several organs, and clinical characteristics that overlap with other severe diseases. Heininger et al. conducted a study that found that approximately 10% of cases could experience severe organ complications due to CMV infection. A comprehensive analysis examining its severe clinical symptoms among immunocompetent patients in the intensive care unit (ICU) showed that the gastrointestinal tract was the region most affected by various conditions. These included hepatitis, gastroenteritis, duodenitis, enteritis, colitis, and proctitis. Consequently, the central nervous system is impacted, causing diseases such as encephalitis, myelitis, encephalomyelitis, meningitis, and meningioradiculopathy. The hematological system can also be impacted, leading to the development of hemolytic anemia, thrombocytopenia, disseminated intravascular coagulation, and pancytopenia. The incidence of multi-organ involvement, including the lungs and eyes, has been reported to be infrequent. The scarcity of recorded cases of myocarditis in immunocompromised patients hinders the recognition of CMV myocarditis as a distinct medical condition. In recent years, there have been recorded cases of vascular symptoms, such as portal or femoropopliteal vascular thrombosis and pulmonary embolism, that are believed to be associated with damage to vascular endothelial cells. The potential immunomodulatory impacts of CMV can heighten susceptibility to subsequent bacterial and fungal infections in a critical care setting [2].

CMV pneumonia is a well-documented manifestation of CMV infection in individuals with compromised immune systems. However, lung involvement is rarely detectable in immunocompetent critically ill patients, specifically when intubated for causes unrelated to lung problems. Several studies have shown that the frequency of the infection can reach up to 50% among individuals with ventilator-associated pneumonia or ICU-acquired acute respiratory distress syndrome (ARDS) [2].

7.7 Diagnosis

Observing symptoms indicative of organ damage and detecting the presence of cytomegalovirus (CMV) infection only in the bloodstream, regardless of the diagnostic techniques used, is insufficient to establish a diagnosis. This limitation arises due to the potential presence of other infectious or non-infectious factors. The enzyme-linked immune assays and anticomplement immunofluorescence assays are commonly used techniques to measure the levels of CMV-specific IgM or IgG antibodies. IgM antibodies are typically detectable during the initial phase of the infection and often remain in the body for a duration of 4–6 months. Given the persistent presence of IgG seropositivity, relying on IgG antibodies as a diagnostic tool is unreliable. In a significant group of patients without additional risk factors, as well as in those with sepsis, extended stays in the critical care unit, or higher severity scores, there was no observed association between CMV serology and a negative outcome. At present, there is insufficient data to support the use of quantitative PCR (qPCR) as a reliable method for confirming CMV infection in tissue samples. In addition, the positive predictive value of quantitative polymerase chain reaction (qPCR) is insufficient, and there are no recognized exact thresholds. Building on this idea, diagnosing CMV pneumonia is often difficult because viral shedding occurs in the airways without any accompanying symptoms. When diagnosing CMV pneumonia, it is important to consider multiple aspects. These include (1) a negative result from a DNA test for CMV in bronchoalveolar lavage (BAL) fluid has a negative predictive value close to 100%, strongly indicating the absence of the condition, (2) the detection accuracy of CMV DNA in BAL fluid as a marker increases with higher quantities of viral DNA in the BAL and with an elevated risk of CMV infection in the patient being examined. The accurate determination of the threshold viral DNA load in the BAL is impeded by multiple factors, such as inter-patient variability, variations in the BAL procedure and processing techniques, discrepancies in the test used for DNA quantification, and the severity of symptoms [3].

7.8 Appropriate Time to Treat

In a case where reactivation of cytomegalovirus (CMV) (confirmed by positive antigenaemia and/or PCR) occurs together with clinical symptoms of infection, especially lung infiltrates, and the presence of risk factors (Fig. 7.1), curative antiviral treatment, specifically ganciclovir, is advised. For certain individuals with weakened immune systems, it is important to consider giving preventive medication for CMV reactivation, even in the absence of obvious signs. This must be made after carefully assessing the potential advantages and disadvantages. In this specific context, unless the amount of virus in the body is very high (more than 10,000 copies/mL), analyzing trends in viral load may offer more meaningful information than concentrating on a specific numerical value [4].

At present, the number of antiviral medications for treating CMV is limited. The implementation of these medications is linked to the occurrence of adverse consequences, which can exacerbate the overall prognosis for patients in the intensive care unit (ICU). In this context, the toxicities of ganciclovir, foscarnet, and cidofovir have been extensively studied and analyzed, leading to substantial exploration and reporting on the subject. The primary factor contributing to the toxicity associated with ganciclovir is mostly associated with hematological adverse effects, specifically neutropenia, thrombocytopenia, and occasionally anemia. Foscarnet primarily exerts its deleterious effects on the renal system. Patients on foscarnet therapy may experience disturbances in electrolyte levels, requiring regular monitoring of calcium, magnesium, phosphate, and potassium. Meanwhile, the use of cidofovir is associated with a significant occurrence of nephrotoxicity as a side effect. Currently, ganciclovir is considered a highly advantageous choice among these medications, mostly due to its comparatively low toxicity. Oral administration of valganciclovir is contraindicated during the initial phases of severe illness due to its poor intestinal

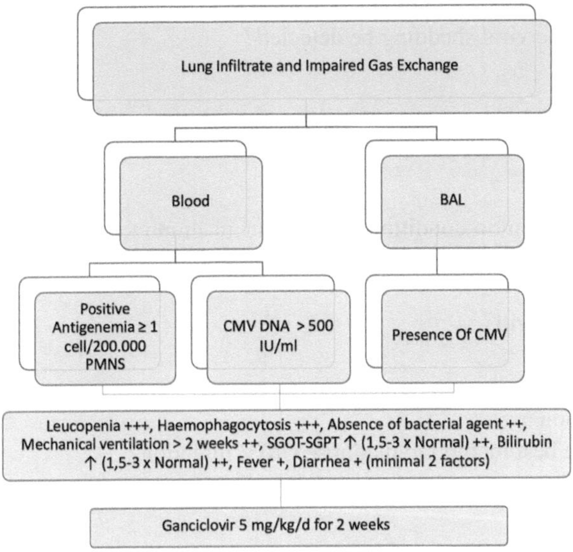

Fig. 7.1 Criteria for Starting Cytomegalovirus Treatment in Critically Ill Patients. (Adapted with permission from Springer-Verlag Berlin Heidelberg and ESICM)

absorption in individuals with ileus. Each of these medications has the potential to induce drug-resistant bacteria by specifically targeting DNA polymerase [4].

7.9 Prognosis

Cytomegalovirus (CMV) reactivation is observed in 35% of patients who test positive for the virus and has been linked to unfavorable outcomes, including an extended duration of stay in the intensive care unit and/or hospital, prolonged requirement for organ support, heightened susceptibility to bacterial infections, and increased mortality [5].

Key Point
In critically ill patients, a CMV infection should always be considered. A positive PCR CMV BAL result is indication for administering Ganciclovir 5 mg/kg/d for 2 weeks.

Question

1. The incidence of CMV steadily increases to 91% at the age of:
   (a) 40–49 years old
   (b) 80 or over years old
   (c) 40 years old
   (d) 49 years old
   (e) 61 years old

2. In immunocompetent individuals with CMV infection, in what specimen can asymptomatic viral shedding be detected?
   (a) Blood
   (b) Saliva
   (c) BAL
   (d) Feces
   (e) Mucosa
3. Below are common conditions that occur in immunocompetent CMV patients treated in the intensive care unit (ICU), except:
   (a) Hepatitis
   (b) Gastroenteritis
   (c) Duodenitis
   (d) Proctitis
   (e) Pneumonia
4. What is the best method to diagnose CMV infection?
   (a) qPCR
   (b) serology
   (c) CMV Antigens
   (d) Viral Culture
   (e) BAL
5. Currently, the excellent drug choice (due to fairly low toxicity) in CMV therapy is?
   (a) Cidofovir
   (b) Foscarnet
   (c) Ganciclovir
   (d) Valganciclovir
   (e) Acyclovir

Answer Keys

1. B
2. B
3. E
4. A
5. C

Acknowledgments Cipta Mahendra, MD, Department of Internal Medicine, Respirology and Critical Illness Division, Universitas Indonesia, Dr. Cipto Mangunkusumo General Central National Hospital, Jakarta, Indonesia.

Ersananda Arlisa Putri, MD, Department of Internal Medicine, Respirology and Critical Illness Division, Universitas Indonesia, Dr. Cipto Mangunkusumo General Central National Hospital, Jakarta, Indonesia.

Ivan Banjuradja, MD, Department of Internal Medicine, Universitas Indonesia, Dr. Cipto Mangunkusumo General Central National Hospital, Jakarta, Indonesia.

Robert Shinto, MD DM, Department of Internal Medicine, Tropical Infectious Diseases Division, Universitas Indonesia, Dr. Cipto Mangunkusumo General Central National Hospital, Jakarta, Indonesia.

References

1. Osawa R, Singh N. Cytomegalovirus infection in critically ill patients: a systematic review. Crit Care. 2009;13:R68.
2. Al-Omari A, Aljamaan F, Alhazzani W, Salih S, Arabi Y. Cytomegalovirus infection in immunocompetent critically ill adults: literature review. Ann Intensive Care. 2016;6:110.
3. Ljungman P, Camara R, Robin C, Crocchiolo R, Einsele H, Hill JA, Ward KN. Guidelines for the management of cytomegalovirus infection in patients with haematological malignancies and after stem cell transplantation from the. Lancet Infect Dis. 2019; https://doi.org/10.1016/s1473-3099(19)30107-0.
4. Schildermans J, Vlieger G. Cytomegalovirus: a troll in the ICU? overview of the literature and perspectives for the future. Front Med Lausanne. 2020;7:188.
5. De Vlieger G, Wijngaerden E. Cytomegalovirus in patients in the intensive care unit. JAMA Intern Med. 2017;177:1541.

Bronchoscopy in Burn Inhalation Injury

8

8.1 Case Illustration

A 40-year-old female patient presented to the hospital with severe burns due to a fire accident. The patient was trapped for approximately 30 min in the burning house, 8 h before hospital admission. Upon arrival, signs of agitation, along with coughs and coarse sounds on speaking were observed. Due to the lack of bronchoscopy resources, the patient was referred from another hospital to the current facility for assessment of airway conditions. Intravenous (IV) fluids were first administered for rehydration after the burn injury at the referring hospital. During the assessment, a history of pre-existing health issues was denied.

On physical examination, the patient was observed to be in full awareness but had limited verbal responsiveness. An endotracheal tube (ETT) was inserted into the airway since admission to the referring hospital and was connected to a ventilator. The blood oxygen saturation and other vital signs were observed to be in the respective normal range. In addition, visible burn injury was found covering the face, back, as well as upper and lower extremities. Several bullae and erythema were found on the surface of the injury. Examination of eyes, ears, mouth, and nostrils revealed the absence of any deformity. On auscultation, the lungs, heart, and abdomen were within normal findings.

Laboratory examinations revealed that several parameters were outside the normal range, including blood leucocyte level (28,140 cells/μL; normal: 4000–10,000), albumin (2.9 g/dL; normal: 3.5–5.2), procalcitonin (4.57 ng/mL; normal: <0.05), and C-reactive protein (127.6 mg/L; normal: <5.0). Meanwhile, all other results were within the respective normal range. Chest X-ray showed infiltrates in the lower right lung field, with no sign of pneumothorax, mediastinal, and subcutaneous emphysema (Fig. 8.1). Based on these findings, the patient was diagnosed with burn injury (covering about 37% of total body surface area) and hypoalbuminemia. IV fluids (including albumin), midazolam, and morphine were then administered as initial therapies. The patient was then urgently planned to undergo bronchoscopy to inspect and examine the airways for any inhalational trauma.

G. Singh, *Challenging Cases in Respirology and Critical Care*,
https://doi.org/10.1007/978-981-96-5002-6_8

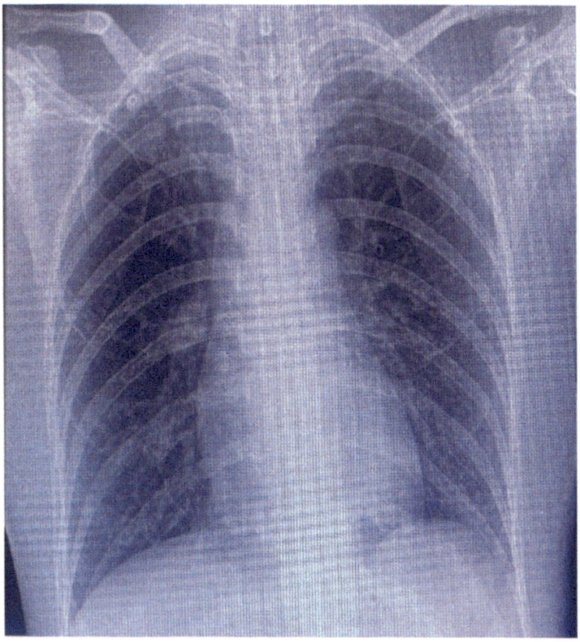

Fig. 8.1 Chest X-ray imaging on initial hospital admission. (Image Courtesy: Reyhan Eddy Yunus MD)

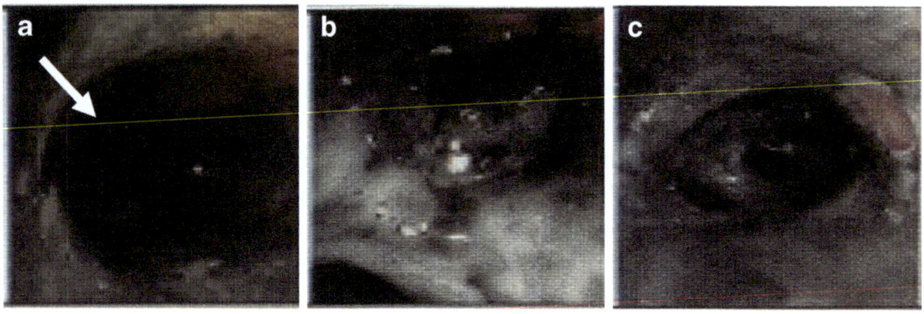

Fig. 8.2 (**a–c**) First bronchoscopy's imaging, showing black mucosal plaques lining the mucosae of the trachea and the bronchi. (white arrow). (Image Courtesy: Erika Marfani MD)

The next day, a bronchoscopy examination was carried out on the patient. The airway showed black mucosal plaques lining the mucosae of the trachea and the bronchi (Fig. 8.2), indicating inhalational trauma. Bronchial washing (BW) procedure was also performed, and the sputum obtained was sampled and sent for examination in the laboratory. The patient was fasted and received parenteral nutrition through IV fluids. Subsequently, a nasogastric tube (NGT), a urinary catheter, and a central venous catheter (CVC) were inserted. Ampicillin-sulbactam was then administered as a precaution against infection.

After several days, the patient became delirious and attempted to withdraw the ETT, leading to the administration of sedatives to achieve calmness. Slimes were found obstructing the ETT and acetylcysteine was given to thin the secretions. The bullae were then swabbed and sampled for laboratory examinations. Corticosteroids were also given to alleviate the resulting pain caused by the burn injury. The patient began to open the eyes but was still unable to make appropriate eye contacts. Undulating fever was experienced but no vomiting was observed, leading to the administration of supportive treatments (IV fluids, multivitamins, symptomatic medicamentosa, bandage replacements) during the treatment.

The patient's blood pressure tended to decline and norepinephrine administration was initiated. The bronchial culture analysis revealed the presence of α-hemolytic streptococci, with approximately 50,000 cells/mL. An antibiotic sensitivity test was ordered and the use of fluoroquinolone was suggested, leading to the administration of levofloxacin along with ampicillin-sulbactam. In addition, sputum analysis showed the presence of a few Gram-positive cocci, while swabbed bullae were found sterile. Blood electrolyte levels were reported to be outside the respective normal range (Na: 133 mEq/L; K: 3.2 mEq/L; Cl: 103.8 mEq/L), and correction was performed using appropriate IV fluid.

In the following week, the first skin debridement was performed in the operating theatre. The bullae were swabbed and sampled again for the second laboratory examination. A follow-up chest X-ray imaging showed nodular consolidation on the right lung field (Fig. 8.3). The patient then underwent a second bronchoscopy procedure, showing an inflamed lower respiratory tract with minimal carbon deposits, particularly on the right and left inferior lobes (Fig. 8.4). Slimes were still covering the airway but reduced in both quantity and thickness. The patient was subjected to extubation but it was unsuccessful due to decreased blood saturation during the attempt. Blood albumin and hemoglobin levels were low (2.30 g/dL and 7.8 g/dL, respectively), necessitating administration of IV albumin and blood transfusion.

Several days later, the bullae swab sample showed the presence of *Pseudomonas aeruginosa* infestation. In this context, an antibiotic sensitivity test revealed that *P. aeruginosa* was resistant to the carbapenem class of antibiotics. Consequently, the patient was medicated with piperacillin-tazobactam instead of meropenem. Ampicillin-sulbactam and levofloxacin administration were also stopped, but norepinephrine was still maintained to support the blood pressure. A second skin debridement procedure was then carried out, and the bullae were swabbed and sampled for the examinations. Nutrition through the NGT and IV fluids were adjusted according to the current clinical status and progress. When questioned, the patient appeared in somnolence but started to perform some affirmatory gestures.

During the third week after admission, there were no signs of coughs and slimes on the ETT. Although sedatives and norepinephrine were still administered, the doses used were reduced and the CVC was finally disconnected. The swab sample results showed the presence of *Enterobacter* bacteria in addition to the existing *P. aeruginosa*, but the antibiotic regimen remained unchanged. Subsequently, the patient underwent a third skin debridement to clear the bullae remnants and undulating fevers were still experienced. A third bronchoscopy was performed (Fig. 8.5), showing mucus hypersecretion

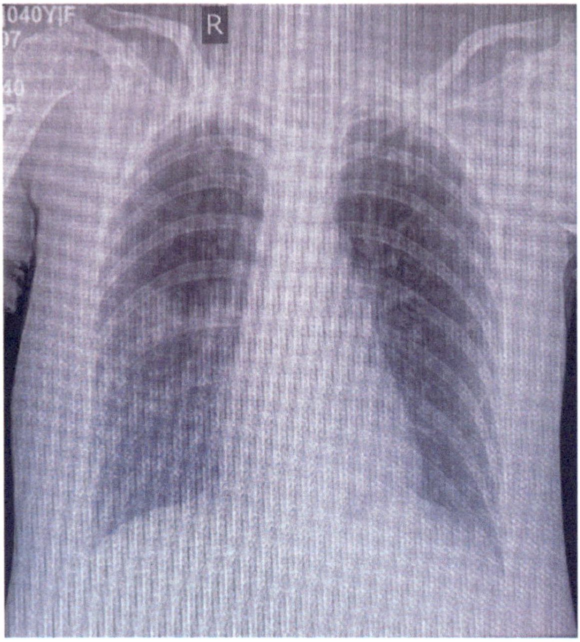

Fig. 8.3 Follow-up chest X-ray imaging, showing nodular consolidation on the right lung field. (~1st week since hospital admission). (Image Courtesy: Reyhan Eddy Yunus MD)

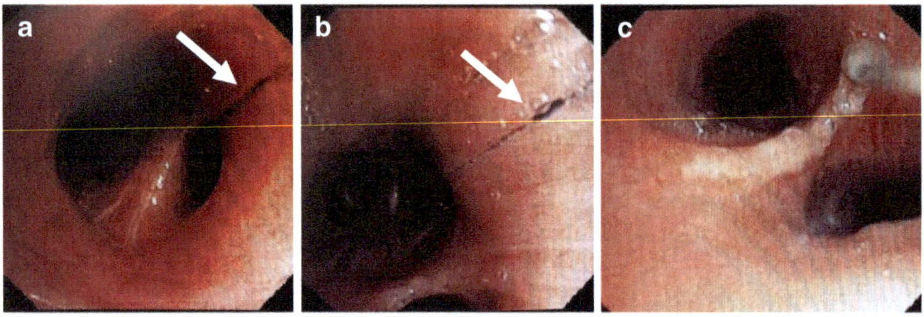

Fig. 8.4 (**a**–**c**) Second bronchoscopy's imaging. Inflamed lower respiratory tract with minimal carbon deposits was found. (white arrow). (Image Courtesy: Erika Marfani MD)

of the airway. Signs of inflammation were also still observed but carbon deposits were cleared from the airway. At this period, rehabilitative measures, including chest physiotherapy, breathing exercises, and joint movements, were being considered.

In the fourth week since admission, the patient was extubated successfully. Sedatives and norepinephrine were also finally stopped after evaluation and deemed clinically stable. Despite the improvement, oxygen supplementation continued through a nasal cannula. The NGT and urinary catheter were also retained with each oral meal being introduced. However, slimes were still felt and complained, prompting the administration of acetylcysteine.

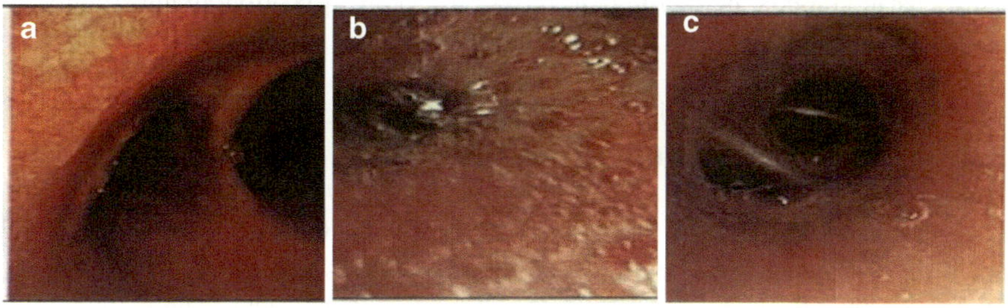

Fig. 8.5 (a–c) Third bronchoscopy imaging. Inflamed lower respiratory tract with no visible carbon deposits. (Image Courtesy: Erika Marfani MD)

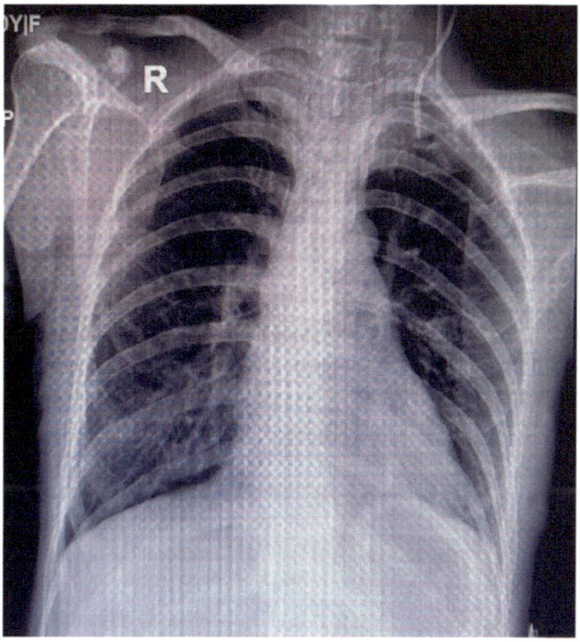

Fig. 8.6 Follow-up chest X-ray imaging on the final week of hospitalization, showing no abnormalities. The patient was lying in bed when the procedure was performed. (Image Courtesy: Vally Wulani MD DM)

During the final week of hospitalization, another skin debridement was performed to clear the remaining bullae and stimulate skin reepithelization. The antibiotic regimen of piperacillin-tazobactam was completed and discontinued. The CVC, NGT, and urinary catheter were finally removed from the patient. The rehabilitation programs and exercises were continued to enable the normal, pain-free movement and walking of the lower extremities. The chest X-ray imaging revealed normal findings, as shown in Fig. 8.6. Consequently, the patient was discharged from the hospital and instructed to visit the outpatient clinic to monitor the skin reepithelization progress and undergo rehabilitation programs. During the whole course of treatments, the swab tests for the presence of SARS-CoV-2 virus were consistently negative.

8.2 What Is the Patient's Problem Focus?

A 40-year-old female patient presented to the hospital with severe burns due to a fire accident. The patient was referred due to a lack of resources needed to perform bronchoscopy procedure and assess the airways. On physical examination, full awareness was observed, with vital signs, body organs, and systems being within normal findings, except the skin. Burn injury and the bullae were found covering the face, back, as well as upper and lower extremities.

The patient was promptly subjected to several bronchoscopy procedures during the first three weeks since admission to examine the airways for any inhalational trauma. In addition, bronchial washing (BW) was performed each time to clear the black mucous residues caused by the fire incident. Clinical improvements were continually observed in the following weeks after the successive washing. At the end of the fifth week, the patient was finally discharged from the hospital.

8.3 Discussion

Although there have been significant improvements in the care of individuals with inhalation injury, particularly in terms of providing assistance, the rates of illness and death remain high. In this context, an inhalation injury refers to the potential harm caused by exposure to heat that damages the upper larynx, irritation of the respiratory tract due to chemical exposure, poisoning of the body from substances, such as carbon monoxide (CO) and cyanide, or a combination of these factors. The induced inflammatory response may lead to elevated levels of fluid resuscitation, advancing pulmonary dysfunction, prolonged durations of mechanical ventilation, heightened susceptibility to pneumonia, and the development of acute respiratory distress syndrome (ARDS) [1].

8.4 Pathophysiology

Inhalation injury is a complex problem that occurs in burns, affecting approximately 10–20% of patients and leading to a significant increase in both illness and death rates. Additional factors that have been found to have a substantial impact on mortality rates include the extent of burn injury and the age of the individuals affected. In addition, the prevalence of this condition has a significant correlation with the extent of burn and age. The recognition of inhalation injury is a critical factor in predicting the mortality rates of those affected by burn. Several studies have also shown that inhalation injury significantly reduces survival rates, even in patients with equal age and burn size characteristics. The thermal airway injury mostly affects the upper airway structures, while the lower airway injury is predominantly chemical in nature. Exposure to steam warrants recognition due to its potential to cause significant harm, affecting the upper respiratory passages and inflicting direct thermal damage to the lungs. The severity of inhalation injury has been reported to vary based on various factors, including the composition of the inhaled gases, the presence of particulate matter (particularly soot), the length of exposure, and host factors, such as pre-existing lung conditions and the inability to escape the incident [1].

The predominant pathophysiological process found in upper airway inhalation injury is produced by microvascular changes caused by direct thermal damage and chemical irritation. High temperatures typically induce protein denaturation, leading to the initiation of the complement cascade and liberation of histamine. Subsequently, the production of xanthine oxidase occurs, causing the formation of reactive oxygen species (ROS). The produced ROS interact with nitric oxide in the endothelium, leading to the formation of edema in the upper airway. This occurs by raising the microvascular pressure and local permeability. Pro-inflammatory cytokines, ROS, and eicosanoids can stimulate the migration of polymorphonuclear cells to the specific location, causing elevated levels of ROS and the activation of signaling proteases. In this context, the microvascular hydrostatic and interstitial oncotic pressure experiences a significant increase, while the interstitial hydrostatic pressure reduces. Burn resuscitation comprises the administration of large amounts of crystalloid solution, which reduces the oncotic pressure of the plasma and affects the pressure difference in the small blood vessels, leading to a significant increase in swelling of the airways. Except for damage caused by inhaling steam and explosions, the upper airway efficiently defends the lower airway by regulating heat transfer to reduce harm to the lower airway [2].

8.5 Diagnosis

Previously, the diagnosis of inhalation injury often relied on both subjective and objective criteria. A thorough history and physical examination are essential components in this context due to their ability to help in predicting the host's response and the existence of co-morbidities. For example, the elderly population, who are unable to escape danger, may endure a prolonged period of being exposed to smoke and toxic substances. Key factors to consider when diagnosing the disease based on the patient's medical background include the precise etiology (such as combustion and fumes or vapor), the length of time of exposure, whether the incidence occurred in an enclosed setting, and any resultant impairment. During the physical examination, the following indications may be observed, including facial burn, scorched nose or facial hair, carbonaceous sputum, soot, stridor, or edema. Initially, chest X-rays at admission may reveal the absence of abnormalities. In addition, pulse oximetry (SpO_2) measurements of oxygen saturation are often unaffected and can be misleading, even in case of carbon monoxide poisoning where the SpO_2 reading typically falls within the normal range. Similarly, arterial blood gases may not be suggestive of a specific diagnosis. Although carbon monoxide poisoning may occur, the level of oxygen in the arterial blood (PaO_2) can remain normal or higher, while only the arterial oxygen saturation decreases [2].

Additional procedures performed to confirm inhalation injury include carboxyhemoglobin tests, chest computed tomography (CT), fiberoptic bronchoscopy (FOB), radionuclide scan using 133 Xenon, and pulmonary function testing. At present, these procedures demonstrate significant divergence both inside and externally among institutions, leading to a lack of discernment. Among the studies discussed, FOB provides the most precise prognostication of the risk of acute lung injury, resuscitative requirements, and mortality [2].

FOB is the typical approach used to diagnose inhalation injury, which is conveniently reachable and allows for a thorough evaluation over time. Signs of hyperemia, edema, and soot observed during FOB are suggestive of inhalation injury. However, there is still a lack of consensus on the methodology for assessing the extent of the injury. The degree of damage depends on the specific substance inhaled, the length of exposure, and the individual's physiological reaction to the injury. To underscore the problem with grading inhalation injury, it is crucial to acknowledge that FOB, the widely accepted diagnostic procedure, cannot access the narrower airways within the lungs. Consequently, several studies have shown that the range of bronchoscopic outcomes and death rates can be ascribed to the harm that occurs in the most distant air passages [3].

The Abbreviated Injury Score (AIS), introduced by Endorf and Gamelli, is the primary approach for evaluating the severity of inhalation injury. The AIS adopts a severity rating ranging from 0 (meaning no injury) to 4 (showing a serious injury) based on the observations made during the initial FOB evaluation. The application of the grading scale for evaluating inhalation injury using bronchoscopy has shown inconclusive results about its capacity to precisely forecast the outcome. In this context, some studies have found a correlation between more severe injury and decreased oxygenation. For example, a study revealed a correlation between a higher grade of inhalation injury and an extended duration of mechanical ventilation. However, other studies have failed to establish this association. Findings also show that there is no documented association between the AIS grade of inhalation injury severity and the need for fluid resuscitation. This indicates that there is no reliable association between the severity and an elevated fatality rate. A recent study revealed that patients with severe inhalation injury, previously classified as grades 3 and 4, showed noticeable trends toward worse oxygenation, longer duration of mechanical ventilation, and higher volumes of fluid resuscitation compared to those with grades 1 and 2. Therefore, further enhancement of the approach is required to achieve optimal results. Conducting numerous bronchoscopic evaluations within the initial 24–48 h following a burn could yield more accurate data compared to a solitary examination upon admission to the hospital [2].

An assessment of the severity of a medical condition can be made by examining laboratory measurements, such as PaO_2/FiO_2 and alveolar-arterial gradients. However, it is crucial to acknowledge that these values can exhibit substantial variations based on different breathing patterns and other clinical attributes [2].

8.6 Management

Inhalation injury typically leads to the formation of blockages, a reduction in the availability of surfactant, an elevation in airway resistance, and a decline in pulmonary compliance. Patients require intensive respiratory care, including chest physiotherapy, airway suctioning, therapeutic serial bronchoscopies, and early mobilization. These alternatives are the current treatment options available [2].

8.7 Bronchodilators

Bronchodilators typically decrease airway resistance and improve airway compliance. β2-adrenergic agonists, such as albuterol and salbutamol, alleviate airway constriction by relaxing smooth muscle and suppressing bronchospasm. This effect leads to an increase in the ratio of arterial oxygen partial pressure to fractional inspired oxygen concentration (PaO_2/FiO_2) [2].

8.8 Muscarinic Receptor Antagonists

Tiotropium, a muscarinic receptor antagonist, decreases airway resistance and mucus production by causing the contraction of smooth muscles and stimulating submucosal glands. In addition, several studies have shown that it restricts the secretion of cytokines [2].

Both beta-agonists and muscarinic receptor antagonists mitigate the inflammatory response following inhalation-induced injury. The respiratory system is anatomically lined with muscarinic and adrenergic receptors. The precise impact of these receptors on the inflammatory and host responses remains largely unknown. However, several studies have demonstrated that the agents can reduce the concentrations of pro-inflammatory cytokines following exposure to stress [2].

8.9 Inhaled (Nebulized) Mucolytic Agents and Anticoagulants

Mucolytic medications, such as N-acetylcysteine (NAC), are often used to alleviate airway obstruction caused by mucus, fibrin cast formation, and cellular debris arising from inhalation injury. NAC is a molecule with anti-inflammatory characteristics that functions as an antioxidant and eliminates free radicals. In addition, it is a powerful agent that breaks down mucus and decreases the detrimental impacts of reactive oxygen species (ROS) [2].

Inhaled anticoagulants are often used to relieve airway congestion caused by fibrin casts. Heparin demonstrates anti-inflammatory properties by obstructing the production of fibrin and inhibiting the creation of casts. However, the available evidence from a limited number of human studies is controversial. Several studies suggest that the administration of nebulized heparin (5000–10,000 units) and 3 mL of 20% NAC every 4 h for 1 week to burn patients with inhalation injury who are undergoing mechanical ventilation can provide benefits. This therapy has also been reported to improve the oxygen levels in the blood and the flexibility of the lungs, decrease the requirement for re-insertion of a breathing tube, and increase the chances of survival. Subsequent studies have revealed that it does not produce any improvements in the end outcome [2].

8.10 Prognosis

Inhalation of smoke or chemical products of combustion can cause respiratory injury, leading to serious illness and death. Prolonged pulmonary dysfunction has also been linked to inhalation injury, even when in isolation. In a previous study, four patients suffering from the condition are extremely prone to encountering difficulties. The primary cause of death in most burn case is respiratory failure, which can occur due to direct injury or complications, such as pneumonia. Severe injury often leads to long-lasting issues, such as bronchiectasis, bronchiolitis obliterans, and the need for artificial airways [4, 5].

Key Point
The usual method for diagnosing inhalation damage is fiberoptic bronchoscopy. It is easily accessible and enables a comprehensive assessment over time. Hyperemia, edema, and soot on FOB are indicative of inhalation injury.

Question

1. The following are the factors that determine the degree of inhalation injury, except:
   (a) Composition of the inhaled gases
   (b) The presence of particulate matter (specifically soot)
   (c) The duration of exposure
   (d) Individual host
   (e) Gender
2. Which one of the additional methods employed to confirm inhalation injury, below:
   (a) Chest X-ray
   (b) PaO_2 in arterial blood
   (c) Fiberoptic bronchoscopy
   (d) MRI
   (e) FiO_2
3. What is the predominant method for assessing the severity of an inhalation injury?
   (a) The Abbreviated Injury Score
   (b) The Revised Baux Score
   (c) The Ryan Model
   (d) BOBI score
   (e) McGwin

4. What is the common thermal airway injury impact?
   (a) Trachea
   (b) Bronchioles
   (c) The upper airway structures
   (d) Lung
   (e) Alveoli
5. The following are the vigorous respiratory care of inhalation injury, except:
   (a) Chest physiotherapy
   (b) Airway suctioning
   (c) Therapeutic serial bronchoscopies
   (d) Early mobilization
   (e) Bronchodilator

Answer Keys
1. B
2. B
3. E
4. A
5. C

Acknowledgments Cipta Mahendra MD, Department of Internal Medicine, Respirology and Critical Illness Division, Universitas Indonesia, Dr. Cipto Mangunkusumo General Central National Hospital, Jakarta, Indonesia.
Ersananda Arlisa Putri MD, Department of Internal Medicine, Respirology and Critical Illness Division, Universitas Indonesia, Dr. Cipto Mangunkusumo General Central National Hospital, Jakarta, Indonesia.
Erika Marfiani MD, Department of Internal Medicine, Respirology and Critical Illness Division, Universitas Indonesia, Dr. Cipto Mangunkusumo General Central National Hospital, Jakarta, Indonesia.
Adi Basuki MD, Department of Plastic Reconstructive, and Aesthatic Surgery, Universitas Indonesia, Dr. Cipto Mangunkusumo General Central National Hospital, Jakarta, Indonesia.

References

1. Walker PF, Buehner MF, Wood LA, Boyer NL, Driscoll IR, Lundy JB, Cancio LC, Chung KK. Diagnosis and management of inhalation injury: an updated review. Crit Care. 2015;19:351.
2. Jones SW, Williams FN, Cairns BA, Cartotto R. Inhalation injury: pathophysiology, diagnosis, and treatment. Clin Plast Surg. 2017;44:505–11.
3. Bai C, Huang H, Yao X, et al. Application of flexible bronchoscopy in inhalation lung injury. Diagn Pathol. 2012;8:174.
4. Shubert J, Sharma S. Inhalation injury, 2023. https://www.ncbi.nlm.nih.gov/books/NBK513261/.
5. Dries DJ, Endorf FW. Inhalation injury: epidemiology, pathology, treatment strategies. Scand J Trauma Resusc Emerg Med. 2013;21:31.

9 Pulmonary Embolism in Ischemic Stroke

9.1 Case Illustration

A 69-year-old male patient was brought to the hospital with one-sided body weakness and unresponsiveness for 6.5 h before arrival, where the right side was observed to be weaker than the left side. The patient could still open the eyes but stayed quiet and was unable to comprehend family members' words and instructions. Gestures showing shortness of breath were shown by the patient. According to accompanying family members, there was no experience of seizures and headaches.

Before admission, the patient was taken to another hospital, where CT scanning and chest X-ray were performed as the initial management. Cardiomegaly was found but there was no sign of any infarct or bleeding. Citicoline, vitamin K, and tranexamic acid were administered, along with medication to manage the cardiomegaly result during the stay at the hospital. After initial management, the patient was referred for further treatments and had a urine catheter, a nasogastric tube (NGT), and a nasal cannula inserted upon arrival.

The patient had been diagnosed with coronary artery disease 5 years ago and was given only oral drugs to manage as well as control the symptoms. Moreover, there was no history of surgery, smoking, and alcohol intake. Hypertension was admitted but not known for the duration, while the patient's mother had heart disease and hypertension. Before arriving at this hospital, several drugs were consumed, including amlodipine, Na-bicarbonate, furosemide, spironolactone, digoxin, cefixime, and candesartan.

Physical examinations showed elevated blood pressure (170/90 mmHg) and heart rate (110 times/min), while blood oxygen saturation was 98% with supplementation of 3 lpm. Body organs were found within normal limits but a sign of barrel chest was observed. Glasgow Coma Scale (GCS) parameter showed a total score of 9 (E4M5Vx; the patient was unable to produce any comprehensible sound or response to a stimulus). Signs of right central facial palsy were observed. Although neck stiffness was not found, motor function tests showed right-side

G. Singh, *Challenging Cases in Respirology and Critical Care*,
https://doi.org/10.1007/978-981-96-5002-6_9

weakness. Physiological reflexes were found to wane and babinski reflex was positive on the right foot. The patient's modified Rankin Scale (MRS) and National Institutes of Health Stroke Scale (NIHSS) score was 4 and 17, respectively. A repeat chest X-ray was performed, showing signs of cardiomegaly that confirmed the previous hospital's imaging expertise.

Laboratory examination showed several abnormalities, including elevation of D-dimer (1400 mg/L; normal: <440) and fibrinogen (506 mg/dL; normal: 200–400) value. Additionally, blood urea (94.2 mg/dL; normal: 18–55) and leucocyte count (12,530 cells/μL) were elevated. eGFR (33.3 mL/min/1.73 m^2) value showed a stage-III kidney failure. Urinary tract infections were suspected based on the urinalysis results, showing a significant presence of leucocytes and erythrocytes, leucocyte esterase, and albumin. The patient was confirmed negative for SARS-CoV-2. Based on the initial result from anamnesis, physical, and laboratory examinations, several diagnoses were made. These included acute ischemic stroke (AIS), global aphasia, and right hemiparesis caused by ischemic stroke, hypertension, acute kidney injury, macroscopic hematuria, hypercoagulable state, and microalbuminuria. Heart failure (HF) due to chronic hypertension was also suspected. The New York Heart Association (NYHA) functional classification was in class II–III, while both CHA_2DS_2-VASc and HAS-BLED scores were 5.

Several medications were administered, including aspirin, furosemide, amlodipine, bisoprolol, and candesartan. Despite the macroscopic hematuria finding, heparin was also given to the patient after the treating physician's consideration. Intravenous fluids were not infused but daily nutritional intake was given through the NGT. Oxygen supplementation was kept at 3 lpm using the nasal cannula. The next day, echocardiography was performed to further examine the heart. The results were poor echo window, global hypokinetic, high normal left ventricle (LV) and dilated left atrium (LA), decreased LV diastolic function, and increased LV filling pressure. The right ventricle (RV) systolic function was within normal results. Therefore, the patient was diagnosed with HF with reduced ejection fraction (HFrEF) and spironolactone was initiated to manage this condition. Additional laboratory examinations found an increase in blood uric acid (hyperuricemia) and cholesterol levels (dyslipidemia), leading to the prescription of allopurinol and atorvastatin.

During the first week of admission, the patient appeared ill and somnolent, showing unresponsive to most instructions, and only reacted briefly to pain stimuli. Grimacing appearance was observed when the patient's lower extremities were moved slightly, along with agitation and signs of restlessness. A carotid Doppler and a transcranial Doppler were performed, showing normal results for the transcranial Doppler. However, high peripheral resistance and bilateral bulb soft plaques were found during the carotid Doppler imaging procedure. The results of a brain CT scan showed infarcts at the cortical and subcortical regions of the left frontal lobe and insula, as well as atherosclerosis of distal right and left internal carotid artery. Gradual physiotherapy training was applied to restore the patient's mobility and motoric functions, leading to the resolution of gross hematuria. The patient did not experience fever, nausea, with breathing difficulty, and plans were made to undergo digital subtraction angiography (DSA) imaging.

During the following week, the clinical conditions fluctuated, as a reddish color reappeared in the urine collected through the catheter. Although eye contacts were maintained, the patient was still unresponsive and unable to produce any comprehensible sound or response. Blood electrolytes were found abnormal and the blood pressure was decreased, leading to temporary cessation of furosemide and candesartan. Intravenous fluids were administered to correct the electrolyte disturbances, resulting in the cancellation of DSA imaging. A kidney and urinary bladder ultrasound imaging was performed to determine the cause of the urine's redness, but the results were within the normal range. Another chest X-ray imaging was obtained and the results were in status quo compared to the previous chest X-ray imaging.

By the end of the second week, the patient's urine color appearance returned to normal. Sudden signs of shortness of breath were observed during the night, characterized by fast-paced breathing, and retraction of the intercostal, and sternocleidomastoid muscle. However, coughs, fever, nausea, and vomitus were not found, including chest pain and night or cold sweat. In the morning, the breathing difficulty ceased without any medication or intervention, but the respiratory rate increased from normal range. The blood pressure finally returned to normal, leading to the resumption of candesartan and furosemide administration. Another chest X-ray image showed heterogeneous opacities at the upper right lung region, indicating pneumonia. Widening of the lung's right and left hilus was also shown, resembling the sign of pulmonary hypertension. Laboratory examination showed elevation of blood C-reactive protein (CRP) and procalcitonin level, resulting in additional diagnosis with high-risk hospital-acquired pneumonia (HAP) and administration of levofloxacin.

Early third week of admission, the patient showed improving clinical conditions, evidenced by simple responses to instructions but breathing difficulty was still felt. Subsequently, a pulmonologist was consulted to manage the HAP. A lung ultrasound imaging was ordered to check for effusion but the result was negative. In response to the result, the pulmonologist requested thoracal and pulmonary CT angiography to further determine the cause of difficult breathing. A critical result was obtained, showing signs of acute emboli on both pulmonary and interlobar arteries, without lung infarction (Fig. 9.1). Calcifications of the coronary artery were found, while D-dimer value was still elevated, and blood albumin level decreased. Based on the CT angiography critical result, the diagnosis was changed

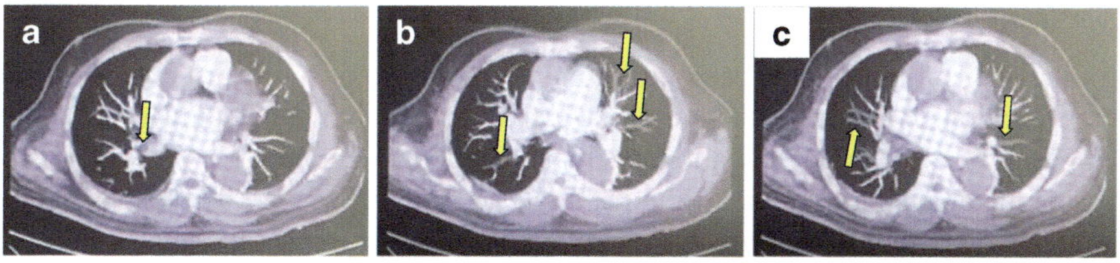

Fig. 9.1 (a–c) The patient's thoracal-pulmonary CT angiography imaging. Signs of acute emboli (pointed by yellow arrows) on both pulmonary and interlobar arteries were found. (Image Courtesy: Sahat Matondang MD DM)

to acute emboli of the lung (Fig. 9.1). Consequently, antibiotics were discontinued and enoxaparin replaced heparin an anticoagulant. The blood oxygen saturation was within normal limits.

By the end of the third week, the patient kept improving clinically, with breathing difficulty almost resolved. Rehabilitations to optimize mobility and restore daily activities were maintained. Theophylline was additionally given to further improve the patient's condition. Eye contact and responses were adequate, although right-sided weakness was complained, showing the need for long-term management post-hospital treatment. Laboratory parameters, including CRP, urea, D-dimer, fibrinogen, electrolytes, and albumin gradually returned to normal level. Before discharge from the hospital, the enoxaparin was switched to rivaroxaban as the take-home medicine. During the hospital stay, the patient did not contract the SARS-CoV-2 virus.

9.2 What Is the Patient's Problem Focus?

A 69-year-old male patient was brought to the hospital with one-sided body weakness and unresponsiveness for 6.5 h before admission, along with shortness of breath. Seizures and headaches were denied and there was no history of surgery, smoking, and alcohol intake. The patient had been diagnosed with coronary artery disease in the last 5 years, with a history of hypertension, which was also found in the mother.

The patient was primarily diagnosed with AIS, achieving a score of 5 for both the CHA_2DS_2-VASc and HAS-BLED scoring system. The carotid Doppler imaging showed high peripheral resistance and bilateral bulb soft plaques. In the second week, difficult breathing was felt, with the intercostal and sternocleidomastoid muscles being retracted. Chest X-ray showed heterogeneous opacities at the upper right lung region, suggesting pneumonia. The result also showed a widening of the right lung and left hilus, indicating pulmonary hypertension. Subsequently, the patient was diagnosed with HAP, but a thoracal-pulmonary CT angiography identified acute emboli on both pulmonary and interlobar arteries as the underlying cause of the respiratory system. Therefore, the final diagnosis was changed to acute emboli of the lung. Management changes were applied, including cessation of antibiotics stoppage and switching of the anticoagulant.

9.3 Discussion

Stroke is a prominent factor contributing to mortality and impairment. Medical complications following ischemic stroke significantly contribute to unfavorable outcomes. One of these complications includes pulmonary embolism (PE), which is a severe medical condition that occurs at a rate of 0.50–0.69 per 1000 persons in the general population annually [1]. Pulmonary embolism has a significant death rate, with a case fatality ranging from 8.6% to 17% within 3 months, and a long-term of 24%. Despite its significance, the prevalence of pulmonary embolism in patients with acute ischemic stroke (AIS) has not been extensively explored. Previous investigations on post-stroke consequences in hospital settings have frequently included the term "venous thromboembolism" (VTE), such as both pulmonary embolism and deep venous thrombosis (DVT). Although this condition is frequently associated with immobility, advanced age, smoking, hypertension, thrombophilia, and cancer in the general medical community, there is a lack of studies examining the specific impact on the incidence of pulmonary embolism in the AIS community. This shows that there is a scarcity of data about the influence of pulmonary embolism on stroke outcomes [2].

9.4 Epidemiology

The estimated occurrence rate of AIS following pulmonary embolism ranges from around 1% to 10%. Pulmonary embolism is the primary factor contributing to mortality within the first 2–4 weeks after stroke, although occurring in rare cases. In a study conducted by Clergeau et al., magnetic resonance imaging (MRI) was used to examine hospitalized patients diagnosed with acute pulmonary embolism for the presence of silent AIS, showed by restricted diffusion on diffusion-weighted imaging (DWI). Among 60 patients, 6 (10%) showed evidence of AIS, and 15 (25%) had a Patent Foramen Ovale (PFO). Out of the patients who showed DWI alterations, five had a quiet stroke with an underlying PFO, while one experienced restricted diffusion in DWI without PFO. A logistic regression analysis was also conducted, showing that PFO was a significant predictor of silent AIS among these patients. The results suggested that distal clots migrate, impacting both pulmonary and cerebral tissue [3].

9.5 Clinical Manifestation

Thromboembolic events, such as AIS and pulmonary embolism, show distinct clinical manifestations. Although neurological impairments and reduced consciousness are commonly observed in pulmonary embolism patients, stroke rarely presents with hemoptysis and dyspnea. This shows that the coexistence of respiratory and neurological symptoms should lead to the suspicion of a concurrent process. The most common neurological symptoms observed were focal paresis/plegia (94.11%), changed mental state (58.82%), and aphasia (47.05%). However, the most prevalent symptoms associated with pulmonary embolism were tachycardia (64.70%), tachypnea (58.82%), dyspnea (47.05%), and hypoxemia (41.17%) [3].

9.6 Imaging

Imaging tests are essential for a conclusive diagnosis of both AIS and pulmonary embolism. Non-contrast brain MRI and CTPA are the established methods for identifying and locating the affected vascular area in both disorders. To determine the cause of AIS, transthoracic echocardiogram (TTE) with agitated saline contrast has been proven effective, identifying the presence of PFO or intra-atrial thrombi through a bubble study. Additionally, it assesses the severity of pulmonary embolism by detecting right heart strain and provides prognostic information. Transesophageal echocardiography also enhances the accuracy in identifying thrombi and PFO when the results of TTE are inconclusive. Additional pertinent examinations include lower extremity ultrasound for the detection of deep vein thrombosis (DVT), which requires significant consideration. Furthermore, there is a need to include occult malignancy workups such as a pan scan and pelvic MR Venogram to evaluate for May-Thurner syndrome (MTS) in senior patients. The scarcity of data regarding the testing frequency for occult malignancy and MTS may account for the presence of PFO and DVTS in several patients [3].

9.7 Management

The management of pulmonary embolism includes prompt administration of anticoagulant medication to impede the advancement of blood clots and prevent the production of new clots. The existing norms are focused on specific specialties without including exceptional scenarios. During the acute phase, treatment options consist of anticoagulation, systemic intravenous thrombolysis, intra-arterial thrombolysis (when there is a high risk of systemic bleeding with intravenous thrombolysis), installation of an IVC filter, and endovascular pulmonary/cerebral embolectomy [3].

A study conducted by Velez S et al. showed that either the brain or the lungs could be targeted as the major focus. Acute thrombolysis has played a substantial role in the therapy of AIS. Neurologically, the results were positive, with 75% of the patients ($n = 3/4$) who received rt-PA either fully recovering or experiencing minor disability symptoms. The patients who received solely IV-heparin showed less favorable neurological results [3].

In the case of AIS, the current stroke guidelines recommend postponing the use of anticoagulation for 2 weeks in patients with atrial fibrillation who will need lifelong anticoagulants. This recommendation contrasts with the treatment for pulmonary embolism, which is to promptly initiate anticoagulation as the standard of care. A delay of more than 24 h in starting anticoagulation treatment for pulmonary embolism is associated with a threefold higher mortality rate. Therefore, there is a challenge in determining whether to immediately begin anticoagulation for pulmonary embolism patients with AIS, due to an increase in the risk of hemorrhagic transformation. The complexity is high when patients are eligible for acute intravenous recombinant tissue plasminogen activator (rt-PA) treatment, as anticoagulation should be delayed by 24 h after rt-PA administration. This shows the need to explore other methods for managing pulmonary embolism, such as catheter-directed thrombolysis. When the potential harm of using rt-PA exceeds the advantages, the recommendation is made to consider using MT and endovascular treatment with a stent retriever [3, 4].

In cases of significant pulmonary embolism, there is a need to alleviate the excessive strain on the right ventricle and prevent sudden cardiac failure. This can be achieved by promptly reopening the blocked blood vessels in the lungs using mechanical or pharmacological methods of dissolving blood clots. For patients with significant AIS and a high potential of hemorrhagic conversion, the use of intravenous rt-PA is considered the first-line treatment. The guidelines for thrombolytic treatment for pulmonary embolism specify that a history of stroke within the past 6 months is an absolute contraindication. Additional consensus guidelines suggest that absolute contraindication should be considered relative when there is a life-threatening situation associated with pulmonary embolism [3].

The simultaneous administration of thrombolysis in two separate and distant vascular regions is a unique phenomenon. The primary concern is in the disparities in recommended dosage, duration, and administration method between AIS and pulmonary embolism. Specifically, the recommended dosage for AIS is 0.9 mg/kg, with 10% administered in 1 min and the remaining 90% infused over 1 h. For pulmonary embolism in patients weighing ≥65 kg, alteplase is administered as a loading bolus of 10 mg over 1–2 min, followed by 90 mg over 2 h. Due to these disparities, the adoption of a customized method is recommended, considering the patient's specific condition and hemodynamic state, rather than relying solely on general standards [3].

9.8 Systemic Anticoagulation

The management of systemic anticoagulation varies significantly between AIS and pulmonary embolism. The precise guidelines for commencing long-term anticoagulant treatment after stroke consider the cause and prevention of future occurrences. The commencement of treatment is typically postponed until the subacute phase due to the potential dangers of hemorrhagic conversion. Anticoagulation is essential for managing acute pulmonary embolism, as previous studies have shown that treatment delay can lead to a negative prognosis and worsened outcomes. According to the latest recommendations, it is advised to start intravenous administration of unfractionated heparin immediately after the incident. This treatment should continue for a minimum of 5–10 days. Subsequently, a transition to a vitamin K antagonist with a desired international normalized ratio (INR) range of 2–3 or a novel oral anticoagulant is recommended. The use of only anticoagulation for AIS has been found to be ineffective in the initial phase. This is attributed to the inability to decrease the potential future occurrences, improve survival rates, or have a significant effect on disability, but increasing the chance of hemorrhagic conversion [3].

9.9 Mechanical Thrombectomy, Catheter-Directed Reperfusion

The Penumbra System, developed by Penumbra Inc. in Alameda, CA, USA, is used for extracting blood clots in cases of pulmonary embolism. Patients who are unable to receive thrombolysis due to absolute contraindications have several interventional options available. These include using pigtail or balloon catheters to fragment the thrombus, hydrodynamic catheters to perform thrombectomy, aspiration catheters for suction thrombectomy, and rotational thrombectomy [3].

Catheter-directed thrombolysis (CDT) includes the direct delivery of thrombolytic medicines into the obstructive blood clot. This method increases the concentration of the medication within the clot while reducing concentration in the overall circulation, compared to the administration of thrombolytic agents through the peripheral system. However, there are no comparative studies on the efficacy of CDT and systemic thrombolysis [3].

9.10 Patent Foramen Ovale Closure

Transfemoral device closure of PFO is often recommended to prevent secondary stroke after a cryptogenic stroke in specific situations. These include patients under the age of 60 who have experienced a cryptogenic non-lacunar stroke, a significant right-left interatrial shunt, or an atrial septal aneurysm. The American Academy of Neurology (AAN) recommends that patients with PFO following ischemic stroke should receive PFO closure after a thorough examination by both a vascular neurologist and cardiologist. These patients should also be informed about the potential risks and benefits associated with the procedure. The likelihood of a subsequent stroke in PFO patients and no other identifiable causes of stroke is exceedingly low (1% per year) when receiving medical treatment. The AAN suggests that patients under the age of 60 who have experienced stroke believed to be caused by PFO can potentially benefit from the closure treatment. Patients should be informed about a 3.4% decrease in the likelihood of experiencing a second stroke within 5 years. Additionally, there should be awareness of the potential dangers associated with atrial fibrillation, including a 3.9% probability of encountering procedural problems. Individual assessment is essential to determine the appropriate method for reducing the likelihood of a subsequent stroke caused by paradoxical embolism. This includes establishing transcatheter closure of PFO on a case-by-case basis [3].

9.11 Prognosis

The mortality related to pulmonary embolism is approximately 24% high but early treatment is significantly effective [1]. Acute pulmonary embolism is associated with a substantial mortality rate, reaching approximately 30%. The death rate for individuals who have been diagnosed and treated for pulmonary embolism is 8%, with only 10% experiencing sudden death. Generally, two out of three patients often pass away within 2 h following their initial appearance. These death rates vary based on the types, showing the need for prompt diagnosis and intervention [5].

Key Point
The risk of Pulmonary Embolism, including fatal cases, in patients with acute ischemic stroke (AIS) is well known but insufficiently examined. Ischemic stroke patients experiencing dyspnea should be suspected for pulmonary embolism.

Question

1. The following are neurological manifestations in Pulmonary Emboly:
   (a) Impaired consciousness
   (b) Seizure
   (c) Tremor
   (d) Disorientation
   (e) Severe headache
2. The standards to identify and localize injured vascular territory in both AIS and pulmonary embolism:
   (a) Brain MRI and CTPA
   (b) TTE and Brain MRI
   (c) Echocardiogram and Brain CT Scan
   (d) TTE
   (e) Brain CT Scan and CTPA
3. An alternative technique to delay anticoagulation for pulmonary embolism patients with concomitant AIS:
   (a) Catheter-directed thrombolysis
   (b) IVC filter placement
   (c) Cerebral embolectomy
   (d) Endovascular pulmonary
   (e) Patent Foramen Ovale
4. Using TTE with agitated saline contrast, we can obtain the following information, except:
   (a) The potential etiology of the AIS
   (b) Assessing for the presence of PFO
   (c) Assessing for the presence of intra-atrial thrombi
   (d) PE severity due to identification of right heart strain
   (e) PE severity due to identification of left heart strain
5. Which of the following is essential in the management of acute pulmonary embolism?
   (a) Anticoagulation, systemic intravenous thrombolysis, cerebral embolectomy
   (b) Anticoagulation, systemic intravenous thrombolysis, antihypertension
   (c) Anticoagulation, antihypertension, intra-arterial thrombolysis
   (d) Antihypertension, intra-arterial thrombolysis, IVC filter placement
   (e) Systemic intravenous thrombolysis, antihypertension, endovascular pulmonary

Answer Keys

1. A
2. A
3. A
4. E
5. A

Acknowledgments Cipta Mahendra MD, Department of Internal Medicine, Respirology and Critical Illness Division, Universitas Indonesia, Dr. Cipto Mangunkusumo General Central National Hospital, Jakarta, Indonesia.

Ersananda Arlisa Putri MD, Department of Internal Medicine, Respirology and Critical Illness Division, Universitas Indonesia, Dr. Cipto Mangunkusumo General Central National Hospital, Jakarta, Indonesia.

Muhammad Kurniawan MD DM PhD, Department of Neurology, Neurovascular Division. Universitas Indonesia, Dr. Cipto Mangunkusumo General Central National Hospital, Jakarta, Indonesia.

References

1. Eswaradass P, Dey S, Singh D, Hill M. Pulmonary embolism in Ischemic stroke. Can J Neurol Sci. 2018;45:343–5.
2. Pongmoragot J, Rabinstein AA, Nilanont Y, Swartz RH, Zhou L, Saposnik G. Investigators of Registry of Canadian Stroke Network (RCSN) and University of Toronto Stroke Program for Stroke Outcomes Research Canada (SORCan [www.sorcan.ca]) Working Group. Pulmonary embolism in ischemic stroke: clinical presentation, risk factors, and outcome. J Am Heart Assoc. 2013; https://doi.org/10.1161/JAHA.113.000372.
3. Saleh Velez FG, Ortiz Garcia JG. Management dilemmas in acute ischemic stroke and concomitant acute pulmonary embolism: case series and literature review. eNeurologicalSci. 2021;23:100341.
4. National Institute of Neurological Disorders and Stroke rt-PA Stroke Study Group. Tissueplasminogen activator for acute ischemic stroke. N Engl J Med. 1995;333(24):1581–7.
5. Bělohlávek J, Dytrych V, Linhart A. Pulmonary embolism, part I: epidemiology, risk factors and risk stratification, pathophysiology, clinical presentation, diagnosis and nonthrombotic pulmonary embolism. Exp Clin Cardiol. 2013;18:129–38.

10 Tuberculosis Associated Chylothorax

10.1 Case Illustration

A 17-year-old female patient came to the hospital with decreased appetite and body weight for 2 months before admission. The patient felt nauseated after every meal, limiting intake to only 2–3 tablespoons before vomiting, with insignificant shortness of breath. Body aches on the lower extremities were reported and particularly painful with movement. Approximately 15 kg of body weight was lost, which was reduced to 35 kg on admission.

A month before admission, the patient visited another hospital and was diagnosed with a gastric problem. A chest X-ray imaging procedure was conducted, showing the presence of fluids in the left lung field, which was referred to a pulmonologist for further management. The next day, the fluids were drained, appearing thick and dense yellow color (Fig. 10.1). Laboratory examination showed that the fluid was rich in lipid content, indicating chylothorax. Following the fluid evacuation, the patient was discharged but returned to the hospital a week after with another shortness of breath. A repeat chest X-ray imaging was performed and fluid accumulation was found on the left lung. Another drainage was conducted, obtaining approximately 1.5 L of fluid with the same dense yellow appearance.

Regarding the recurrent presence and characteristics of fluid, the treating pulmonologist suspected cancer. After a month, the patient was referred to this hospital to receive further treatments, consulting hematologist oncologist. Based on the previous history of recurrent presence of the fluid, the patient was suspected of lymphoma. However, there was no detectable or significant lump present. The treating hematologist oncologist ordered PET scan imaging to confirm the diagnosis and evaluate the extent of the lymphoma, with the result suggesting extensive lymphadenopathy. A chest CT scan imaging was obtained, showing massive fluid accumulation on the left lung field (Fig. 10.2). In response to the results, the patient was referred to a cardiothoracic surgeon to perform supraclavicular lymph node biopsy and insert a chest tube on the left lung region to evacuate chylothorax.

G. Singh, *Challenging Cases in Respirology and Critical Care*,
https://doi.org/10.1007/978-981-96-5002-6_10

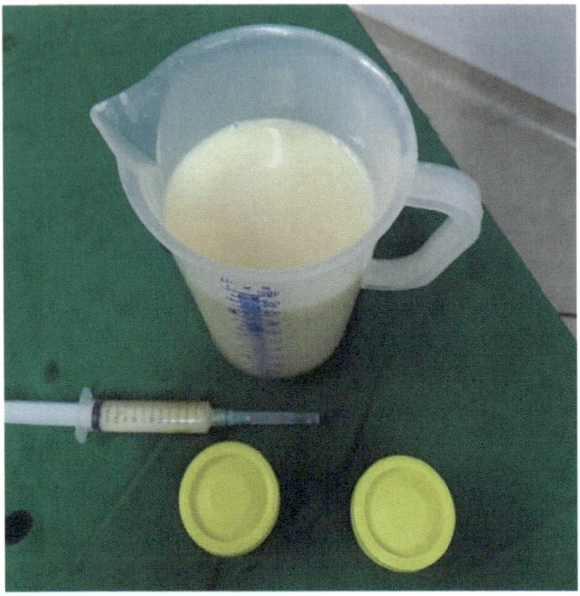

Fig. 10.1 The patient's aspirated left lung fluid gross appearance. The fluid was thick and had a dense yellow color

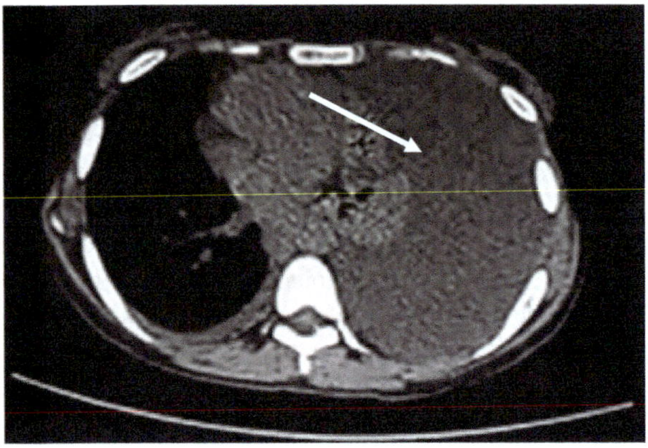

Fig. 10.2 The patient's CT scan imaging on hospital admission. Accumulation of near-water fluid density was found on the left lung field. (Image Courtesy: Rio Hermawan MD)

The biopsy result came out after several days, and the patient was diagnosed with TB lymphadenitis (Fig. 10.3). Combining the PET scan and the biopsy results, a robust diagnosis was finally made, namely, pulmonary TB and TB lymphadenopathy with chylothorax. The patient was consulted by the pulmonologist to manage the infection. Additionally, the performing surgeon decided to insert an indwelling pleural catheter (IPC) into the left hemithorax and kept installed until the infection had been cleared from the lungs. Antituberculosis drugs were subsequently administered, supplemented with vitamin D to stimulate the immune response. The initial planned treatment duration was 12 months, followed by discharge and counseling to preserve the inserted IPC.

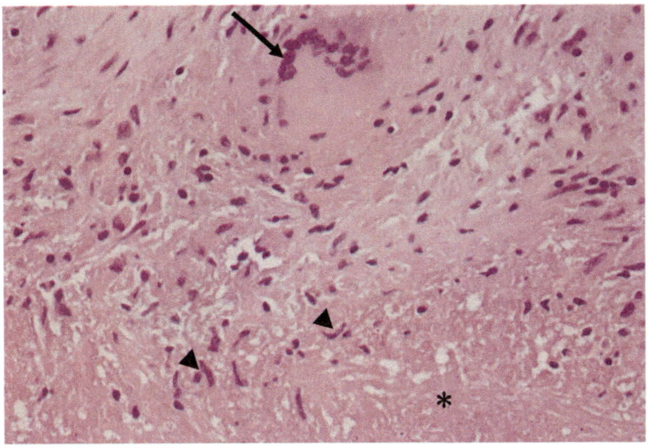

Fig. 10.3 The patient's biopsy tissue histopathology imaging. The lymph node tissues' shapes are hardly recognizable. Caseous necrotic areas (asterisk) were found, surrounded by epithelioid cells (▲) and Langhans giant cells (arrow). The stromal tissues are fibrotic; small blood vessels are seen between these tissues. No signs of malignancy are found. (Magnification: 40×). (Image Courtesy: Stella Marleen MD)

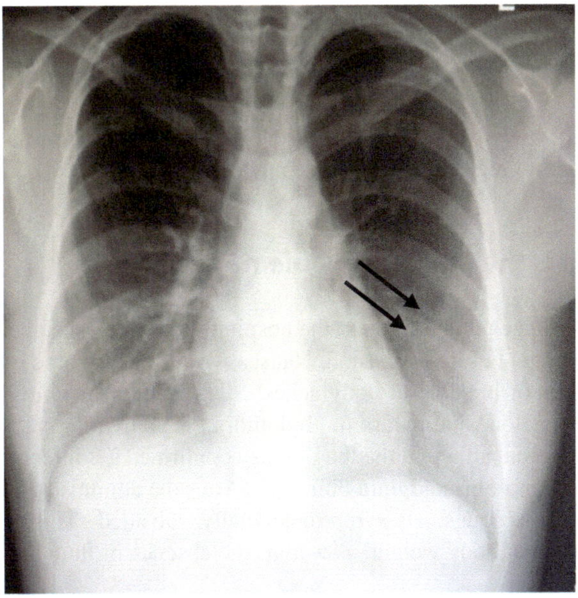

Fig. 10.4 The patient's chest X-ray imaging was obtained after 6 months since antituberculosis treatment. Minimal opacities were found on the left lung field (black arrow). (Image Courtesy: Rio Hermawan MD)

The patient started to show adequate clinical response since the commencement of the antituberculosis treatment, followed by improved left lung appearance 6 months after (Fig. 10.4). After 12 months of treatment initiation and completion of the antituberculosis drug, both lungs showed no significant anomalies on a repeat chest X-ray imaging (Fig. 10.5). Breathing difficulty had resolved, appetite was

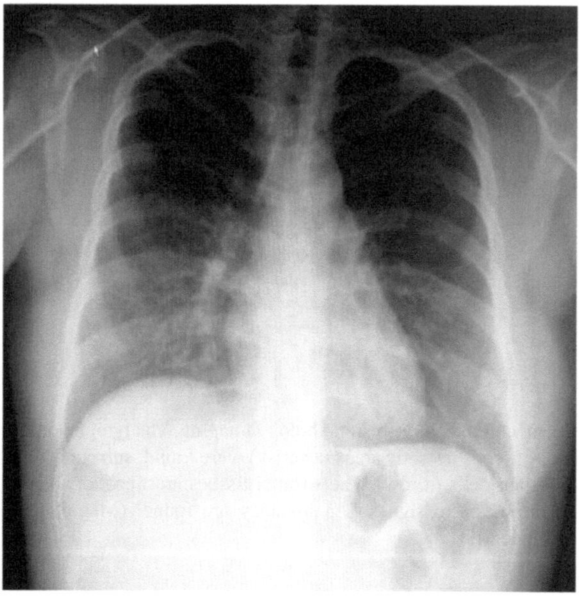

Fig. 10.5 The patient's chest X-ray imaging was obtained after completion of the antituberculosis treatment. No significant abnormality was found. (Image Courtesy: Rio Hermawan MD)

restored, and the body weight was increased. Additionally, there was no more fluid build-up in the left lung, leading to the removal of IPC.

10.2 What Is the Patient's Problem Focus?

A 17-year-old female patient came to the hospital with decreased appetite and body weight for 2 months before admission. Nausea was felt every time after meal, with a slight shortness of breath and body aches. Significant reduction in body weight was experienced, alongside recurrent chylothorax. The treating physician initially suspected lymphoma, although the lung biopsy confirmed TB infection as the cause of the patient's symptoms and fluid build-ups. After the administration of appropriate antituberculosis drugs, all symptoms finally subsided. This was shown by restored appetite and body weight, as well as the absence of fluid build-ups.

10.3 Discussion

10.3.1 Tuberculosis

Tuberculosis (TB) annually impacts approximately 10 million individuals with a range of 8.9–11.0 million. Furthermore, it is among the primary causes of death from infectious diseases worldwide. TB causes approximately 1.2 million fatalities in individuals without HIV, ranging from 1.1 to 1.3 million, and an additional 208,000 deaths in those with HIV, varying between 177,000–242,000 [1]. Among the anticipated 10 million cases, approximately 70% are detected, treated, and reported to the World Health Organization (WHO), leading to 7.1 million notifications by National TB Programs. Out of the 7.1 million individuals, who were informed in 2019, 5.9 million (84%) were diagnosed with pulmonary tuberculosis (PTB). Specifically, PTB includes all cases of TB that have been proven through bacteriological testing or diagnosed based on clinical evaluation, engaging the lung tissue or tracheobronchial tree [2].

10.4 Evaluation

10.4.1 Tuberculin Skin Testing: Mantoux Test (Skin Testing with PPD)

The Mantoux reaction is the conventional screening test for TB exposure, which includes injecting a dose of PPD (purified protein derivative). The interpretation of the result is based on the overall risk of exposure. Generally, patients are categorized into three groups according to the level of exposure risk, with three matching threshold values, as described below [3].

Low Risk

- Patients with a low likelihood of being exposed are classified as having a positive Mantoux test only when there is a substantial amount of swelling after the injection of PPD into the skin. The threshold for this particular group of individuals is considered to be 15 mm [3].

Intermediate Risk

- Patients with a moderate likelihood are classified as positive when the induration exceeds 10 mm [3].

High Risk

- Patients with a high likelihood of being exposed are classified as positive when the induration exceeds 5 mm [3].

Examples of Patients in the Different Risk Categories

- Low Risk/Probability: The group of patients who are unexposed to TB and have a minimal chance of contracting the disease. These include patients who have not traveled, served in the military, tested positive for HIV, contact with someone having a persistent cough, been exposed to any occupational hazards, used steroids in the past, and are non-resident of TB-prevalent areas [3].
- Intermediate Risk/Probability: This category includes patients residing in areas with a high prevalence of TB such as Latin America, Sub-Saharan Africa, and

Asia. Others include those working or living in shelters, and staff in medical or microbiology departments [3].
- High Risk/Probability: The group consists of HIV-positive patients, with evidence of previous TB such as a healed scar on an X-ray, and contact with those experiencing persistent cough [3].

A Mantoux test is used to detect whether an individual has been exposed to or has latent TB. This test is not sufficiently specific, requiring further visits for result interpretation and confirmation with a chest X-ray. Although Mantoux reaction is sensitive, it lacks specificity and can produce false-positive results in individuals who have received the BCG vaccine [3].

10.4.2 Interferon Release Assays (IGRA, QuantiFERON Assays)

Interferon is TB screening test that shows comparable sensitivity and higher specificity compared to Mantoux. It measures the concentration of the inflammatory cytokine, particularly interferon-gamma [3]. Several benefits are associated with antigen-specific stimulation to induce the release of IFN-γ, particularly in those who have already received the BCG vaccine. These include the requirement of one blood sample and elimination of the need for multiple visits to interpret the results. Other examinations, such as HIV testing, could be conducted with patient approval using the same blood sample. However, the limitations of QuantiFERON are high cost and the need for specialized technical skills to carry out the test [3].

10.4.3 Screening in Immunocompromised Patients

Immunocompromised individuals show reduced responsiveness to PPD or false-negative Mantoux results due to cutaneous anergy. When evaluating negative TB screening tests in HIV-positive persons, there is a need to maintain a high level of suspicion [3].

10.5 The Significance of Screening

A positive screening test signifies TB exposure and a high likelihood of developing active TB in the future. The occurrence of this condition in patients with a positive Mantoux test ranges from 2% to 10% in the absence of treatment.[3] Patients who test positive should have a chest X-ray as the minimum required diagnostic test, occasionally requiring supplementary diagnostic examinations. Moreover, those who fulfill the requirements for latent TB should be administered isoniazid as a preventive measure [3].

10.6 Screening Questionnaires for Resource-Poor Settings

Multiple validated screening questionnaires exist to facilitate TB screening for healthcare personnel operating in rural and resource-limited settings [3]. These questionnaires use an algorithm that integrates multiple clinical indicators and symptoms of TB, including [3]

- Chronic cough,
- Weight loss,
- Fever and night sweats,
- History of contact,
- HIV status,
- Blood in sputum.

Several studies have substantiated the efficacy of using multiple criteria instead of solely emphasizing chronic cough or weight loss [3].

10.7 Confirmatory and Diagnostic Tests

1. A chest X-ray is essential to confirm or exclude the existence of active illness in all instances that test positive during screening.
2. Acid Fast Staining-Ziehl-Neelsen.
3. Culture.
4. Nuclear amplification and gene-based tests are advanced diagnostic methods for TB. These tests use DNA-based molecular methods to identify bacteria or bacterial particles.

The novel molecular-based methods are more achievable and provide prompt diagnosis with exceptional accuracy. Confirmation of TB can be achieved within hours, compared to the typical waiting period of days or weeks for a normal culture. This is crucial, particularly among patients with weakened immune systems, where there is a significant incidence of inaccurate unfavorable outcomes. Molecular-based assays can also be used to identify cases of multidrug-resistant TB [3].

10.8 Chylothorax Due to TB

Nontraumatic chylothorax can be caused by various factors, although the majority of cases are not attributed to TB. Despite being uncommon, chylothorax has been a well-documented consequence of TB. This medical condition can be distinguished from a pseudochylothorax by the presence of a sudden accumulation of fluid in the pleural space, with smooth and unthickened pleural surfaces. Chylothorax is characterized by elevated levels of triglyceride ($\geq$110 mg/dL), low cholesterol (pleural/serum cholesterol <1), or the presence of chylomicrons as shown by lipoprotein electrophoresis. In the initial case, the relationship between TB and chylothorax is confirmed by several factors. These include the lack of pre-existing pleural effusion, clear biochemical evidence, conclusive demonstration of chylomicrons, radiological features, and microbiological evidence of Mycobacterium TB. The cause of the pleural thickening was attributed to TB and empyema due to Candida albicans, as reported in previous studies [4, 5].

Various processes have been identified in the formation of chylothorax in TB. The manifestations of this condition occur in three main aspects, namely, (1) the presence of enlarged lymph nodes in the mediastinum, which can cause blockage or erosion of the thoracic duct leading to leakage of chyle into the pleural space. (2) The occurrence of enlarged lymph nodes in the abdomen, which can obstruct the cisterna chyli and create an opening for lymphaticovenous anastomosis. (3) The development of constrictive pericarditis, characterized by elevated pressures in the left subclavian vein, leading to increased production of lymph and reduced drainage. In this study, the presence of exudates in all cases of chylothorax associated with TB shows that the pleura and lymphatic ducts are directly affected by TB or the immunological response of the host, serving as the main cause in the majority of patients. Additional processes are essential in this systematic analysis, such as the erosion of the thoracic duct by spinal abscesses, the presence of severe pleural disease with lymphatic exudation, and the damage to the duct caused by immunological reconstitution syndrome (IRS) [4].

10.9 Treatment Recommendation

1. New patients with pulmonary TB (PTB) should be treated with a 6-month regimen containing rifampicin: 2HRZE/4HR (strong recommendation, high certainty of evidence) [2].
2. The optimal dosing frequency for new PTB patients is daily throughout the entire treatment period (strong recommendation, high certainty of evidence) [2].
3. For patients with drug-susceptible PTB, thrice-weekly dosing is not recommended in either the intensive or continuation phases of treatment. Daily dosing remains the preferred frequency (conditional recommendation, very low certainty of evidence) [2].
4. The use of fixed-dose combination (FDC) tablets is recommended over separate drug formulations for treating patients with drug-susceptible TB (conditional recommendation, low certainty of evidence) [2].
5. In new PTB patients treated with rifampicin-containing regimens, if a positive sputum smear is found at the completion of the intensive phase, extending the intensive phase is not recommended (strong recommendation, high certainty of evidence) [2].

Chylothorax associated with TB is managed by combining antituberculosis medications with therapeutic thoracentesis. In cases of severe breathing difficulty, the use of a pleuroperitoneal shunt or chest tube to drain the fluid is recommended. Recurrent pleural fluid discharge may indicate malnutrition and underlying immunological issues. Chyle is typically characterized by elevated levels of protein, lipids, electrolytes, and lymphocytes. Octreotide has been suggested for therapeutic use in specific cases. In cases of acute thoracic duct injury, the defect usually resolves spontaneously. However, if chylothorax persists beyond 4 weeks, surgical intervention, such as thoracic duct ligation during exploration, may be considered [2].

10.10 Prognosis

TB-associated chylothorax generally has a favorable prognosis with conservative management. Even though a higher proportion of patients present with disseminated disease at the time of diagnosis and may have additional comorbidities, the survival rate remains high at 94.4% [4].

Key Points

Chylothorax should be considered as one of the etiologies of PTB, as not all cases are caused by malignancy. Prognosis of this condition is good, specifically when diagnosed and treated early.

Question

1. The following statements concerning several mechanisms for the development of chylothorax in TB are true, except:
   (a) Mediastinal adenopathy with obstruction or erosion into the thoracic duct, leading to leakage of chyle into the pleural space.
   (b) Abdominal lymphadenopathy causing obstruction of the cisterna chyli.
   (c) Opening of lymphatic-venous anastomoses.
   (d) Constrictive pericarditis associated with elevated left subclavian venous pressures, resulting in increased lymph production.
   (e) Constrictive pericarditis with elevated left subclavian venous drainage of lymph
2. Which of the following established the association of chylothorax with TB in the indexed case?
   (a) The observation of exudates in all cases of TB-related chylothorax.
   (b) The unclear biochemical evidence and suggestive of TB.
   (c) The microbiologic demonstration of non-TB mycobacterium.
   (d) The long-standing pleural effusion before the current illness.
   (e) The definitive demonstration of chylomicrons along with radiological features.
3. Below are clinical manifestations of chylothorax, except:
   (a) Fatigue.
   (b) Weight loss.
   (c) Pleural effusion.
   (d) Intermittent fever.
   (e) Shortness of breath.

4. The following differentiates chylothorax from a pseudochylothorax except:
   (a) Elevated triglyceride levels (≥110 mg/dL) and low cholesterol levels (pleural/serum cholesterol <1).
   (b) Low triglyceride levels (≤110 mg/dL) and low cholesterol levels (pleural/serum cholesterol <1).
   (c) Low triglyceride levels (≤110 mg/dL) with the presence of chylomicrons demonstrated by lipoprotein electrophoresis.
   (d) Low triglyceride levels (≤110 mg/dL) and elevated cholesterol levels (pleural/serum cholesterol >1).
   (e) Elevated cholesterol levels (pleural/serum cholesterol >1) with the presence of chylomicrons demonstrated by lipoprotein electrophoresis.
5. What is the best treatment combination for chylothorax TB?
   (a) Antituberculosis treatment with therapeutic thoracentesis.
   (b) Antituberculosis treatment with mediastinoscopy.
   (c) Antituberculosis treatment with chest tube insertion.
   (d) Chest tube insertion with therapeutic thoracentesis.
   (e) Chest tube insertion with mediastinoscopy.

Answer Keys
1. E
2. D
3. B
4. A
5. B

Acknowledgments Cipta Mahendra MD, Department of Internal Medicine, Respirology and Critical Illness Division, Universitas Indonesia, Dr. Cipto Mangunkusumo General Central National Hospital, Jakarta, Indonesia.

Ersananda Arlisa Putri MD, Department of Internal Medicine, Respirology and Critical Illness Division, Universitas Indonesia, Dr. Cipto Mangunkusumo General Central National Hospital, Jakarta, Indonesia.

Hariadi Hadibrata MD, Department of Cardiovascular and Thoracic Surgery, Mochtar Riady Comprehensive Cancer Center (MRCCC) Siloam Hospital, Jakarta, Indonesia.

Jeffry Beta Tenggara MD DM PhD, Department of Internal Medicine, Medical Hematology and Oncology division, Mochtar Riady Comprehensive Cancer Center (MRCCC) Siloam Hospital, Jakarta. Indonesia.

References

1. Singh S, Girod JP, Ghobrial MW. Chylothorax as a complication of tuberculosis in the setting of the human immunodeficiency virus infection. Arch Intern Med. 2001;161:2621.
2. WHO. WHO consolidated guidelines on tuberculosis, module 4: treatment - drug- susceptible tuberculosis treatment in 2022, 2022.

3. Adigun R, Singh R. Tuberculosis, 2023. https://www.ncbi.nlm.nih.gov/books/NBK441916/.
4. Rajagopala S, Kancherla R, Ramanathan RP. Tuberculosis-associated Chylothorax: case report and systematic review of the literature. Respiration. 2018;95:260–8. https://doi.org/10.1159/000484694.
5. Kutlu O, Demirbas S, Sakin A. Chylothorax due to tuberculosis lymphadenitis. North Clin Istanb. 2017;3:225–8. https://doi.org/10.14744/nci.2015.52714. PMID: 28275756; PMCID: PMC5336629.

11 Severe Pneumonitis in Lung Cancer

11.1 Case Illustration

A 56-year-old female patient presented to the hospital with a chief complaint of shortness of breath persisting over the last 3–4 months. This complaint was intermittent and particularly pronounced at night, thereby disrupting sleep. Initially, the patient did not seek medical attention, but approximately a month later (2 months before the hospital admission), the breathing difficulty worsened, leading to the consultation of an internist. A prescription for gastric medication was given, which caused slight and temporary improvement of the symptom. However, after several days, the condition deteriorated, prompting another visit to the internist. Alongside the breathing difficulty, there were also complaints of dry coughs. A chest X-ray revealed signs of pneumonia, leading to the administration of several drugs, including antibiotics. During the treatment period, significant fluctuations were observed in the symptoms. After the consumption of the drugs, the symptoms recurred, with breathing becoming increasingly difficult and the patient could neither speak nor walk normally. In addition, the difficulty also persisted at rest, with the occurrence of occasional vomiting.

Due to the severity of the condition, the patient was brought to a nearby hospital the following day. Another chest X-ray imaging was obtained, revealing massive pleural effusions in both lungs. Despite the finding, the patient declined to undergo a chest tube placement procedure to drain the effusions, leading to the administration of a diuretic drug as an alternative. Hospital discharge was then granted but returned the next day due to the same symptoms. An echocardiography examination was performed, indicating signs of pericardial tamponade caused by effusions. Subsequently, a thoracic computed tomography (CT) scan was performed to evaluate the conditions further and the results confirmed the presence of pleural and pericardial effusions. Mediastinal lymphadenopathy and lung edema were also observed on the imaging. Concerning the presence of pericardial effusions, pericardiocentesis was performed, with the fluid being found to be voluminous, thick in

G. Singh, *Challenging Cases in Respirology and Critical Care*,
https://doi.org/10.1007/978-981-96-5002-6_11

consistency, and appeared dark red. Histopathological examination of the fluid revealed the presence of atypical mesothelial cells. The pleural effusions were also drained out and sent to the laboratory yielding similar outcomes. Based on these findings, the patient was referred to another hospital to receive further treatment.

Upon arrival, another pericardial effusion emerged, which was later drained. The fluid appeared red, similar to the appearance of the previous pericardial effusions. Subsequently, an abdominal CT scan was performed, which showed several findings, including multiple hepatic cysts, a simple cyst on the kidney, multiple vertebral osteoblastic lesions, pericardial effusions, and consolidations on the lung fields. In response, peritoneal washing was conducted and the washing fluid was sent for a cancer antigen 125 (CA-125) examination, which revealed an abnormally high level. In line with these results, the managing physician suspected the presence of metastasized ovarian cancer, and chemotherapies were suggested as the treatment. Due to a lack of appropriate resources, the patient was then referred to a national hospital (i.e., this hospital) for further management.

At admission, the patient's family requested a positron emission tomography (PET)-scan imaging procedure to confirm the presence of cancer. The PET-scan showed no sign of suspicious metabolic activities in the ovarium but revealed an increase in activities of the lungs as well as femoral, scapula, and thoracic bones. Another echocardiography was conducted, which indicated slight enlargement of the heart, dilation of the pulmonary artery, and signs of pericardial effusions. Bronchoscopy was also performed, revealing normal intrabronchial tracts. During bronchoscopy, a rapid on-site evaluation (ROSE) method was implemented, and the result was positive for lung adenocarcinoma (see Fig. 11.1). The patient was then ultimately diagnosed with advanced lung cancer with bone metastases.

Several further tests were subsequently conducted to characterize the malignant cell's molecular traits. These traits included the expression of anaplastic lymphoma

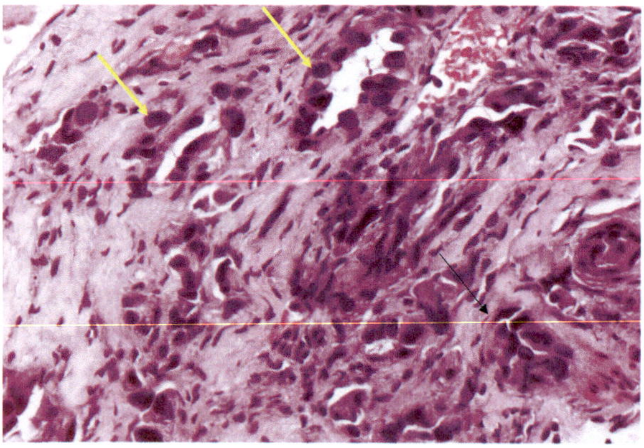

Fig. 11.1 The patient's histopathologic imaging obtained from ROSE. The tumor cells are arranged in a glandular pattern (pointed by arrows), with pleomorphic nuclei, hyperchromatic and coarse chromatin. The cytoplasm is eosinophilic. (Magnification: 40×). (Image Courtesy: Stella Marlen MD)

kinase (ALK), programmed death-ligand 1 (PD-L1), and epidermal growth factor receptor (EGFR) mutational analysis. The ALK and PD-L1 testing yielded negative results, while the EGFR analysis indicated the presence of deletion of exon 19. Based on the results, the patient was scheduled for a combination therapy of chemotherapy (i.e., dacomitinib) and radiotherapy. Additional medications were also administered, including vitamins, antioxidants, antinauseants (omeprazole, ondansetron), cardiopulmonary-supporting drugs (bisoprolol, ivabradine, sildenafil, spironolactone, enoxaparin), and colchicine.

In the initial days, following the start of the combination therapy, the patient showed clinical improvements. In this context, a decrease in the signs and symptoms of shortness of breath was observed, but relapse occurred the following week. Laboratory examinations were then carried out for further evaluation, including the blood serum electrolytes, albumin, and interleukin-6 (IL-6). Galactomannan serum level, pericardial effusions, and blood culture were also examined to determine the presence of any microorganism. Albumin level showed a significant decrease (2.66 g/dL; normal: 3.50–5.20), while IL-6 level was increased to 23.73 (normal: $\leq$7.00 pg/mL). The electrolytes were within normal range, but the galactomannan level was below the normal limit. The pericardial effusions' culture was sterile, while the blood culture revealed the presence of *Staphylococcus epidermidis*. A chest X-ray imaging was also obtained, with inhomogeneous opacities and bilateral pleural effusions being observed in both lungs.

In response to the condition, snakefish extracts were given to increase serum albumin, while methylprednisolone was administered to reduce the IL-6 level. Dacomitinib and radiation therapy were temporarily stopped to allow recovery, but all other medications were continued. After a week, the patient's breathing was improved, leading to the resumption of dacomitinib and radiotherapy. However, approximately about 2 weeks later, a relapse occurred. The regimen was again halted to allow another recovery, but this time, the patient never recuperated from the breathing difficulty. The symptoms worsened despite the regimen's discontinuation and the supportive treatments. About a week later, the patient had apnea and was finally declared dead after unsuccessful resuscitation attempts.

The patient had no history of hypertension and diabetes mellitus before the first hospital admission. A family member reported the occurrence of cardiomegaly, but the duration was unknown because a doctor was not consulted. In addition, the patient's father had a history of colon cancer with lung metastasis.

11.2 What Is the Patient's Problem Focus?

A 56-year-old female patient presented to the hospital with shortness of breath for the last 3–4 months. Despite consulting a doctor approximately 2 months before admission and receiving several drugs to alleviate the symptom, the condition persisted. Further diagnostic investigations, including computed tomography (CT) scan imaging, revealed pleural and pericardial effusions, lung edema, and mediastinal lymphadenopathy. After a series of examinations and medical consultations, the patient was diagnosed with lung cancer with bone metastases. The diagnosis was confirmed by both positron emission tomography (PET) scan imaging and bronchoscopy using the rapid on-site evaluation (ROSE) method.

Several molecular characteristics of the malignant cells were examined, revealing negative expression of anaplastic lymphoma kinase (ALK) and PD-L1, while the epidermal growth factor receptor (EGFR) mutational analysis showed deletion of exon 19. Consequently, the patient was scheduled for chemotherapy with dacomitinib and radiotherapy as the regimen was based on the molecular traits found. A reduction in breathing difficulty occurred initially during the first days of treatment, but the condition was reversed in the next week. Subsequent assessments revealed a decrease in albumin level, while interleukin-6 (IL-6) level increased. The chest X-ray imaging showed opacities across the lung fields and bilateral pleural effusions were found on the image. Several medications were then administered to enhance the patient's recovery. In the following week, the work of breathing was restored, leading to the resumption of the regimen. However, the patient relapsed again 2 weeks after and the regimen was postponed to allow recuperation. The patient never recovered from the relapse and the condition continued deteriorating despite the regimen's discontinuation and the supportive treatments. After a week, the patient had apnea and was finally declared dead shortly.

Based on findings, a history of cardiomegaly was reported but the duration was unknown because a doctor was not consulted. In addition, the patient's father had a history of colon cancer with lung metastases. All other significant medical histories were denied by the patient's family members.

11.3 Discussion

The incidence of cancer is projected to increase from approximately 9 million in 2017 to 26 million new cases by 2030. A total of 30–50% of affected patients have been reported to undergo radiation therapy, either as a standalone treatment or in combination with chemotherapy and surgery. Consequently, more than 7 million individuals undergo radiation annually on a global scale. The increased success rates in treating all types of cancer have led to a higher number of healthcare professionals encountering a large population of patients who have survived for a long time but later experienced various chronic conditions. Therefore, all clinicians must possess knowledge regarding the prevalent negative consequences of radiation therapy [1].

Lung cancer is an aggressive malignancy marked by rapid progression and a poor prognosis. The primary cause of death in affected individuals is distant metastasis, with the skeletal system being a common site for bone-related complications. Bone metastases, which occur in about 30–40% of patients with advanced lung cancer, often develop as the disease progresses. Bone metastases in lung cancer carry considerable clinical implications, including bone pain, pathological fractures, spinal instability, spinal cord compression, and hypercalcemia. Understanding the mechanisms underlying the spread of lung cancer to the bone, alongside the available diagnostic techniques and treatment options, is crucial for effective management. In the case presented, the diagnosis was established using positron emission tomography (PET) imaging and bronchoscopy coupled with the rapid on-site evaluation (ROSE) technique [2, 3].

In line with previous studies, the susceptibility and reaction to radiation damage may differ among different organ tissues, including the lung. The primary clinical signs of lung irradiation consist of congestion, cough, dyspnea, fever, and chest pain, which occur due to the onset of radiation pneumonitis. Radiographic examination often reveals the existence of infiltrates in the region that has been subjected to the treatment. Hypoxia in severe cases often leads to subsequent right-sided heart failure. Under specific circumstances, when the lung is partially exposed to radiation, it can result in the occurrence of bilateral immune-mediated pneumonitis. This condition usually recovers naturally without requiring medical treatment. Pneumonitis often follows a natural progression, with the acute phase gradually resolving and giving way to a chronic phase characterized by inflammation and fibrosis. The chronic phase of the condition usually becomes apparent over a few months to several years. Several studies have shown that the degree of fibrosis is directly proportional to the region that has been exposed. Consequently, when a large area is exposed, patients may develop restrictive lung disease, which is characterized by symptoms, such as cough, difficulty in breathing, chest pain, and significant reductions in the ability to exchange gases and the volume of air inhaled or exhaled. The use of PET-scan enables the differentiation between a tumor and a radiation injury, as the manifestations of these disorders are similar. To effectively manage early radiation pneumonitis, it is necessary to perform a comprehensive evaluation to rule out other potential causes of initial breathing difficulty. In addition, the administration of systemic steroids with a progressive reduction in dosage is recommended [4, 5].

11.4 Mechanism of Radiation-Induced Inflammatory Responses and Fibrosis

Fibrosis frequently occurs as a consequence of persistent inflammation or damage in any part of the body. In this context, it refers to the reparative mechanism that occurs after the acute inflammatory response, which is often known as classical radiation pneumonitis. This leads to the deposition of collagen, causing the formation of a localized fibrotic area on a chest X-ray, which is directly visible beneath the irradiated region. The etiology of fibrosis remains inadequately elucidated, but irradiation has been reported to induce chromosomal aberrations and cellular demise, leading to the substitution of cells with scar tissue and fibrotic lesions. However, a specific mechanism for fibroblast recruitment, collagen deposition, and concurrent vascular impairment has not been proposed [4].

Although the specific cell responsible for radiation-induced lung damage remains unidentified, the overall process of injury and repair following tissue damage—whether caused by radiation, surgery, chemotherapy, or infection—largely depends on the activation of cells to produce essential biological substances, including cytokines and growth factors.

In this context, the substances help to coordinate various aspects of the inflammatory response. Therefore, a significant portion of the morbidity associated with radiation-induced tissue inflammation is not solely attributable to tissue damage. Several aspects can be explained by a highly intricate mechanism that involves the local generation of cytokines, which is triggered by tissue irradiation, both directly and indirectly [4].

At present, there is empirical data in the scientific literature suggesting that irradiation can stimulate the production of inflammatory gene products. Building on this idea, gene transcription, a crucial requirement for protein synthesis, is regulated by a set of proteins known as promoters or transcriptional factors [4]. A specific objective of these transcription factors is to regulate the expression of the gene encoding tumor necrosis factor-alpha (TNF-a), a crucial cytokine involved in inflammation and fibroblast proliferation. The production of the substance is significantly enhanced after exposing a human sarcoma cell line and peripheral blood monocytes to radiation. Since fibrosis is a consistent and predictable result of radiation exposure in the entire body, it is expected to be accompanied by the release of cytokines that have been identified in chronic inflammatory investigations as crucial in the fibrogenic response. This process comprises the attraction of fibroblasts to areas of inflammation, subsequent replication of fibroblasts to augment their population, and the stimulation of fibroblasts to produce higher quantities of collagen [4].

Fibroblast recruitment is driven by chemotactic factors such as transforming growth factor-beta (TGF-β) and fibronectin. Key growth factors that support fibroblast function include platelet-derived growth factor (PDGF), with PDGF-β derived from macrophages and endothelial cells, and PDGF-α from fibroblasts, as well as insulin-like growth factor-1 (IGF-1) and tumor necrosis factor-alpha (TNF-α). Among these, TGF-β is widely recognized as the primary driver of collagen synthesis. Fibroblast growth factors, including platelet-derived growth factor-B (PDGF-B) and insulin-like growth factor-1 (IGF-1), along with chemotactic factors such as monocyte chemotactic protein-1 (MCP-1) and transforming growth factor-beta (TGF-β), inflammatory cytokines like tumor necrosis factor-alpha (TNF-α) and interleukin-1 (IL-1), and fibrogenic factors such as TGF-β, have been identified in both spontaneous and experimental cases of inflammatory lung disorders [4].

The macrophage, which is abundant in the lung, is a significant source of these cytokines. Consequently, irradiation can be expected to cause the release of the cytokines. The secretion of fibroblast growth factors was evaluated in three types of mononuclear phagocytes, including culture-derived, alveolar macrophages from bronchoalveolar fluid, and the myelomonocytic cell line U-937. The three fibroblast growth factors were released in response to in vitro irradiation, with the amount and timing of release being dependent on the dose and duration of irradiation. The primary stimulatory effect on growth was attributed to PDGF-ß, but minor quantities of IGF-1 and TNF-a were also generated in certain situations. In addition, the irradiation technique did not have any effect on the viability of the cells, as determined by tryphan blue exclusion. The release of PDGF-ß was associated with an upregulation of PDGF-ß mRNA and protein expression. However, cycloheximide, a protein synthesis inhibitor, significantly but not completely suppressed protein release. These observations suggest that irradiation directly stimulates the production and secretion of growth factors [4].

Cells acquired by bronchoalveolar lavage from patients were irradiated in vivo, both before and 4–6 weeks after undergoing thoracic irradiation. The results revealed the presence of a basal level of growth factor activity, which can be attributed to TNF-a. However, after the technique, substantial quantities of growth factor activity associated with PDGF-ß were liberated. The results suggest that PDGF-ß is generated in response to both irradiation in living organisms and laboratory settings. This provides substantial evidence in favor of the concept that the release of fibroblast growth factors from macrophages is a significant contributor to the development of fibrosis caused by irradiation in individuals [4].

In line with previous findings, Rubin et al. have shown the local release of the fibrogenic cytokine, TGF-B, in a rabbit model. TGF-ß was solely secreted into the bronchoalveolar lavage fluid on the irradiated side of the thorax in vivo. Other cells besides macrophages have been reported to possess the ability to secrete cytokines that promote inflammation and fibrosis. Additional cell types, such as fibroblasts, pneumocytes, and endothelial cells, are also expected to contribute to the inflammatory response triggered by local irradiation. In the endothelium, there is compelling evidence that irradiation can stimulate the production of PDGF [4].

When a significant number of the characteristics are caused by inflammation, affected individuals are often affected by a wide range of substances that have been utilized to regulate other long-term inflammatory processes. Consequently, it is feasible to "counteract" certain undesirable consequences of irradiation and avert several adverse effects of radiotherapy. This enables the administration of higher quantities of radiation, and ideally improves modifying the therapeutic ratio in the treatment of cancer [4].

The evaluation of Bronchoalveolar Lavage and Gallium Lung Scan can predict lung function. In a healthy lung, the interstitium consists of a combination of cells, with lymphocytes constituting 30–40% of the total population and B cells being the most abundant. However, in lungs with acute pneumonitis, lymphocytes account for 60–70% of the total population, with recently activated T lymphocytes being the majority. In this context, the Gallium lung scan is commonly used to evaluate inflammatory alterations in the pulmonary parenchyma [4].

11.5 Sporadic Radiation Pneumonitis

The clinical manifestation of radiation pneumonitis cannot be fully accounted for by the mechanisms discussed earlier. Several factors remain unclear, including (a) its unpredictable and sporadic onset, (b) its occurrence in only a minority of patients, (c) the disproportionate severity of dyspnea relative to the volume of lung irradiated, and (d) the resolution of symptoms without lasting complications in most cases (Fig. 11.2) [4].

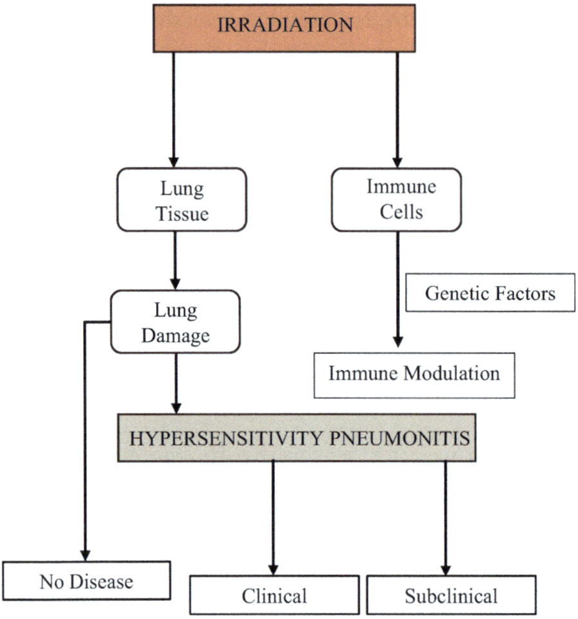

Fig. 11.2 Mechanism of interaction of irradiation, immunological, and genetic factors in the pathogenesis of radiation induced sporadic pneumonitis. (Adapted from: Morgan GW, Breit SN. Radiation and the lung: a reevaluation of the mechanisms mediating pulmonary injury)

Hypersensitivity pneumonitis can manifest as acute, subacute, or chronic, depending on the frequency, intensity, and length of inhalational exposure, as well as other factors that determine the immunopathogenesis in the host. Several studies have also shown that both systemic and respiratory symptoms may manifest. The acute form of the disease is characterized by symptoms similar to those of influenza, including chills, fever, sweating, muscle pain, fatigue, headache, and nausea. These symptoms usually appear 2–9 h after exposure, reach their highest intensity between 6 and 24 h, and can last for a few hours to several days. Cough and dyspnea are often observed respiratory symptoms, but are not present in every case. The subacute manifestation of the condition may gradually take over many days to weeks. In addition, it is characterized by signs, such as cough and difficulty breathing, and can potentially escalate to a severe state of breathing difficulty accompanied by bluish discoloration of the skin, necessitating immediate hospitalization. The chronic form of the condition manifests gradually over several months, characterized by a progressive cough and difficulty breathing during physical activity. Prominent symptoms may include fatigue and weight loss [6].

Several studies have shown that the physical examination can reveal either normal findings or the presence of crackles in the lower parts of the lungs or throughout the lungs in any of the different ways the condition presents. Pyrexia is a frequent occurrence following immediate exposure, while Cyanosis can be observed in case of severe illness. In addition, right heart failure can further aggravate situations involving significant fibrosis, with clubbing not being anticipated [6].

The symptoms, signs, and other indications of hypersensitivity pneumonitis are typically associated with a relatively short period, ranging from days to weeks or even months, in the majority of patients, provided there is no further exposure to the substance causing the condition. Although chronic fibrosis may develop in individuals continuously exposed to an antigen, there is currently no evidence to support the notion that idiopathic pulmonary fibrosis represents a "burned out" or end-stage hypersensitivity pneumonitis [6].

11.6 Epidermal Growth Factor Receptor-Tyrosine Kinase Inhibitors (EGFR-TKI)

According to previous studies, the occurrence rate of interstitial lung disease (ILD) caused by gefitinib was found to be between 3.5% and 5.8% in Asian patients. ILD has been reported to be associated with a greater occurrence of radiation pneumonitis of a higher grade (grade > 2) in patients undergoing irradiation. The precise mechanisms remain unclear, but pulmonary interstitial changes are recognized as a key factor in the development of radiation pneumonitis following radiotherapy and EGFR-TKI treatment. In a cohort of 145 patients with oligometastatic Non-Small Cell Lung Carcinoma (NSCLC) harboring EGFR mutations, 7% developed radiation pneumonitis after undergoing consolidation radiotherapy followed by EGFR-TKI therapy. In addition, several studies have reported the occurrence of life-threatening pneumonitis. A phase II report investigating the simultaneous use of EGFR-TKIs and irradiation (54–60 Gy) in patients with advanced NSCLC and EGFR mutations revealed that 10% of participants experienced grade 3 radiation pneumonitis, which in some cases led to fatality.

A previous prospective study also investigated the frequency of radiation pneumonitis in patients diagnosed with NSCLC who had simultaneous treatment with radiotherapy and erlotinib. The results revealed that 37.5% (9/24) of patients experienced radiation pneumonitis of grade 2 or above, while 8.7% and 12.5% had grades 3 and 5, respectively. However, three patients with fatal pneumonitis experienced bilateral imaging alterations that were not limited to the radiation output. The lung-related radiation dose characteristics of the deceased patients was not above the standard dose limits. The aforementioned analyses revealed that the rates of grade 3 pneumonitis ranged from 1.3% to 11.1%, while the incidence of grade 4 or higher was between 2.2% and 12.5%. Based on the stringent dosage limitations in the present study, 37.7% of patients experienced symptomatic radiation pneumonitis (grades 2 or higher), while 6.7% suffered from severe (grade 3) forms. In addition, pneumonia of grades 2 or higher was detected in 8.9%, but no severe adverse events of grades 4 or 5 were observed, and there were only limited instances of late lung damage. These findings unequivocally established the importance of physicians being vigilant regarding pulmonary toxicity when administering a combination of radiation and EGFR-TKIs for the treatment of NSCLC. Additional study of the risk variables associated with severe pneumonitis must be conducted in prospective trials. All generations of EGFR-TKIs exhibit comparable side-effect profiles, but the incidence and severity of Adverse Events (AEs) differ across the specific medications. These medications hinder the activity of both mutated and normal forms of EGFR, hence, the "target effect" negatively affects normal tissues with EGFR expression. Occasionally, all generations of EGFR-TKIs can cause major adverse events, including drug-induced lung injury, such as ILD [7, 8].

Key Points

Radiation and certain types of TKIs can worsen pneumonitis in lung cancer. Special attention toward pulmonary toxicity should be given in lung cancer patients during treatment with radiotherapy and EGFR-TKIs.

Question

1. The following are the initial clinical manifestations of lung irradiation, except:
   (a) Congestion
   (b) Cough
   (c) Dyspnea
   (d) Hemoptysis
   (e) Chest pain
2. In patients receiving radiotherapy, ILD is associated with radiation pneumonitis of what grade?
   (a) Grade 1
   (b) Grade 2
   (c) Grade 1 and Grade 2
   (d) Grade 1 and Grade 3
   (e) Grade 4 and Grade 5
3. Which of the following is a type of mononuclear phagocyte?
   (a) Culture-derived macrophages
   (b) Alveolar macrophages from Pleural fluid
   (c) The myelomonocytic cell line U-933
   (d) Secreting proinflammatory and
   (e) Fibrogenic cytokines
4. The following determines hypersensitivity presentation of pneumonitis:
   (a) Duration of inhalational exposure
   (b) Grade of lung carcinoma
   (c) Onset
   (d) Medication history
   (e) Type of lung carcinoma
5. Clinical manifestations of radiation pneumonitis are often indistinguishable due to the following, except:
   (a) The unpredictable and sporadic onset
   (b) The occurrence in only a minority of patients
   (c) The degree of dyspnea that is out of proportion to the volume of lung irradiated

(d) The resolution of symptoms without sequelae in the majority of patients diagnostic indication of thoracoscopy procedure
(e) The resolution of symptoms without sequelae in the minority of patient diagnostic indication of thoracoscopy procedure

Answer Keys
1. D
2. E
3. A
4. A
5. E

Acknowledgments Cipta Mahendra MD, Department of Internal Medicine, Respirology and Critical Illness Division, Universitas Indonesia, Dr. Cipto Mangunkusumo General Central National Hospital, Jakarta, Indonesia.
Ersananda Arlisa Putri MD, Department of Internal Medicine, Respirology and Critical Illness Division, Universitas Indonesia, Dr. Cipto Mangunkusumo General Central National Hospital, Jakarta, Indonesia.
Ralph Girson Gunarsa MD DM, Department of Internal Medicine, Medical Hematology and Oncology division, Mochtar Riady Comprehensive Cancer Center (MRCCC) Siloam Hospital, Jakarta, Indonesia.

References

1. Majeed H, Gupta V. Adverse effects of radiation therapy. In: StatPearls Publ; 2023. https://www.ncbi.nlm.nih.gov/books/NBK563259/.
2. Jamil A, Kasi A. Lung Metastasis. In: StatPearls Publ; 2003. https://www.ncbi.nlm.nih.gov/books/NBK553111/.
3. Wu S, Pan Y, Mao Y, Chen Y, He Y. Current progress and mechanisms of bone metastasis in lung cancer: a narrative review. Transl Lung Cancer Res. 2021;10:439–51. https://doi.org/10.21037/tlcr-20-835. PMID: 33569325; PMCID: PMC7867745.
4. Morgan GW, Breit SN. Radiation and the lung: a reevaluation of the mechanisms mediating pulmonary injury. Int J Radiat Oncol Biol Phys. 1995;31:361–9.
5. McDonald S, Rubin P, Phillips TL, Marks LB. Injury to the lung from cancer therapy: clinical syndromes, measurable endpoints, and potential scoring systems. Int J Radiat Oncol Biol Phys. 1995;31:1187–203.
6. Richerson HB, Bernstein IL, Fink JN, Hunninghake GW, Novey HS, Reed CE, Salvaggio JE, Schuyler MR, Schwartz HJ, Stechschulte DJ. Guidelines for the clinical evaluation of hypersensitivity pneumonitis. Report of the Subcommittee on Hypersensitivity Pneumonitis. J Allergy Clin Immunol. 1989;84:839–44. https://doi.org/10.1016/0091-6749(89)90349-7. PMID: 2809034.
7. Xu K, Liang J, Zhang T, Zhou Z, Chen D, Feng Q. Clinical outcomes and radiation pneumonitis after concurrent EGFR-tyrosine kinase inhibitors and radiotherapy for unresectable stage III non-small cell lung cancer. Thorac Cancer. 2021;12:814–23.
8. Ohmori T, Yamaoka T, Ando K, Kusumoto S, Kishino Y, Manabe R. Molecular and clinical features of EGFR-TKI-associated lung injury. Int J Mol Sci. 2021;22:792.

Coinfection of Invasive Aspergillosis with Pulmonary Tuberculosis

12

12.1 Case Illustration

A 72-year-old male patient presented to the hospital with a chief complaint of shortness of breath that had persisted for several days. The patient experienced increasing breathing difficulty and decided to seek medical attention. An initial chest X-ray was performed to evaluate the lungs, revealing consolidation of the upper right lung (Fig. 12.1) and a collapsed right lung, suggesting pneumothorax. The patient was then admitted to manage the breathing symptoms, followed by the administration of two antibiotics, each from the cephalosporin and quinolone groups. After 2 days of treatment, there was significant improvement in breathing, leading to a request for discharge. The treating physician, an internist-pulmonologist, recommended the continuation of the antibiotics treatment and a computed tomography (CT) scanning procedure to evaluate and determine the underlying cause. However, the patient declined the recommendation, opting instead to wait for the α1-antitrypsin testing result as some of the family members had previously suffered from α1-antitrypsin deficiency disease. The treatment was later discontinued, and the patient was discharged from the hospital.

The next day, the patient returned to the hospital with the same breathing symptoms, and another pulmonologist was consulted with the administration of the same antibiotic regimen. After several days, the condition improved, and a request to be discharged home was presented. The treating pulmonologist also suggested that the patient undergo a CT scanning procedure to evaluate the lungs further, but the suggestion was again rejected. The patient insisted on waiting for the α1-antitrypsin testing result and was later discharged as requested.

Approximately 2 days after the discharge, the patient returned again to the hospital with the same breathing difficulty and finally agreed to undergo the CT scanning procedure as suggested on the first hospital visit. The CT scan imaging showed irregular opacities with an air bronchogram in the superior medial lobe of the right lung, while pleural effusions were seen on the right lung (Fig. 12.2). Multiple lymphadenopathies were also found on the CT images, leading to the diagnosis of

G. Singh, *Challenging Cases in Respirology and Critical Care*,
https://doi.org/10.1007/978-981-96-5002-6_12

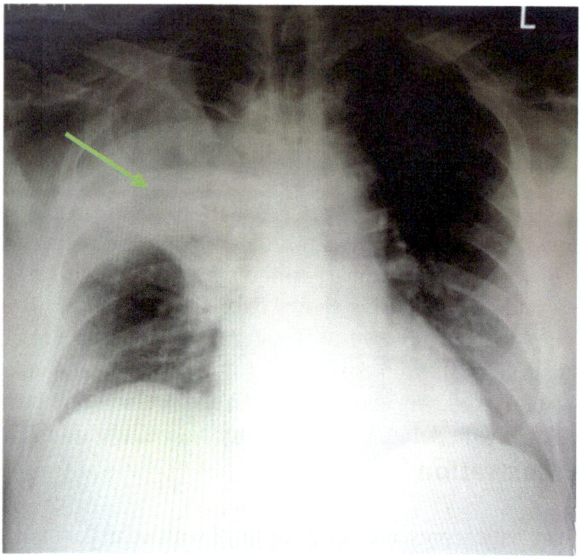

Fig. 12.1 Initial chest X-ray image on hospital admission. Consolidation on the upper right lung was found (green arrow). (Image Courtesy: Nungky Kusumaningtyas MD)

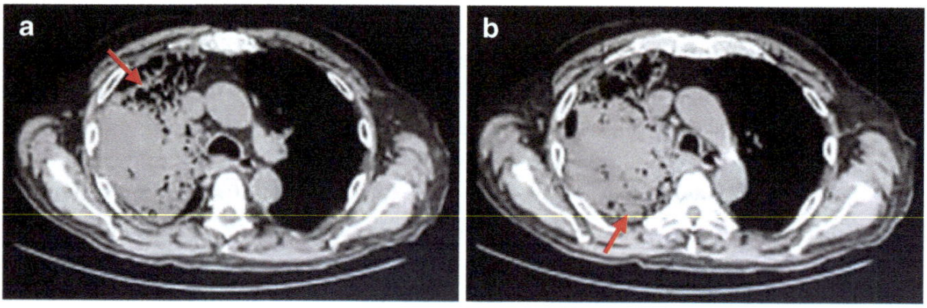

Fig. 12.2 (**a**, **b**) The patient's CT scan images on second hospital admission. Irregular opacities with air bronchogram were observed in superior medial lobe of the right lung (red arrow). Loculated pleural effusion with air-fluid level was also found in the superolateral lobe of the right lung (red arrow). (Image Courtesy: Nungky Kusumaningtyas MD).

hydropneumothorax based on the findings. Subsequently, a chest tube was then inserted into the right hemithorax to inflate the collapsed right lung. Pleural effusions were drained out, and approximately a liter of the fluid was obtained.

A week after the chest tube insertion, the patient underwent another chest X-ray imaging to evaluate the right lung. The results showed that the lung had not returned to its normal size and had further collapsed (Fig. 12.3), with persistent breathing difficulty. In response, a cardiothoracic surgeon was consulted and the patient was scheduled for a thoracic surgery to investigate the right lung abnormalities observed on the images. The patient agreed to the suggestion and underwent the surgery the following day. A big cavity was found on the superomedial lobe, which was disseminated with granulomas (Fig. 12.4). Massive adhesions occurred between the

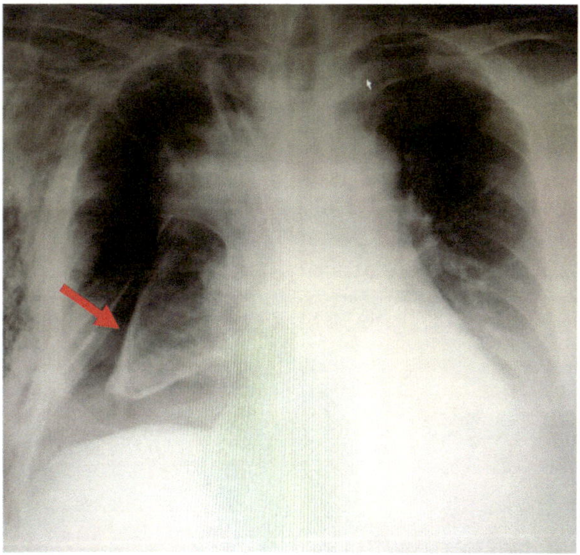

Fig. 12.3 Follow-up chest X-ray image after about a week since the last–third–hospital admission. An increased right lung pneumothorax was observed despite the chest tube insertion into the right lung cavity (red arrow). (Image Courtesy: Nungky Kusumaningtyas MD)

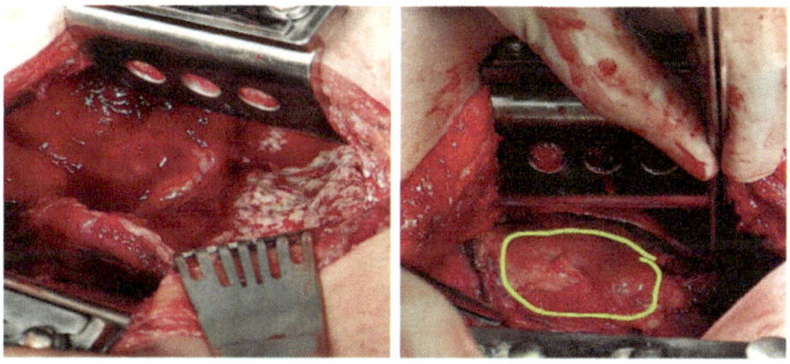

Fig. 12.4 (Left) The cavity was found on the superomedial lobe of the right lung. (Right) Granulomas were found disseminating the cavity (yellow circle). (Image Courtesy: Hariadi Hadibrata MD)

right lung's superior and middle lobes, eliminating the demarcating line, while the inferior lobe was found unaffected. The granulated right lung tissues were subsequently sampled for histopathology examination, with the chest tube kept in place.

The following day, the patient underwent bronchoscopy to evaluate the airways, and there was no observable abnormality in the bronchi (Fig. 12.5). A transbronchial lung biopsy was conducted to obtain a bronchial tissue sample, which was sent to the histopathology laboratory to be examined, and empiric antibiotics were continued to be administered. The bronchial tissue examination result showed emphysematous tissues and low-grade inflammation. In addition, there was no sign of malignancies, and the presence of acid-fast bacilli, fungal hyphae, and spores was also absent in the examined bronchial tissues.

Several days later, the histopathology examination of the granulated right lung tissues revealed necrotic areas surrounded by epithelioid cells (Fig. 12.6), and a Langhans

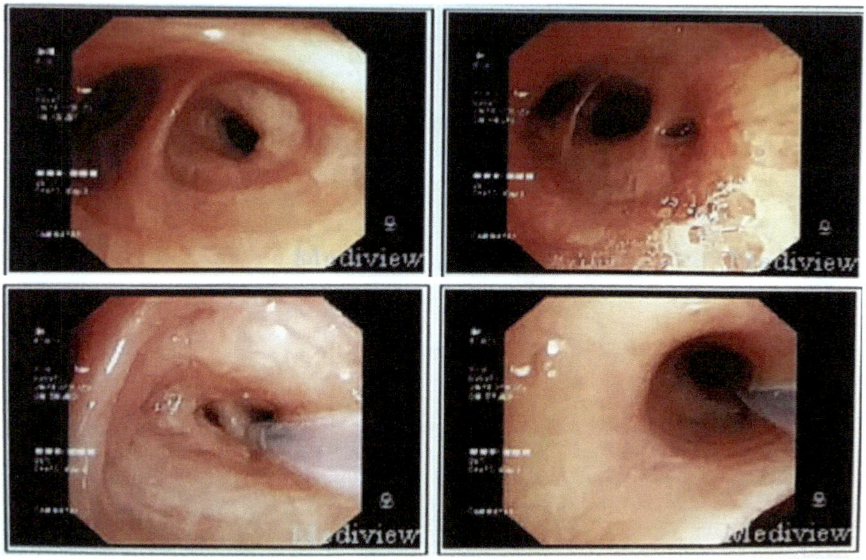

Fig. 12.5 The patient's bronchoscopy imaging. No observable abnormalities were found on the visualized bronchi. (Image Courtesy: Gurmeet Singh MD DM PhD)

giant cell was found (Fig. 12.7). In addition, there was no sign of malignancies and certain specific findings were observed. Acid-fast bacilli, fungal hyphae, and spores were also absent, with galactomannan (GM) level in the blood being determined through a blood test. The results revealed a below-threshold level, indicating no aspergillosis infection. Gram staining of the sampled tissues was also performed but yielded no presence of acid-fast bacilli. However, the patient was still diagnosed with pulmonary tuberculosis (PTB) due to the hallmark findings associated with tuberculosis (TB) infection in the lung tissue, as shown in Figs. 12.6 and 12.7. A standard antituberculosis drug regimen was then administered to treat the disease.

Despite the antituberculosis drugs given, the patient did not improve significantly and continued to experience shortness of breath. A follow-up chest X-ray imaging obtained about 3 weeks after the surgery and 2 weeks since the antituberculosis treatment initiation, showed that the right lung was in status quo, with no significant inflation (Fig. 12.8). A culture was then performed on the obtained granulated tissues during the thoracic surgery to determine the presence of any infectious microorganism. Several days later, the culture had grown *Aspergillus niger* and α1-antitrypsin testing result returned negative. The patient was subsequently diagnosed with PTB and aspergillosis. Treatment was performed with antifungal drugs in addition to the antituberculosis medications. After the completion of both the antituberculosis and antifungal regimens, the patient was finally relieved from the breathing symptoms.

The patient had a history of regular exercise and admitted to a history of smoking but had quit approximately 30 years ago. In addition, there was no prior history of any surgery or hospitalization, and an annual influenza vaccination was previously received.

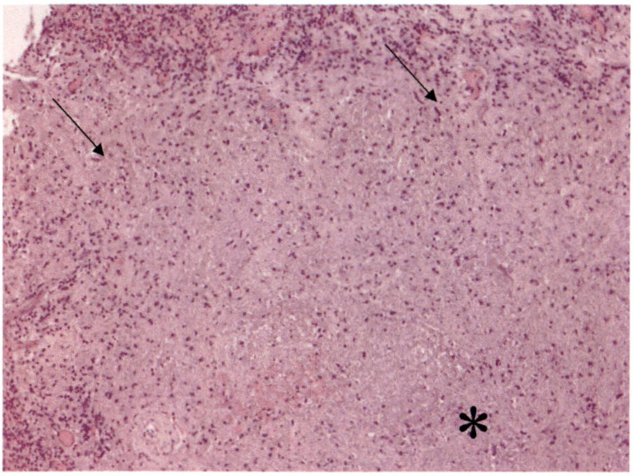

Fig. 12.6 The patient's right lung biopsy through VATS histological appearance. A large necrotic area (*) surrounded by epithelioid cells (arrows) was spotted. (Magnification: 10x) (Image Courtesy: Stella Marleen MD)

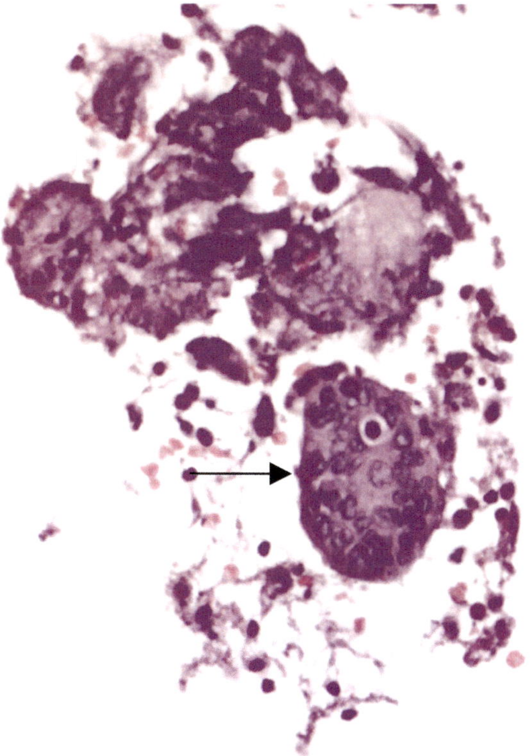

Fig. 12.7 A Langhans giant cell (arrow) found on the patient's right lung tissues. (Magnification: 40x). (Image Courtesy: Stella Marleen MD)

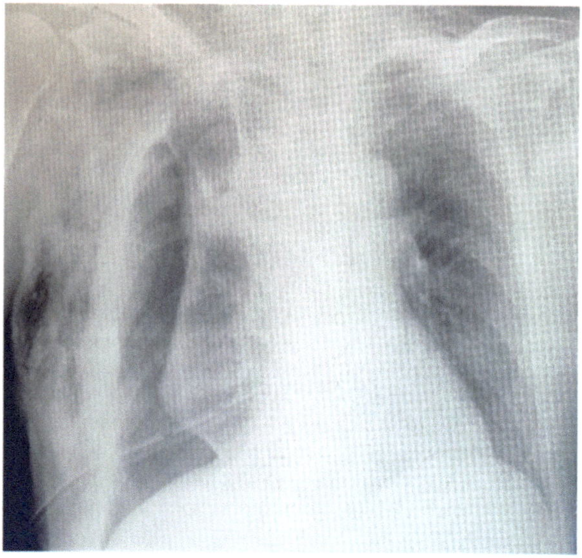

Fig. 12.8 Post-surgery chest X-ray imaging. The patient's right lung was seen relatively unchanged compared to the pre-surgery chest X-ray imaging (see Fig. 12.3). (Image Courtesy: Nungky Kusumaningtyas MD)

12.2 What Is the Patient's Problem Focus?

A 72-year-old man presented to the hospital with a chief complaint of breathing difficulty that had persisted for several days. An initial chest X-ray and computed tomography (CT) scan imaging showed pleural effusions, consolidations, and collapse of the right lung, indicating right-sided hydropneumothorax. In response to the findings, empiric antibiotics were given, and a chest tube was inserted to restore the right lung but no significant improvement was observed.

A thoracic surgery was later performed to sample the granulated right lung tissues found during the operation. The histopathology examination reported necrotic areas surrounded by epithelioid cells and the presence of Langhans giant cells. Signs of malignancies and the presence of infectious microorganisms were absent. The transbronchial lung biopsy procedure revealed no abnormalities other than emphysematous tissues and low-grade inflammation. Galactomannan level of the blood and Gram staining test of the lung tissues also did not indicate infectious microorganisms. However, the patient was diagnosed with pulmonary tuberculosis (PTB) due to the associated histopathology findings, leading to the administration of antituberculosis.

Approximately 2 weeks later, the patient was still experiencing shortness of breath despite the antituberculosis medications. Another chest X-ray imaging revealed the right lung's status quo and a culture of the granulated tissues was ordered. The culture test aimed to detect the presence of any infectious microorganisms affecting the right lung, with the result showing the isolation of *Aspergillus niger*. The patient was finally diagnosed with PTB and aspergillosis infection, leading to the administration of antifungal drugs. After all the treatment had been completed, the patient was finally relieved from the breathing symptoms.

12.3 Discussion

Pulmonary tuberculosis (PTB) is a significant health issue and a severe infection with lasting consequences. Affected patients typically exhibit constitutional symptoms, including fever, night sweats, and weight loss, along with cough and hemoptysis. In this context, tuberculosis (TB) infection can lead to lung damage, which increases the development of a fungal infection, specifically aspergillosis. This condition presents as aspergilloma in the form of cavities in the lungs. Several studies have shown that aspergillosis is occasionally ignored due to its ability to imitate TB infection. In addition, acute invasive aspergillosis (IA) co-infection with TB in a young and healthy patient is uncommon [1]. Pulmonary fungal infections have been reported to possess clinical and radiological features that closely resemble TB, thereby increasing the likelihood of misdiagnosis as TB [2]. Chronic pulmonary aspergillosis (CPA) is a common complication that arises after treating PTB, and it is associated with a high mortality rate over 5 years [2].

12.4 Pulmonary Tuberculosis

Tuberculosis is the primary cause of mortality caused by an infectious agent on a global scale, particularly affecting individuals with impaired immune systems. Recent reports revealed that one-third of the global population has been infected with the bacteria that causes the disease. The global annual incidence of Mycobacterium Tuberculosis infections is estimated to be ten million. In addition, tuberculosis is responsible for approximately 24% of the global illness burden, which has significant socioeconomic consequences. The disease is primarily characterized by necrotizing granulomatous inflammation, with the lungs being the principal organs affected in around 87% of patients. Building on this idea, virtually every physical organ can serve as a location for the disease. Several studies have shown that it frequently impacts individuals residing in densely populated environments, such as institutionalized patients, immigrants from countries with a high incidence of tuberculosis, immunocompromised patients, and healthcare personnel [3].

12.5 Aspergillosis

Aspergillus is an airborne/saprophytic agent that typically does not cause any condition. However, in individuals with compromised immune systems or damaged lungs, such as those with tuberculosis (TB), it can lead to the development of diseases. Compared to other fungal infections, Aspergillus is also usually not pathogenic, but it can escalate into an active infection with severe consequences. In the case of Pulmonary Tuberculosis (PTB), specifically secondary TB, patients develop hollow areas known as cavitary lesions that are susceptible to its infection. The presence of tiny cavitary lesions facilitates the colonization and proliferation of Aspergillus spores, which leads to the enlargement or formation of more cavities, causing tissue damage. Aspergillus infection can be ignored in patients who have TB since the symptoms are similar, such as coughing blood, weight loss, fever, and night sweats. Moreover, the absence of clinical suspicion can lead to incorrect diagnosis, and the long-lasting nature of the infection poses challenges in its differentiation from PTB. The majority of Aspergillus infections are characterized by a chronic nature requiring a pre-existing lung injury, which commonly arises in PTB patients. This highlights the critical importance of promptly identifying fungal infections in the management of patients [1].

12.6 Tuberculosis Coinfection of Pulmonary Fungal Infection

The incidence of opportunistic fungal infections has recently increased in recent years despite their usual inability to cause disease in individuals with good health. However, fungi have the potential to cause infections in individuals with weakened immune systems, such as those with underlying disorders, extensive use of antibiotics, and impaired immunity in patients with pulmonary tuberculosis (PTB). The occurrence and frequency of respiratory fungal diseases in numerous poor nations have predominantly been uninvestigated and disregarded. This has led to pervasive misconceptions over their genuine significance in public health. Given its profound impact, similar to that of other respiratory diseases, this disregard must be seen as a significant cause for alarm. According to the Centers for Disease Control and Prevention (CDC), the death rate linked to Invasive Aspergillosis (IA) has increased by 35.7% since 1980, and the death rate for untreated invasive respiratory aspergillosis (IRA) is almost 100%. However, Candida is frequently identified as the predominant fungal pathogen and can lead to serious secondary infections in those with weakened immune systems, such as patients with tuberculosis (TB) [4].

12.7 Clinical Features

Aspergillus, similar to other fungal infections, typically lacks pathogenicity. However, in individuals with impaired immune systems or lung damage, it can develop into an active infection with severe effects. Patients with secondary tuberculosis (TB), especially in the pulmonary tuberculosis (PTB) form, exhibit the formation of cavitary lesions that are susceptible to Aspergillus infection. The presence of tiny cavitary lesions facilitates the colonization and proliferation of Aspergillus spores, which leads to the enlargement or formation of more cavities and causes tissue damage. In addition, Aspergillus infection is often ignored in TB patients due to similarity in symptoms, including coughing up blood, weight loss, fever, and night sweats. Building on this idea, the absence of clinical suspicion can lead to misdiagnosis, and its long-term nature poses challenges during differentiation from PTB. The majority of Aspergillus case are characterized by a chronic nature requiring a pre-existing lung injury, which commonly arises in PTB [1].

12.8 Diagnosis

12.8.1 Radiological Features

Chest radiographs are considered outdated for diagnosis when a chest computed tomography (CT) scan is available. While contrast agents are typically not required for diagnosis, they can be helpful in evaluating the likelihood of hemoptysis when a lesion is close to a major blood vessel. Studies have shown that Invasive Aspergillosis (IA) can present with two distinct CT scan patterns, depending on its mode of extension: angio-invasive and airway-invasive (Fig. 12.9).

The angio-invasive pattern refers to the radiological appearance of hyphae penetrating the walls of blood vessels, leading to the formation of fungal thrombi that cause tissue necrosis and the spread of infection through the bloodstream. This pattern is traditionally associated with a significant decrease in neutrophil count. It typically presents as nodules, often surrounded by hazy lung tissue, indicating bleeding around the nodules and the presence of a distinctive halo sign. The halo sign is strongly suggestive of neutropenia-related invasive aspergillosis (IA), but it lacks specificity and can also be seen in various other conditions, such as invasive mold disease (IMD), bacterial infections, primary or metastatic cancers, granulomatosis with polyangiitis, bronchiolitis obliterans organizing pneumonia, or focal lung injury. Therefore, it is important to consider the potential evolution of this finding over time. Initial CT scans may reveal small nodules, while follow-up scans may not show the characteristic hazy lung tissue, which typically resolves within 5–10 days [5].

The airway-invasive trend is predominantly observed in patients who are not neutropenic. The CT-scan shows the spread of infection within the bronchial tubes, with thicker walls and numerous nodules in the central parts of the lobes, creating a characteristic tree-like pattern. The observed pattern is commonly observed in several lung diseases, including mycobacteria and viruses. Therefore, it is not compelling evidence for IA until additional supporting material is provided, specifically considering the high occurrence of coinfections. This pattern has also been linked to a more unfavorable functional trajectory, necessitating artificial ventilation [5].

12.9 Bronchoscopy

Bronchoscopy can identify the unique and relatively rare presentation of invasive tracheobronchial aspergillosis (ITBA), occurring in about 7% of aspergillosis patients within the chest cavity. ITBA often presents with inflammation and excessive mucus production, ulcerations, plaque-like lesions, or pseudo-membranous necrosis, primarily affecting the lower airways. This condition is closely associated with AIDS, radiation therapy, or lung transplantation, and typically involves the area immediately beyond the bronchial anastomosis, leading to damage of the surrounding scar tissue. Furthermore, bronchoscopy is valuable in evaluating the extent of these lesions, which are often poorly defined by CT scans [5].

12.10 Microbiology

Respiratory samples differ in their sensitivity and specificity, and not all are equally reliable. The gold-standard method for diagnosing Invasive Aspergillosis (IA) is the analysis of bronchoalveolar lavage fluid (BALF). However, this procedure is not always feasible due to the patient's physical condition and their willingness to undergo a potentially risky procedure. Sputum is generally more accessible, but obtaining high-quality samples may require physiotherapy interventions in patients with non-productive coughs. Tracheal aspirates or brushes serve as valuable intermediate samples in intubated patients. It is crucial, however, to interpret both sputum and tracheal aspirates with caution to avoid misinterpreting colonization as true infection [5].

Although Aspergillus species have the ability to invade blood vessels, it is rare to find blood samples that test positive for this fungus. Blood samples are often included in the diagnosis process of IA to identify biomarkers and fungal DNA. Manufacturer instructions indicate that tests can be conducted on whole blood, plasma, or serum. The thresholds for determining positive may vary based on the characteristics of the samples [5].

1. **Direct Microscopy**

Conducting microscopic analysis on all respiratory samples that are available (such as BALF, tracheal aspiration, or sputum) is essential despite the potential for varying and unproductive results. Several studies have also shown that the use of calcofluor-white can improve performance. In this context, Aspergillus is characterized by septate hyphae that exhibit dichotomous acute angle branching [5].

2. **Culture**

The typical medium used for cultivating Aspergillus includes Sabouraud-dextrose, brain-heart-infusion, or potato-dextrose agar. Chloramphenicol is commonly added to prevent bacterial contamination, while cycloheximide can help reduce fungal contamination, though it may lead to slightly lower fungal yield. Specialized media can be used to specifically identify different Aspergillus species. The culture should be maintained at a temperature of 30 °C for 21 days in an environment with controlled humidity. If microscopy fails to determine the species, positive culture samples can be further analyzed using mass spectrometry identification Matrix-Assisted Laser Desorption/Ionization Time-of-Flight (MALDI-TOF) or genomic sequencing. Additionally, a good culture allows for the evaluation of the strain's susceptibility to antifungal medications [5].

3. **Antibodies**

Since immunosuppression is linked to Invasive Aspergillosis (IA), the absence of antibodies specifically targeting Aspergillus cannot be utilized as diagnostic evidence compared to case of ABPA or Chronic pulmonary aspergillosis (CPA). Certain individuals continue to have a humoral reaction, leading to the identification of these antibodies approximately 10 days after the commencement of invasive respiratory aspergillosis (IRA). Anti-Aspergillus antibodies can potentially reduce the sensitivity of the galactomannan detection test [5].

4. **Galactomannan**

Galactomannan (GM) is a polysaccharide found in the cell wall of Aspergillus fungi. Its detection can be performed in serum, BALF, and cerebrospinal fluid, showing higher sensitivity compared to culture. However, its applicability in sputum and tissue biopsies has not been established. The results are typically expressed as an index relative to a control, with the threshold for positivity in serum still a matter of debate. The manufacturer recommends a single value above 0.5, while experts suggest a threshold of 0.7 for a single test or two consecutive tests exceeding 0.5. In bronchoalveolar lavage fluid (BALF), there is no consensus on the cut-off value, with some studies proposing >0.5 and others suggesting >1.0. Despite these discrepancies, a recent meta-analysis reviewing 19 studies found evidence supporting the >0.5 cut-off, which showed a sensitivity of 89% and a specificity of 79% [6].

The high sensitivity of GM detection has made it a key tool in diagnosing suspected invasive aspergillosis (IA) in neutropenic patients. In hematology patients, its success rate ranges from 60 to 80%, but it is less effective in non-neutropenic individuals and yields poor outcomes when anti-mold prophylaxis is used [5].

5. **(1,3)-β-D-Glucan**

Incorporating the detection of β-D-glucan (BDG) in serum can improve the sensitivity of the diagnostic evaluation. However, due to its presence in the cell walls of several fungi, such as Aspergillus, Candida, and Pneumocystis, BDG's utility is limited by a lack of specificity. Although BDG is not synthesized by Mucorales or Cryptococcus, it can still help differentiate between various fungal infections. Bronchoalveolar lavage fluid (BALF) can also be used to detect BDG, though its limited specificity restricts its broader diagnostic applications [5].

6. **Polymerase Chain Reaction**

The availability and standards of Aspergillus PCR have been limited, leading to its less advanced development compared to the use of GM. These challenges have been successfully resolved, and PCR is now included in standard diagnostic procedures using commercially available kits that utilize serum, plasma, or BALF samples. Additional specimens that can be examined include recently obtained tissue or samples that have been preserved via formalin fixation and paraffin embedding [5].

Previous reports indicate that PCR sensitivity is notably high, potentially exceeding 90% in routine blood samples. When combined with GM detection in BALF, PCR can achieve a sensitivity of up to 96%. The specificity of PCR is exceptionally high, reaching 100% in certain cases. However, there have been instances of cross-reactivity with other molds, such as Penicillium spp., Fusarium spp., and Rhizopus oryzae. Additionally, PCR offers the advantage of using probes to detect mutations associated with antifungal resistance, including azole resistance [5].

7. **Point of Care Tests**

Point-of-care diagnostics, often referred to as "bedside testing," play a crucial role in the timely initiation of appropriate antifungal therapy. Currently, two options with European conformity (CE-mark) certification are available. The first is the AspLFD lateral flow device, developed by OLM Diagnostics in Newcastle-upon-Tyne, UK. This device detects an extracellular glycoprotein associated with Aspergillus growth. The second option is the lateral flow assay developed by IMMY in Norman, OK, USA, which detects galactomannan (GM) with a sensitivity and specificity exceeding 70% [5].

12.11 Diagnostic Criteria

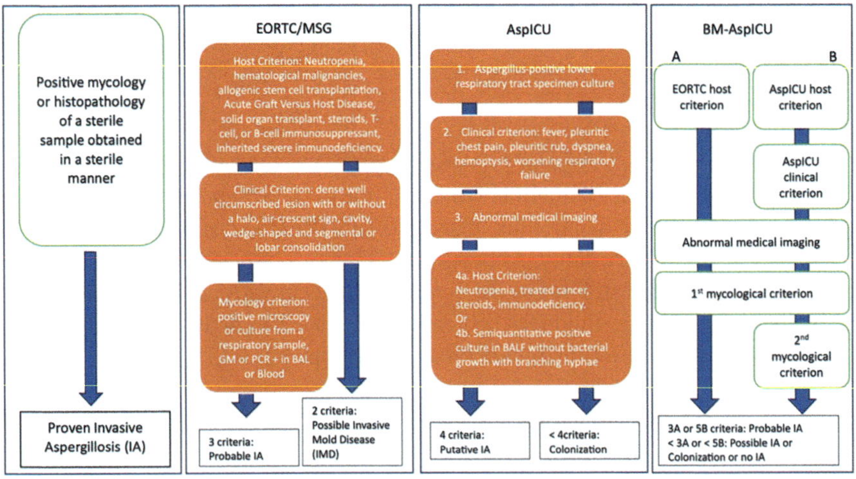

Fig. 12.9 Invasive pulmonary aspergillosis diagnostic criteria. Abbreviations: *EORTC-MSG* European Organization for Research and Treatment of Cancer/Mycosis Study Group, *AspICU* Aspergillosis in Intensive Care Unit diagnostic algorithm, *BM-AspICU* Biomarkers-based Aspergillosis in Intensive Care Unit diagnostic algorithm

12.12 Management

12.12.1 Antituberculosis Agent

Antituberculosis therapy remains the cornerstone for managing pulmonary tuberculosis (PTB), even in the presence of invasive aspergillosis. Newly diagnosed pulmonary tuberculosis (PTB) patients must receive a standard treatment regimen of 6 months with rifampicin: 2HRZE/4HR (strong recommendation, high certainty of evidence). This regimen consists of 2 months of intensive therapy with isoniazid, rifampicin, pyrazinamide, and ethambutol, followed by 4 months of continuation therapy with isoniazid and rifampicin. Where feasible, daily dosing throughout both phases is strongly recommended due to its superior efficacy compared to thrice-weekly dosing (strong recommendation, high certainty of evidence). For drug-susceptible PTB patients, the use of thrice-weekly dosing is not recommended in either the intensive or continuation phases, as daily dosing remains the preferred frequency (conditional recommendation, very low certainty of evidence). The use of fixed-dose combination (FDC) tablets is recommended over separate drug formulations for patients with drug-susceptible TB, as FDCs simplify administration, improve adherence, and reduce the risk of missed doses (conditional recommendation, low certainty of evidence). In new PTB patients receiving rifampicin-containing regimens, extending the intensive phase is strongly discouraged, even when a positive sputum smear is detected at the end of this phase. High-certainty evidence indicates that this practice does not improve treatment outcomes (strong recommendation, high certainty of evidence) [6].

12.12.2 Antifungal Agent

1. **Amphotericin B and Lipid Formulations**

Historically, the polyene deoxycholate amphotericin B is the first antifungal to demonstrate efficacy against Aspergillus. Due to its unfavorable toxicity profile, several studies have recommended the non-use of the drug, currently recommended to avoid its use. However, it remains beneficial in environments with limited resources [5].

Significant progress has been achieved with the introduction of lipid-based formulations of amphotericin B, including liposomal amphotericin B (L-AmB), amphotericin B lipid complex (ABLC), and amphotericin B colloidal dispersion (ABCD). These formulations are associated with reduced kidney toxicity and are equally effective as deoxycholate amphotericin B. Among these, L-AmB has become the most widely used lipid formulation due to its excellent safety profile. Extensive studies have confirmed its efficacy against invasive respiratory aspergillosis (IRA). The standard dosage for Aspergillus infections is 3 mg/kg/day, although increasing the dose in highly immunocompromised patients has not significantly improved antifungal outcomes. L-AmB is particularly advantageous in managing breakthrough infections during azole prophylaxis or as salvage therapy. Furthermore, converting amphotericin B and L-AmB into aerosol formulations offers a preventive strategy for invasive aspergillosis (IA), with L-AmB demonstrating better tolerance in this application [5, 7].

2. **Azoles**

Azoles, by impeding the production of ergosterol, a vital component of cell membranes, are crucial in the treatment of numerous fungal diseases. Fluconazole, which has little effectiveness against Aspergillus, was not effective in treating IRA. The first azole used for this purpose was itraconazole, which led to a complete or partial response in 39% of patients after treatment. However, it had limitations due to toxicity and concerns about how well it might be absorbed by the body [5].

The introduction of voriconazole represented a significant milestone in managing invasive respiratory aspergillosis (IRA). A landmark randomized trial comparing voriconazole to amphotericin B demonstrated favorable outcomes in 52.8% of patients treated with voriconazole, compared to 31.6% receiving amphotericin B. While generally well-tolerated, voriconazole's use is often limited by adverse effects, including liver toxicity, ocular and neurological disturbances, and drug–drug interactions, particularly with hematologic agents such as cyclosporine, midostaurine, or venetoclax. Long-term use has been associated with rare complications like phototoxicity, skin carcinomas, peripheral neuropathy, and periostitis. To mitigate these risks, therapeutic drug monitoring (TDM) is recommended and readily accessible. The standard dosing protocol involves 6 mg/kg twice daily for the first 24 h, followed by 4 mg/kg twice daily. Voriconazole is endorsed as the first-line treatment by the Infectious Diseases Society of America (IDSA), the European Conference on Infections in Leukemia (ECIL), and the European Society of Clinical Microbiology and Infectious Diseases (ESCMID) [5].

Posaconazole, initially used as salvage therapy for patients who failed to respond to or tolerate traditional antifungal treatments, demonstrated a success rate of 42%, which was deemed clinically significant. With superior tolerability compared to voriconazole, posaconazole has gained favor, particularly for prophylaxis. Delayed-release tablet formulations have resolved prior concerns regarding bioavailability, enhancing its practicality. Moreover, posaconazole provides a unique advantage over voriconazole with its efficacy against Mucorales, a pathogen often indistinguishable from Aspergillus. A recent study comparing posaconazole to voriconazole for invasive aspergillosis (IA) found it to be non-inferior while offering a better safety profile. The recommended dosage is 300 mg twice daily on the first day, followed by 300 mg once daily thereafter, with TDM targeting trough levels of 0.7 mg/L for prophylaxis and 1.0 mg/L for treatment [5].

Isavuconazole, the most recent azole to receive approval, has shown promising efficacy against Aspergillus with an excellent safety profile. A randomized, double-blind trial established its non-inferiority to voriconazole, with comparable survival rates at 6 and 12 weeks. Notably, isavuconazole exhibited improved tolerability, with fewer liver, ocular, and skin-related adverse effects, making it an appealing option for patients at risk of hepatic dysfunction. Its pharmacological profile allows for better control of drug interactions, reducing the need for dosage adjustments in concurrent therapies. A meta-analysis comparing isavuconazole to voriconazole and liposomal amphotericin B (L-AmB) confirmed similar efficacy. Additionally, isavuconazole demonstrates robust activity against Mucorales, further enhancing its therapeutic utility [5].

3. **Echinocandins**

Echinocandins, which inhibit β-D-glucan synthesis, have limited efficacy against *Aspergillus* compared to voriconazole. Among these, caspofungin was initially employed as a salvage therapy for patients who could not tolerate or failed to respond to prior treatments for invasive aspergillosis (IA), achieving a promising 45% success rate. However, trials evaluating its use as first-line therapy in neutropenic and allogeneic stem cell transplantation patients showed suboptimal outcomes, with survival rates of 53% and 50% at week 12, respectively. As a result, current guidelines do not recommend caspofungin for primary treatment of IA.

Micafungin and anidulafungin also demonstrate limited efficacy against *Aspergillus* and are not suitable for treating invasive respiratory fungal infections associated with IA. In contrast, rezafungin, a newer echinocandin, has shown promising activity against *Aspergillus* in preclinical studies, including laboratory and animal models, offering potential for future therapeutic applications [5].

12.13 Drug Interaction

The rifampicin-induced activation of CYP3A4, mediated by the Pregnane X Receptors (PXR), is influenced differently by several azole antimycotics. The drug interaction study reported both additive and antagonistic interactions between certain azole antimycotics and rifampicin. Oxiconazole is a highly effective substance that stimulates the expression of the CYP3A4 gene through the PXR pathway. Several studies have shown that the activation of CYP3A4 by oxiconazole can be competitively blocked by rifampicin. Econazole and Miconazole are powerful activators of the PXR and also induce the activity of the enzyme CYP3A4. When taken together with rifampicin, these drugs enhance the activation of the CYP3A4 promoter greatly than the sum of their individual effects. Itraconazole induced the activation of the CYP3A4 promoter and the recruitment of SRC-1 to PXR. However, it did not interact with the ligand binding domain (LBD) of PXR. Clotrimazole, a very strong PXR ligand, did not have any impact on the activation of CYP3A4 caused by rifampicin, nor did it interact with rifampicin on PXR LBD. Ketoconazole also inhibited the activation of CYP3A4 by rifampicin, prevented the recruitment of SRC-1 to PXR, and disrupted the interaction between rifampicin and PXR LDB. Although the drug does not function as an agonist of PXR, it stimulated the production of CYP3A4 mRNA by acting on CYP3A4 promoter response elements. Rifampicin stimulated the interaction of CYP3A4, CYP2C9, and CYP2C19, leading to an increased rate of metabolism of Voriconazole [8]. Fluconazole did not exhibit binding to the ligand-binding domain (LBD) of the PXR and did not induce any changes in the activation of the CYP3A4 promoter [9]. In vitro, amphotericin B and rifampicin demonstrated a synergistic effect against specific yeasts. The study revealed that amphotericin B modified the permeability barrier of the cytoplasmic membrane of the organism, enabling enhanced penetration of rifampicin. This leads to the suppression of fungal RNA polymerase. In vitro, the combination of amphotericin B and rifampicin exhibited fungicidal activity at achievable doses, although each drug individually did not possess fungicidal properties. The concurrent administration of caspofungin and rifampicin led to an elevation in caspofungin levels. However, this effect diminished within the initial 2 weeks of treatment [10].

12.14 Prognosis

The prognosis for individuals with Tuberculosis Coinfection of Pulmonary Fungal Infection is unfavorable. The infection can progress gradually and without detection for several years, and successful treatment becomes challenging when initiated late. Among these patients, a range of 25–60% may exhibit a positive response to antifungal treatment. However, the death rate remains elevated due to the seriousness of the underlying condition and the necessity of ongoing administration of immunosuppressants and steroids. When patients exhibit a positive response, there is a minimum probability of 50% for relapse to occur during successive sessions of immunosuppression [1, 11, 12].

Key Points
Patients with TB are often immunocompromised, thus are more susceptible to contract fungal infections. Early screening for fungal infection in TB patients is beneficial for a better patient outcome.

Question

1. The following are TRUE about the clinical features of Aspergillosis:
   (a) Protein Aspergillus usually pathogenic but in immunocompromised patients and those with lung damage, can progress to active infection.
   (b) Most Aspergillus cases are Acute, as it needs a damaged lung, which typically occurs in PTB.
   (c) The clinical features are similar (hemoptysis, cough, fever, and night sweats).
   (d) The small cavitary lesions allow the Aspergillus spores leading to the expansion or creation of new cavities without destruction.
   (e) Particularly secondary TB, patients develop cavitary lesions which are vulnerable to not only Aspergillosis infection, but also Candidiasis infection.

2. The following are TRUE about the Tuberculosis Coinfection of Pulmonary Fungal Infection, except?
    (a) Candida also is the most commonly isolated fungal pathogen beside Aspergillosis and may cause severe secondary infections in the immunocompromised population, including TB patients.
    (b) Invasive Aspergillosis (IA) has increased by 35.7% with the mortality of untreated invasive respiratory aspergillosis (IRA).
    (c) The mortality of Invasive Aspergillosis (IA) is nearly 100%.
    (d) The incidence and prevalence of respiratory fungal infections in many developed countries have remained largely unexplored and neglected.
    (e) Opportunistic fungal infections have recently increased in patients with broad consumption of antibiotics.
3. In radiological feature of invasive aspergillosis (IA), the halo sign is highly suggestive of:
    (a) Focal lung injury.
    (b) Neutropenia-related IA.
    (c) Invasive mold disease (IMD).
    (d) Primary or metastatic cancers.
    (e) Granulomatous with polyangiitis.
4. The following is the first antifungal to show activity against Aspergillus in PTB:
    (a) Clotrimazole.
    (b) Amphotericin B.
    (c) Echinocandin.
    (d) Miconazole.
    (e) Itraconazole.
5. In Aspergillosis infection, antibodies are often undetected or of low count because:
    (a) Chronic infection.
    (b) Similar symptom with PTB.
    (c) Anti-Aspergillus antibodies decrease the sensitivity of the galactomannan detection test.
    (d) Anti-Aspergillus antibodies decrease the specificity of the galactomannan detection test.
    (e) Similar symptom with Candida infection.

Answer keys

1. A
2. D
3. B
4. B
5. C

Acknowledgments Cipta Mahendra MD, Department of Internal Medicine, Respirology and Critical Illness Division, Universitas Indonesia, Dr. Cipto Mangunkusumo General Central National Hospital, Jakarta, Indonesia.

Ersananda Arlisa Putri MD, Department of Internal Medicine, Respirology and Critical Illness Division, Universitas Indonesia, Dr. Cipto Mangunkusumo General Central National Hospital, Jakarta, Indonesia.

Hariadi Hadibrata MD, Department of Cardiovascular and thoracic surgery, Mochtar Riady Comprehensive Cancer Center (MRCCC) Siloam Hospital, Jakarta, Indonesia.

Hartanto Wijaya MD, Department of Internal Medicine, Mochtar Riady Comprehensive Cancer Center (MRCCC) Siloam Hospital, Jakarta, Indonesia.

References

1. Ahmed AO, Ali GA, Goravey W. Concomitant pulmonary tuberculosis and invasive aspergillosis infection in an immunocompetent host. Eur J Case Rep Intern Med. 2022;9:003249.
2. Amiri MRJ, Siami R, Khaledi A. Tuberculosis status and coinfection of pulmonary fungal infections in patients referred to reference laboratory of health centers Ghaemshahr City during 2007–2017. Ethiop J Health Sci. 2018;28:683–90.
3. Alzayer Z, Al Nasser Y. Primary lung tuberculosis. In: StatPearls Publication; 2023. https://www.ncbi.nlm.nih.gov/books/NBK567737/
4. Hosseini M, Shakerimoghaddam A, Ghazalibina M, Khaledi A. Aspergillus coinfection among patients with pulmonary tuberculosis in Asia and Africa countries; a systematic review and meta-analysis of cross-sectional studies. Microb Pathog. 2020;141:104018.
5. Ledoux MP, Herbrecht R. Invasive pulmonary aspergillosis. J Fungi Basel. 2023;9:131.
6. WHO. WHO consolidated guidelines on tuberculosis, module 4: treatment – drug- susceptible tuberculosis treatment in 2022.
7. Beggs WH. Synergistic action of Amphotericin B and Rifampin against Candida species. J Infect Dis. 1976;133:206–9.
8. N.A. Rifampicin/voriconazole interaction React Wkly NA1287. 2010. https://doi.org/10.2165/00128415-201012870-00110.
9. Svecova L, Vrzal R, Burysek L, Anzenbacherova E, Cerveny L, Grim J, Pavek P. Azole Antimycotics differentially affect rifampicin-induced Pregnane X receptor-mediated CYP3A4 gene expression. Drug Metab Dispos. 2007;36(2):339–48. https://doi.org/10.1124/dmd.107.018341.
10. Ribner B, Keusch GT, Hanna BA, Perloff M. Combination amphotericin B-rifampin therapy for pulmonary aspergillosis in a leukemic patient. Chest. 1976;70(5):681–3. https://doi.org/10.1378/chest.70.5.681.
11. Fontalvo DM, Jiménez Borré G, Gómez Camargo D, Chalavé Jiménez N, Bellido Rodríguez J, Cuadrado Cano B, Navarro Gómez S. Tuberculosis and pulmonary candidiasis co-infection present in a previously healthy patient. Colomb Med Cali. 2016;47:105–8.
12. Kaya S, Gençalioğlu E, Sönmez M, Köksal I. The importance of risk factors for the prediction of patients with invasive pulmonary aspergillosis. Rev Assoc Med Bras (1992). 2017;63:764–70.

Disseminated *Histoplasma capsulatum* Infection with Prolonged Fever 13

13.1 Case Illustration

A 61-year-old male was brought to the hospital with shortness of breath for a week before admission. The symptom was continuously felt and started to worsen a day before admission. In addition, the patient had been experiencing intermittent fever over the past 7 months.

About 3 months before admission, symptoms of severe chills with fever and thrombocytopenia were reported at another hospital. The following month, the patient returned due to COVID-19, accompanied by cough and phlegm. Although COVID-19 resolved after 1 month, the cough with phlegm persisted and the patient was discharged.

Two weeks after, which was 2 weeks before admission to the current hospital, there was still intermittent fever but with increased frequency. Readmission was carried out to manage the fever and laboratory assessment indicated the same result as in the first admission, namely, decreased thrombocyte. The patient was referred and hospitalized in a second hospital to receive further treatment. An antibiotic was given during the hospitalization, leading to a slight improvement in the symptoms, but thrombocytopenia persisted. However, transfusion was not initiated to increase the thrombocyte level. Initially, bone marrow puncture (BMP) procedure was scheduled but this was postponed due to the fluctuating fever and persistent coughs. After a week, the patient was discharged from the hospital.

There was no history of drinking and smoking habits, as well as significant body weight decrease. History of surgery was admitted, specifically endoscopy and colonoscopy procedure 9 years ago to remove a polyp found in the gastrointestinal tract. Fatty liver disease was acquired 25 years ago, but the disease has been declared resolved. Several weeks ago, the patient had been tested for the presence of HBsAg and anti-HCV antibodies in the blood, with both returning negative. Hypertension had been diagnosed 7 years before and amlodipine was given as the treatment. About 5 months ago, heart ablation procedure was performed for supraventricular

G. Singh, *Challenging Cases in Respirology and Critical Care*,
https://doi.org/10.1007/978-981-96-5002-6_13

tachycardia (SVT). Furthermore, the treadmill stress test and echocardiography examination showed no heart abnormality. The father only suffered from diabetes mellitus but there was no history of heart attack, hypertension, kidney disease, and malignancy.

On physical examination, the patient was found to be obese with a body mass index (BMI) = 31.7, a blood pressure of 170/96 mmHg, and oxygen saturation of 99% with 4 lpm of oxygen flow using a nasal cannula. All other vital signs were within normal limits, including the body temperature. Wet crackles were heard in both lung fields, edema was observed at both feet, and thoracic computer tomography (CT) scan imaging showed residual signs of pneumonia on the lower lobe of the left lung. In addition, mild cardiomegaly with pericardial effusion was suspected based on the imaging. On blood examination, some abnormalities were found, including decreased hemoglobin (Hb) and platelet count at 7.9 g/dL and 63,000/dL, respectively, as well as elevated aspartate aminotransferase (AST) (184 units/L) and alanine aminotransferase (ALT) (245 units/L) level. The peripheral blood smear revealed pancytopenia, microcytic hypochromic anemia was observed, and the SARS-CoV-2 infection test was negative.

Based on the history, clinical results, and examinations conducted, the patient was initially diagnosed with community-acquired pneumonia (CAP), pancytopenia, hypertension, and obesity. Several initial medications were planned using levofloxacin, N-acetylcysteine, and bisoprolol. The diet regimens were adjusted according to the obese condition, and a nasogastric tube (NGT) was inserted to support enteral nutrition, with the patient hospitalized.

The following week, productive coughs and fevers were still observed, with fluctuations in body temperature. Paracetamol was given to manage the fever but shortness of breath remained fluctuating. Subsequently, two bags of packed red cells (PRC) were transfused to increase the Hb levels. Another SVT was reported on electrocardiography (ECG) and then adenosine was infused. The patient's phlegm was sampled and cultured, showing the presence of *Enterococcus faecalis*. Based on the bacteria sensitivity test result, levofloxacin was stopped and replaced by ampicillin-sulbactam. Echocardiography was performed to rule out infective endocarditis, but it showed aortic dilatation, mild tricuspid and pulmonary valve regurgitation, as well as mild pericardial effusion. Another blood examination was performed to monitor the treatment progress, with the results showing reduced ALT-AST level (61 and 224 units/L, respectively), and slightly increased Hb level (8,6 g/dL). The platelet count was relatively unchanged in number compared to initial hospital admission. The CD4 and CD8 count was assessed, with both showing a decrease in number, while IgA and IgG serum levels were within normal limits.

Two weeks after admission, signs of clinical improvements were observed although with fluctuating fevers and productive coughs. The patient was able to lift the body and tried to stand up individually. Chest physiotherapy was subsequently initiated to improve expansion, endurance, mobility, and deep breathing. Abdominal CT-scan imaging was obtained to evaluate the bulging abdomen and the results showed hepatosplenomegaly, mediastinal lymphadenopathy, and thyroid nodule. Furthermore, laboratory tests were conducted, showing hypoalbuminemia (1.85 g/dL) and reduced Hb level (7.8 g/dL) despite the PRC transfusions performed the previous week. Quantitative cytomegalovirus (CMV) polymerase chain reaction (PCR) result was negative, but the anti-CMV IgG was positive. Serum lactate dehydrogenase (LDH) was elevated (440 units/L) and protein electrophoresis results showed reversed albumin:globulin ratio, elevation of α-1, β-2, and γ-globulin serum level. Immunofixation and immunophenotyping were subsequently ordered to further clarify whether there was any presence of monoclonality and/or dominance of certain markers. Sputum acid-fast bacilli (AFB) and rapid molecular sputum test were negative, while interferon-gamma release assay (IGRA) test was indeterminate. A throat swab culture was performed, showing the presence of *Streptococcus α-hemolyticus* and *Staphylococcus saprophyticus*.

In the third week, the coughs and fevers were still observed, accompanied by shortness of breath. Another SVT event was recorded and adenosine failed to reverse the tachycardia, necessitating amiodarone infusion. Consciousness was starting to fluctuate with the patient sometimes unable to comprehend an instruction, giving irrelevant responses. The blood pressure dropped below 100 mmHg (systole) despite the discontinuation of bisoprolol. Subsequently, epinephrine was infused to maintain the blood's mean arterial pressure (MAP). Four PRC bags and one thrombocyte concentrate (TC) were transfused to raise the Hb and platelet levels. BMP was performed to examine the cytomorphology and existence of infectious microorganisms. The results showed the presence of a yeast element, *Histoplasma capsulatum* as presented in Fig. 13.1. Culture for *M. avium* complex (MAC) was ordered and cardiomegaly was observed on chest X-ray imaging, with no sign of pneumonia. Blood T4 and thyroid-stimulating hormone (TSH) levels were normal, while the

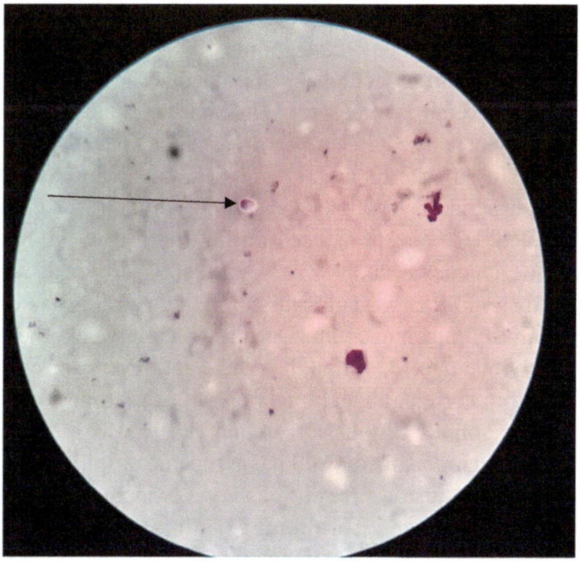

Fig. 13.1 The yeast element found in the patient's bone marrow puncture (BMP) specimen (arrow). The specimen was visualized using Wright-Giemsa staining. (Magnification: 1000x). (Image Courtesy: Robiatul Adawiyah MD DM PhD)

presence of human immunodeficiency virus (HIV), as well as hepatitis B and C virus, were negative. Galactomannan serum level was within normal limits, the ALT-AST level fluctuated, and bilirubin increased (2.81 mg/dL). Urea and Estimated Glomerular Filtration Rate (eGFR) values were within normal range, while disseminated histoplasmosis was diagnosed based on the BMP results. Ursodeoxycholic acid was given to restore the liver profile, and itraconazole was administered to manage the disseminated histoplasmosis. Additionally, albumin 20% was infused to normalize the blood albumin level.

Four weeks after admission, epinephrine was stopped and the patient suffered tachycardia. The blood pressure remained relatively low (90–110/55–60 mmHg), phlegmatic coughs and fevers were still observed, then the sputum was sampled and sent to the laboratory. Shortness of breath and chest pain occurred, along with fluctuations in consciousness. Incomprehensible words were sometimes heard, and the patient appeared agitated or irritated. SVT occurred twice during the week, leading to the administration of bisoprolol, with carotid massage. A decubitus wound was found at the sacrum region and treated using Vaseline with olive oil. Furthermore, erythematous plaques and patches were found at the perianal and groin area, along with fungal elements, namely, blastospores, and pseudohyphae. Miconazole and fusidic acid cream were applied to eradicate the fungal infection.

The Hb and thrombocyte levels remained unchanged despite several PRC and TC transfusions. ALT, AST, and bilirubin increased compared to the previous week's level, at 86, 284 units/L, and 2.91 mg/dL, respectively. Urinalysis examination showed the presence of urobilinogen in significant amounts (66 μmol/L; normal: <16 μmol/L), low albumin level (2.40 g/dL), and increased blood lactic acid (4.7 mmol/L; normal: <2.5 mmol/L). Furthermore, the sputum culture showed the presence of *Staphylococcus epidermidis* and *Klebsiella pneumoniae*. Immunofixation and immunophenotyping procedure showed no sign of monoclonal gammopathies and there was no dominant marker. Based on the overall laboratory results and the clinical impressions, it was postulated that the patient had acquired sepsis due to disseminated histoplasmosis. Two PRC bags were transfused, and the itraconazole dose was reduced in response to the ALT-AST increase. In addition, levofloxacin was infused and meropenem was initiated.

Multiple PRC and TC were transfused during the fifth week or final week of hospitalization. The leucocyte count was significantly dropped to below critical value (510 cells/μL), and then granulocyte colony-stimulating factor (GCSF) was infused in an attempt to raise the count. During the early week, the clinical conditions were relatively unchanged, although coughs and fevers were still fluctuating. Vital signs were within normal range, blood pressure was around 120/80 mmHg but respiration was still supported by nasal cannula. There was no incidence of SVT event and blood examination still showed pancytopenia despite numerous PRC and TC, as well as GCSF transfusion. Urea level started to increase to 211.9 mg/dL and the eGFR value was lowered to 29.5 mL/min/1.73m^2. Reticulocyte count was significantly decreased (9700 cells/μL) and the presence of *Acinetobacter* bacteria was detected in the blood. A repeat chest X-ray imaging showed heterogeneous opacities on the right lung field, hence, tigecycline and imipenem were initiated.

During the last days of the week, consciousness started to dwindle and the Glasgow comma scale (GCS) was lowered. High fever was also observed, SVT event only occurred once, while hemodynamic was unstable and blood pressure decreased to below 50 mmHg despite administration of intravenous epinephrine, norepinephrine, dobutamine, and vasopressin. The patient was then intubated and the bilirubin level was further increased (3.79 mg/dL). Another chest X-ray imaging depicted increased opacities on the right lung field compared to the last obtained imaging, with signs of right lung pleural effusion. The patient finally had cardiac arrest at the end of the day and failed to be resuscitated, leading to death.

13.2 What Is the Patient's Problem Focus?

A 61-year-old male was admitted to the hospital with shortness of breath that had persisted for a week. Seven months before, the patient started to experience intermittent fever, leading to hospitalization several times due to severe chills and thrombocytopenia, as well as previous history of COVID-19. Physical examination showed signs of obesity and hypertension, while wet crackles were heard in the lungs. Furthermore, edema was observed at both feet and the initial thoracic CT-scan imaging indicated residual signs of pneumonia on the left lung and mild cardiomegaly with pericardial effusion. On blood examination, decreased hemoglobin and platelet count, as well as increased serum ALT-AST were found. The peripheral blood smear showed pancytopenia with microcytic hypochromic anemia, while the SARS-CoV-2 infection test was negative.

During the whole hospitalization weeks, the patient suffered supraventricular tachycardia (SVT) several times. Fevers were recorded despite the antipyretics given and coughs remained unchanged. Abdominal CT-scan imaging showed hepatosplenomegaly, mediastinal lymphadenopathy, and thyroid nodule. The bone marrow puncture (BMP) specimen discovered the yeast element of *H. capsulatum,* which established the diagnosis of disseminated histoplasmosis leading to the initiation of itraconazole to treat the infection. Despite numerous packed red cells (PRC) and thrombocyte concentrate (TC) transfusions, the Hb and platelet counts were not raised. Hypoalbuminemia also persisted despite repeated albumin infusions and the liver function was compromised, as shown by the eventual rise of the serum ALT-AST and bilirubin.

On the last week of the hospitalization period, the clinical conditions deteriorated. The consciousness and hemodynamics were unstable, while the leucocyte count dropped significantly to below critical level and the kidney function started to worsen. Increased opacities and effusions on the lung fields were observed on serial chest X-ray imaging. The patient eventually had a cardiac arrest and resuscitation attempts failed, leading to death.

13.3 Discussion

Histoplasmosis, a prevalent fungal infection worldwide, is caused by the dimorphic environmental fungus *H. capsulatum*. The acquisition of the fungus by mammals can either be asymptomatic or lead to a potentially fatal systemic disease. This may occur in hosts with normal or weakened immune systems, although severe disease is more common in those with reduced cellular immunity. *H. capsulatum* yeast cells possess a high level of adaptation to the mammalian host, enabling survival within internal niches of specific phagocytic cells. Frequently, the infections do not show symptoms, but a granulomatous inflammation leads to a lung condition that closely resembles pulmonary tuberculosis. Immunocompromised individuals are at risk of developing disseminated histoplasmosis, which may result in significant morbidity and mortality [1, 2].

13.4 Etiology

Histoplasma capsulatum is a member of the *Ascomycetes* family and exhibits two distinct mating types, designated (+) and (−), based on phenotypic traits. While these mating types are usually present in equal proportions in nature, clinical isolates predominantly belong to the (−) mating type. The underlying reason for this observed predominance in patient specimens remains unclear. Microscopic examination of the mycelial phase reveals two forms of conidia: macroconidia and microconidia. Macroconidia are larger, measuring 8–15 μm in diameter, whereas microconidia are smaller, ranging from 2–5 μm. Microconidia are considered the primary infectious particles, with their small size enabling deep deposition in the alveoli following inhalation [2, 3].

13.5 Epidemiology

Histoplasmosis is the most common endemic fungal infection in the United States, though it is not classified as a reportable disease. Its geographical distribution in the U.S. is predominantly limited to the Midwest and Southeastern regions. Globally, endemic areas are present on every continent. In Europe, cases have been documented in Italy, while significant regions of endemicity exist across North, Central, and South America. In Africa, histoplasmosis has been reported in countries such as Congo, Zimbabwe, and South Africa. In Asia, it is found in regions including India, China, Malaysia, and Taiwan, and it is also present in Australia. It is estimated that over 50% of the global population may reside in areas where *Histoplasma capsulatum* is endemic [2].

13.6 Clinical Symptom

13.6.1 Acute Pulmonary Histoplasmosis

Some patients may remain asymptomatic while exhibiting granulomatous changes on chest X-rays. The lungs serve as the primary entry point for infectious particles or conidia. Granulomas form as a tissue response to the fungal invasion, which can be either caseating or noncaseating, often with calcium deposition. These granulomas function to encapsulate fungal growth, and in self-limited cases, they are characterized by organized granulomatous inflammation. However, the absence of a well-coordinated inflammatory response indicates a compromised cellular immune system, increasing the risk of developing progressive disseminated histoplasmosis (PDH) [2]. Individuals who come into contact with highly infectious strains or those having a compromised immune system may acquire symptomatic disease, either with or without the spread to other parts of the body. Within a period of 7–21 days after inhaling microconidia, individuals may develop flu-like symptoms such as fever, general discomfort, headache, weakness, dry cough, and chest pain. The majority of patients experience fast improvement within 30 days, while a few may have lingering problems for several months. The diagnosis of acute pulmonary histoplasmosis is frequently delayed due to frequent misidentification of other diseases, particularly bacteria community-acquired pneumonia (CAP). A recent study indicated that there was an average delay of 39.5 days before the correct diagnosis of pulmonary histoplasmosis was made [4].

13.6.2 Chronic Pulmonary Histoplasmosis

Chronic pulmonary histoplasmosis can present as either cavitary or noncavitary disease. Early observations from outbreaks in Indianapolis revealed that approximately half of the women diagnosed with chronic pulmonary histoplasmosis exhibited cavitary disease, whereas only 20% had coexisting chronic obstructive pulmonary disease (COPD). Overall, about 40% of patients with chronic pulmonary histoplasmosis developed cavitations, a finding strongly linked to underlying immunosuppression and COPD. Smoking is also a significant risk factor, likely due to its association with chronic pulmonary conditions. This disease rarely occurs in individuals without pre-existing chronic lung conditions.

The clinical presentation of chronic pulmonary histoplasmosis closely resembles that of pulmonary tuberculosis (TB), with symptoms including cough, weight loss, loss of appetite, increased sputum production, fever, chills, night sweats, and hemoptysis. These symptoms are typically mild but persistent, warranting careful differentiation from other chronic pulmonary infections [2, 4].

13.6.3 Progressive Disseminated Histoplasmosis

Progressive disseminated histoplasmosis (PDH) refers to a medical condition that does not show improvement after a minimum 3-week observation period. This condition is characterized by physical or radiographic abnormalities and/or laboratory evidence indicating the role of tissues outside the lungs. Immunocompromised individuals have a significantly greater risk, approximately ten times higher, of acquiring PDH compared to those with a normal immune system [4].

Typically, symptoms are nonspecific and may include fever, exhaustion, and weight loss. Pulmonary symptoms, although not always dominant, can manifest as a dry cough and dyspnea, while imaging may show widespread reticulonodular infiltrates of a miliary-type nature. Patients may have enlarged liver and spleen, swollen lymph nodes outside the lungs, lesions in the central nervous system, and skin abnormalities. Furthermore, gastrointestinal role is frequently observed and may resemble a cytomegalovirus (CMV) infection. Symptoms may include diarrhea, thickening of the mucosal lining, and the formation of ulcers. Laboratory analysis often shows cytopenia, elevated hepatic enzymes, and increased lactate dehydrogenase (LDH) levels. Pseudohypoparathyroidism (PDH) also manifests as a significant disturbance in electrolyte levels, potentially caused by the adrenal glands being affected. It is an uncommon factor leading to hypercalcemia mediated by 1,25-dihydroxy vitamin D. Certain individuals may experience the development of hemophagocytic lymphocytosis syndrome, macrophage activation syndrome, septic shock, or acute hypoxemic respiratory failure, underscoring the need for therapy [4].

13.7 Diagnosis

13.7.1 Serological Test

The detection of antibodies specific to *H. capsulatum* can assist in diagnosing some histoplasmosis syndromes where the presence of antigen may not be positive, such as mediastinal granuloma and fibrosis. Additionally, it can enhance sensitivity when used in combination with antigen detection [1]. Significant drawbacks include the duration of antibody generation after an infection (4–8 weeks) and the incapacity of specific immunocompromised individuals to generate a noticeable humoral response. The three predominant antibody testing methods are complement fixation (CF), immunodiffusion (ID), and enzyme immunoassay (EIA) [4].

The majority of individuals with histoplasmosis show a CF titer of 1:8 or above, with titers of >1:32 or higher indicating a higher possibility of current infections. Furthermore, the presence of an acute infection can be determined by a significant increase in antibody titers, with a minimum fourfold rise, when measured at least 2 weeks apart. The ID test identifies antibodies specific to the antigens H and M. The H band shows limited sensitivity, as it is discovered in only 20% of patients. However, the discovery serves as a confirmation of acute infection. The M band is detectable in around 80% of patients with histoplasmosis, although it is not a good indicator for detecting current or past infection [4]. EIA-based antibody testing, which detects both IgG and IgM, provides greater sensitivity compared to the ID and CF methods in diagnosing acute pulmonary histoplasmosis in patients [4].

13.7.2 Antigen Culture

An extensive multicenter study assessed the efficacy of antigen detection in individuals diagnosed with histoplasmosis. Immunocompromised patients, specifically those with advanced HIV, had a greater sensitivity to antigen testing compared to immunocompetent recipients. Moreover, the test results showed significant variation based on the extent of the disease [4].

Antigen testing can be conducted using various bodily fluids and during an examination of pulmonary histoplasmosis, the presence of antigen was identified in 93% of bronchoalveolar lavage (BAL) samples, but only discovered in 79% of urine and 65% of serum samples. In addition, the sensitivity of combining BAL antigen and cytopathology was 97%. CSF testing yielded positive results in 78% of patients diagnosed with CNS histoplasmosis, demonstrating a specificity of 97%. The incorporation of the CSF immunoglobulin G anti-histoplasma antibody detection test led to a detection rate of 98% for the patients. Moreover, the use of quantitative analysis of antigen levels is beneficial for tracking the effectiveness of treatment, as well as evaluating the outlook and recurrence of the condition [4]. There is 100% cross-reactivity between Histoplasmosis and Blastomycosis as both contain the same galactomannan [4].

13.7.3 Culture

The gold standard for diagnosing histoplasmosis is the isolation of *H. capsulatum* from clinical specimens. However, histopathologic or direct microscopic identification is also considered a reliable diagnostic method [3].

Clinical samples, when delivered to the laboratory for culture, are placed on a nutrient-deficient medium such as Sabouraud agar and kept in an incubator at a temperature ranging from 25 to 30 °C. The mycelial growth typically manifests during a period of 2–3 weeks, although it can occasionally extend up to 8 weeks. The lactophenol cotton blue test is used to examine the mycelia's maturity level and detect septated hyphae, microconidia, or macroconidia under a microscope. The presence of tuberculate projections on the surface, resembling a ship's wheel, strongly indicates the presence of *H. capsulatum*. However, similar projections may be observed on fungi belonging to the genus *Sepedonium* [3].

13.8 Management

The Infectious Disease Society of America (IDSA) has issued guidelines for the management of histoplasmosis. Treatment is unnecessary for acute lung infections that show symptoms lasting less than 4 weeks. However, when symptoms continue beyond this duration, a 3-month regimen of itraconazole is recommended. Patients diagnosed with chronic pulmonary histoplasmosis (CPH) and noncavitary disease are adequately treated with a 6-month therapy, while those with cavitary disease may require treatment for a duration of 1 year. Progressive disseminated histoplasmosis (PDH) patients typically require initial treatment using amphotericin-B for a duration of 2–4 weeks, followed by a year-long course of itraconazole. Empirical data demonstrate that liposomal amphotericin B yields superior results compared to alternative formulations of amphotericin B. At present, the IDSA has not endorsed any other antifungal medication. However, there have been accounts of patients receiving posaconazole in place of itraconazole during the maintenance phase and as a replacement for amphotericin B during the inductive phase [2].

13.9 Prognosis

Acute pulmonary histoplasmosis is often a non-malignant disease, although the number of examples covered in this compilation is limited and clinically severe, significant improvement in health was achieved after receiving treatment. Chronic pulmonary histoplasmosis is distinguished by the presence of cavities in the upper lobes of the lungs. The disease often advances slowly over a span of several years, with occasional periods of improvement and worsening. When the patients are not treated, the prognosis is unfavorable. Progressive disseminated histoplasmosis (PDH) carries a bleak prognosis, leading to death within a year, although there are rare instances where a patient manages to survive [5].

Key Points
In patients with prolonged fever, disseminated fungal infection should be suspected and diagnosis can be made through bone marrow puncture (BMP).

Questions

1. The following are true about histoplasmosis, except:
   (a) The acquisition of the fungus by mammals can either go unnoticed clinically or result in a potentially fatal systemic disease
   (b) *Histoplasma capsulatum* infection can occur in hosts with weakened immune systems
   (c) The infections do not show symptoms, but a granulomatous inflammation leads to a lung condition that closely resembles pulmonary tuberculosis
   (d) *Histoplasma capsulatum* yeast cells possess a high level of adaptation to the mammalian host, enabling them to successfully survive within specific phagocytic cells' internal niches
   (e) Immunocompromised individuals are at risk of developing disseminated histoplasmosis
2. In *Histoplasma capsulatum* infection, microconidia are considered to be infectious particles trapped in:
   (a) Bronchus
   (b) Bronchiole
   (c) Alveoli
   (d) Mucosal lining
   (e) Mucosa gland

3. Below are clinical manifestations of Progressive Disseminated Histoplasmosis, except:
   (a) Lesions in the central nervous system
   (b) Dry cough
   (c) Enlarged liver
   (d) Swollen lymph nodes
   (e) Chest and neck pain
4. How long is the management of histoplasmosis with cavitary disease?
   (a) One year
   (b) Six months
   (c) One month
   (d) Three months
   (e) Two years
5. What is the gold standard for diagnosing histoplasmosis?
   (a) CT-Thorax
   (b) Antigen Culture
   (c) Culture
   (d) Serological test
   (e) Enzyme immunoassay (EIA)

Answer keys
1. B
2. C
3. E
4. A
5. C

Acknowledgments Cipta Mahendra MD, Department of Internal Medicine, Respirology and Critical Illness Division, Universitas Indonesia, Dr. Cipto Mangunkusumo General Central National Hospital, Jakarta, Indonesia.

Ersananda Arlisa Putri MD, Department of Internal Medicine, Respirology and Critical Illness Division, Universitas Indonesia, Dr. Cipto Mangunkusumo General Central National Hospital, Jakarta, Indonesia.

Robiatul Adawiyah MD DM PhD, Department of Parasitology Clinic, Universitas Indonesia, Dr. Cipto Mangunkusumo General Central National Hospital, Jakarta, Indonesia.

Nadia Ayu Mulansari MD DM, Department of Internal Medicine, Medical Hematology and Oncology Division, Universitas Indonesia, Dr. Cipto Mangunkusumo General Central National Hospital, Jakarta, Indonesia.

Adityo Susilo MD DM PhD, Department of Internal Medicine, Tropical Infectious Diseases Division, Universitas Indonesia, Dr. Cipto Mangunkusumo General Central National Hospital, Jakarta, Indonesia.

References

1. Mittal J, Ponce MG, Gendlina I, Nosanchuk JD. Histoplasma capsulatum: mechanisms for pathogenesis. Curr Top Microbiol Immunol. 2019;422:157–91.
2. Akram SM, Koirala J. Histoplasmosis. StatPearls Publication; 2023. https://www.ncbi.nlm.nih.gov/books/NBK448185/
3. Barros N, Wheat JL, Hage C. Pulmonary histoplasmosis: a clinical update. J Fungi. 2023;9(2):236. https://doi.org/10.3390/jof9020236.
4. Bubnick M, Smulian AG. The MAT1 locus of Histoplasma capsulatum is responsive in a mating type-specific manner. Eukaryot Cell. 2007;6:616–21.
5. Rubin H, Furcolow ML, Yates JL, Brasher CA. The course and prognosis of histoplasmosis. Am J Med. 1959;27:278–88.

14 Complicated Lung *Mycobacterium abscessus* Infection

14.1 Case Illustration

A 37-year-old female was brought to the hospital with shortness of breath accompanied by phlegmatic coughs, itchy throat, and fever. The shortness of breath was fluctuating but it was not worsened by certain activities or positions. The fever had persisted for 2 months and was undulating with no certain pattern. In addition, slight pain was experienced in both knees and ankles.

About 6 years ago, the patient had similar symptoms and was diagnosed with tuberculosis (TB), leading to the administration of anti-TB drugs including rifampicin, isoniazid, ethambutol, and streptomycin but generalized rashes and itchiness occurred. The TB treatment was continued using pyrazinamide and moxifloxacin for 2 years. The patient was finally declared TB-free after the therapy completion.

One year before the current hospital admission, the same symptoms reoccurred and chest X-ray imaging depicted signs of TB but no sputum test was ordered. The patient was diagnosed with relapsed TB based on the radiological results, then pyrazinamide, co-amoxiclav, and moxifloxacin were administered. However, the regimen was stopped after 6 months as there were no significant clinical improvements, leading to the suspicion of Non-tuberculous mycobacteria (NTM) infection.

The following month, a sputum test confirmed the presence of NTM complex. Administration of rifampicin, isoniazid, and levofloxacin was attempted but discontinued shortly after because the patient reported vomitus and skin rashes on the whole body after consuming the drugs. A sputum PCR test conducted several weeks after showed the presence of *M. abscessus*. One month later, rifampicin and isoniazid were re-administered and there was no sign of allergies. The treatment was then continued for about 3 months until the hospital admission.

The patient contracted COVID-19 a year ago before admission and hyper-IgE 10 years ago, along with frequent itchy skin rashes, joint pain, and fevers. Treatment was performed with methylprednisolone and mycophenolate sodium but

G. Singh, *Challenging Cases in Respirology and Critical Care*,
https://doi.org/10.1007/978-981-96-5002-6_14

dexamethasone was also consumed without being prescribed. Five years ago, esophagogastroduodenoscopy (EGD) examination was carried out due to erosive pangastritis and hernia hiatal. In addition, colonoscopy was performed the same year due to suspected colitis.

History of hypertension, diabetes mellitus, heart, lung, and liver diseases were denied. There was no recognized food allergy and no similar histories were found in the family. In addition, history of cancer was denied by both the patient and the family. Smoking, drinking, and HIV infection were also denied. The patient was a married private-sector employee and had reported decreased body weight in the last 6 months.

On physical examination, the patient appeared fully conscious, with the Body Mass Index (BMI) and vital signs remaining within normal limits. The blood oxygen saturation (SpO_2) was 99% in room air, body organs were observed normal except for the lungs, and wet crackles were heard on both lung fields. A chest X-ray (Fig. 14.1) examination was performed, showing nodular opacities throughout the lung fields and a cavitary lesion with air crescent sign on the upper left side.

Further examination with a thoracic CT-scan using contrast (Fig. 14.2) suggested TB lung with possible fungal coinfection.

Laboratory investigations showed decreased hemoglobin (11 g/dL) and increased leucocytes (11.69 cells/μL). An NTM secondary infection diagnosis was performed, then rifampicin and isoniazid regimen was prescribed along with ceftriaxone and azithromycin. The patient was hospitalized to monitor the clinical progress.

During the first days, greenish sputum was produced when coughing and the fever was fluctuating. There was no bloody sputum found and laboratory

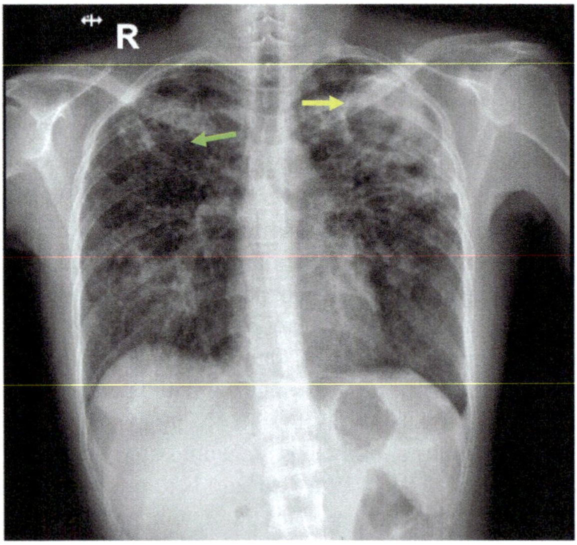

Fig. 14.1 Chest X-ray showed nodular opacities (green arrow) and a cavitary lesion with air crescent sign (yellow arrow). (Image Courtesy: Mohammad Yanuar Amal MD)

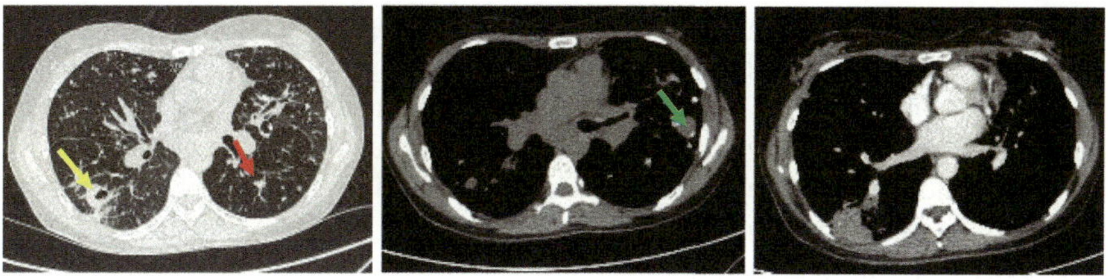

Fig. 14.2 CT-scan using contrast showed thickening cavity with calcified consolidation (yellow arrow), tree in bud opacity as well as multiple irregular (red arrow), and partially calcified nodules scattered in almost all segments (green arrow). (Image Courtesy: Vally Wulani MD)

examination reported the presence of acid-fast bacilli in moderate amounts (1–10 cells/field of view [FOV]). Leucocytes were present in large amounts (>50 cells/FOV) along with a small amount of Gram (+) cocci and *Candida* fungus. Blood laboratory investigation showed normalized leucocyte count but decreased lymphocyte proportion (9.2%; normal: 20–40). Methylprednisolone and paracetamol were added to the medicamentosa regimen. After several days, phlegmatic coughs were still produced but the greenish color subsided. Shortness of breath and fever decreased in occurrence and intensity, while the blood IgE level increased significantly (664.3 IU/mL; normal: <100). The patient was discharged from the hospital after 1 week to continue the treatment as an outpatient.

The following month, the patient was brought again to the hospital with shortness of breath. Physical examination showed normal results except for the lungs, while wet crackles were also heard. Vital signs were normal, with the SpO_2 reaching 99% on free air, but the BMI value reduced (17.5 kg/m^2; normal: 18.5–22.9). Laboratory investigation showed increased total bilirubin and Antimicrobial Susceptibility Testing (AST, 1.79 mg/dL and 203 U/L, respectively), slightly decreased albumin (3.10 g/dL), and elevated D-dimer (21,520 μg/L; normal: <440), while peripheral blood smear indicated eosinophilia. In addition to NTM infection, the patient was additionally diagnosed with community-acquired pneumonia (CAP). Based on previous history of hyper-immunoglobulin E, Churg-Strauss syndrome was also suspected. Several medications were recommended including rifampicin-isoniazid (continued), azithromycin, ethambutol, and streptomycin/amikacin. Heparin was also administered in response to the elevated blood D-dimer value. In addition, vitamin B complex was given and the patient was re-hospitalized.

During the first week, the patient appeared lethargic and had an undulating fever. The coughs were often accompanied by greenish sputum but no abnormalities were found in the urination and defecation process. Drug provocation testing was conducted for ethambutol due to the history of drug allergy. Rifampicin and isoniazid were postponed to normalize the AST and bilirubin values, while the sputum was taken and sent to the laboratory. The presence of *Acinetobacter* and *Streptococcus viridans* was positive in the sampled sputum. An antibiotic sensitivity test conducted on the sputum suggested amikacin and levofloxacin as effective drugs to eradicate the infective NTM. Due to a previous history of suspected allergy to levofloxacin, the patient was subjected to a desensitization period to determine suitability.

Abdominal Ultrasound Sonography (USG) was also performed and the imaging results indicated signs of chronic liver disease (Fig. 14.3).

In the second week, the patient showed no allergic reaction to levofloxacin. The medicamentosa regimen was subsequently finalized, leading to the prescription of five antibiotics, namely, levofloxacin, azithromycin, doxycycline, rifampicin, and isoniazid. Amikacin and imipenem were not selected because *Acinetobacter* was reportedly resistant to both antibiotics. The hemoglobin and leucocyte counts were relatively unchanged compared to the first hospital admission, while mild anemia and slight leukocytosis remained persistent. The clinical conditions were slightly improved, fever decreased in frequency, but productive coughs were still experienced. A blood serology test for the presence of aspergillosis was ordered and the result was positive.

In the third week, the patient felt nauseated after receiving the antibiotics, and an antinausea drug was administered to alleviate the symptoms. Voriconazole was administered to treat the aspergillosis, while levofloxacin was switched to moxifloxacin to better eradicate *M. abscessus*. Lung auscultation indicated decreased wet crackles sound compared to initial admission. The total bilirubin level returned to normal, but the AST level was still above the normal range (120 U/L). The clinical conditions were relatively unchanged compared to the previous week and the feeling of nausea was attenuated.

The clinical progress improved in the fourth week, as the cough turned dry and little sputum was produced throughout the week. However, the bilirubin and AST-ALT levels were increased to 2.51 mg/dL and 138–95 U/L, respectively, leading to the postponement of rifampicin and isoniazid regimens. The ECG recording showed normal results and the patient was tested for the presence of anti-neutrophil cytoplasmic antibody (ANCA), with the result being negative. Methylprednisolone intake frequency was reduced to once weekly and the patient was finally discharged to continue the treatment as an outpatient. Sachets of probiotic-prebiotic supplementation consisting of *L. acidophilus, B. longum, S. thermophilus*, B complex vitamins, dextrose, and zinc oxide were additionally given as take-home prescriptions.

The patient returned to the hospital the next month with the same complaint, including shortness of breath, productive cough, and hoarseness. Wet crackles were heard on both lung fields and a repeat chest X-ray imaging (Fig. 14.4) showed

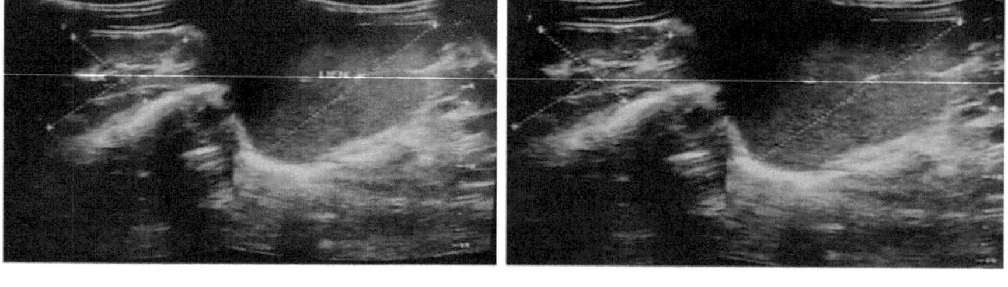

Fig. 14.3 Abdominal USG showed signs of chronic liver disease. (Image Courtesy: Mohammad Reynalzi Yugo MD)

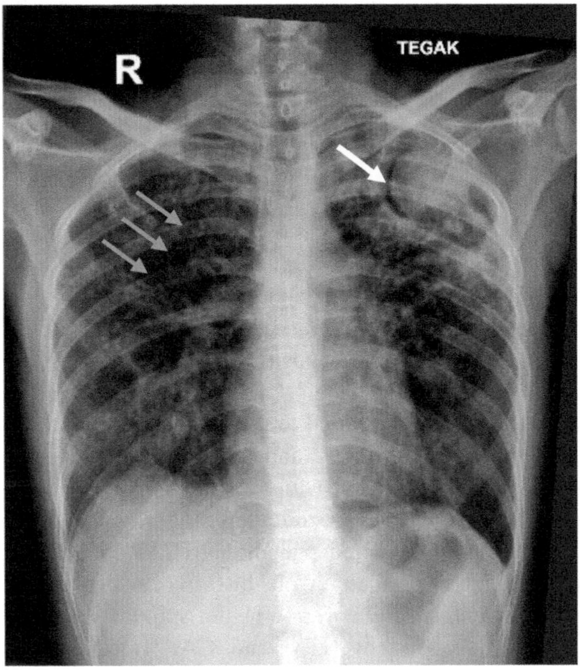

Fig. 14.4 Chest X-ray showed nodular opacities (brown arrow) throughout the lung fields and a cavitary lesion (white arrow) on the upper left lung field, generally showing the same results compared to the last imaging. (Image Courtesy: Rahmad Mulyadi MD PhD)

relatively the same results compared to the last imaging on previous hospital admission. Additionally, signs of fibrosis were found on the upper lung fields.

Laboratory examination showed marked eosinophilia, reaching approximately 12.8% (normal: 1–6%). In addition to continuing the last medicamentosa regimen, salbutamol-budesonide nebulization was recommended to alleviate the shortness of breath symptom. Oxygen supplementation was also given and the patient was hospitalized.

A repeat electrocardiogram (EKG) recording was obtained showing the presence of T-wave inversion on lead aVR and V1. The vital signs were indicative of early shock (BP: 80/50 mmHg; HR: 80 x/min; RR: 28 x/min), then the patient was infused with 0.9% normal saline and gelatin to expand the intravascular volume. Blood examination showed hyper-IgE (1454 IU/mL; normal: <100) and urinalysis indicated the presence of erythrocytes and hemoglobin in high concentration. The sputum examination discovered the existence of *Pseudomonas aeruginosa* and *Klebsiella oxytoca* in the sampled sputum. Cefoperazone-sulbactam was administered in response to the results, while Chest physiotherapy and breathing exercises were implemented to improve breathing. The clinical conditions improved after, with breathing normalized, hoarseness subsided, and the patient was subsequently discharged from the hospital. Any specific drug intended to manage the hyper-IgE condition was not given during the whole hospital admissions and the patient was managed as an outpatient.

14.2 What Is the Patient's Problem Focus?

A 37-year-old female was brought to the hospital with shortness of breath, phlegmatic cough, and fever, as well as slight pain in both knees and ankles. Diagnosis indicated non-tuberculous mycobacterium (NTM) infection after a thorough history-taking, as well as physical and laboratory examination. Previous histories included TB infections, COVID-19, and hyper-IgE alongside decreased body weight, as well as a history of esophagogastroduodenoscopy (EGD) and colonoscopy examination.

The patient was repeatedly admitted to the hospital, during the first admission, rifampicin, isoniazid, ceftriaxone, and azithromycin were administered. Methylprednisolone was also given, while coinfection with Gram (+) cocci and *Candida* fungus occurred. On the second admission, the patient was additionally diagnosed with community-acquired pneumonia (CAP) and Churg-Strauss syndrome was suspected based on the previous history of hyper-IgE. The presence of *Acinetobacter* and *Streptococcus viridans* in the sputum was found, along with aspergillosis. Due to the current NTM and CAP infection, coinfection with *Acinetobacter* and *Streptococcus viridans*, as well as the aspergillosis condition, the given medications were adjusted to include moxifloxacin, azithromycin, doxycycline, rifampicin, isoniazid, and voriconazole. Furthermore, elevation of AST-ALT level warranted the dosage adjustment of the administered rifampicin and isoniazid. Prebiotic-probiotic supplementation was given as a take-home prescription on hospital discharge.

On the third admission, the lungs appeared worsened with signs of fibrotic lesions on the upper lung fields. The presence of T-wave inversion on lead aVR and V1 during an EKG examination was also observed, while the urine contained erythrocytes and hemoglobin in high concentration. Cefoperazone-sulbactam was given after the discovery of *Pseudomonas aeruginosa* and *Klebsiella oxytoca* in the sputum. The patient was finally discharged after a week of hospitalization.

14.3 Discussion

Non-tuberculous mycobacteria (NTM) are a group of microorganisms distinct from *Mycobacterium tuberculosis* (Mtb) and its closely related species, such as *M. africanum*, *M. bovis*, *M. canetti*, *M. caprae*, *M. pinnipedii*, and *M. leprae*. Commonly referred to as environmental, atypical, or anonymous mycobacteria, NTM are ubiquitous in nature and have been isolated from various sources, including air, soil, dust, plants, natural and treated water, biofilms, wild animals, milk, and food products. Structurally, NTM have a thin peptidoglycan layer surrounded by a thick lipid-rich outer coat, which enhances their ability to adhere to rough surfaces and resist antibiotics and disinfectants. This adaptation enables their survival in harsh environments with limited oxygen and carbon availability. In regions with a high burden of tuberculosis (TB), NTM diagnoses are rare, largely due to limited awareness among healthcare providers and insufficient access to advanced diagnostic tools, such as mycobacterial culture and molecular techniques for species identification [3].

Hyper Immunoglobulin E Syndrome: A Unique Predisposition to Infections and NTM. Hyper Immunoglobulin E Syndrome (HIES), or Job's syndrome, is characterized by an increased susceptibility to infections, largely due to the development of bronchiectasis. This structural lung abnormality impairs airway clearance, creating a predisposition to recurrent respiratory infections. Nontuberculous mycobacteria (NTM) are frequently identified in patients with compromised airway clearance, such as those with cystic fibrosis (CF), primary ciliary dyskinesia (PCD), or in asthenic postmenopausal women with scoliosis, pectus deformities, and mitral valve prolapse. [3].

In HIES, which is caused by autosomal dominant mutations in the signal transducer and activator of transcription 3 (STAT3) gene, patients often experience recurrent pyogenic respiratory infections, frequently accompanied by complications such as pneumatoceles and bronchiectasis. The predisposition to pulmonary NTM infections in HIES is primarily linked to airway dysfunction, with immune dysfunction playing a secondary, albeit important, role. The recurrent infections associated with immunological deficits exacerbate structural lung damage, further increasing susceptibility to NTM disease [3].

Given that respiratory tract infections remain a leading cause of mortality in HIES, regular screening for NTM infections is essential for timely diagnosis and management. Early identification and treatment of NTM can significantly mitigate the progression of structural lung disease and improve clinical outcomes in this vulnerable patient population [3].

14.4 Epidemiology

The burden of Non-Tuberculous Mycobacteria (NTM) disease refers to its prevalence, distribution, and the environmental presence of various NTM species. While there is no definitive evidence of person-to-person transmission, recent studies strongly suggest indirect transmission of *Mycobacterium abscessus* and *Mycobacterium massiliense* among cystic fibrosis (CF) patients. The lack of systematic reporting is primarily due to NTM's non-notifiable status in many countries, complicating accurate epidemiological tracking [2].

The incidence of NTM pulmonary disease (NTM-PD) increases with age and varies widely across nations. Over the past 40 years, multiple studies have documented a significant rise in NTM occurrences. In the United States, the prevalence of NTM-positive cultures is estimated between 1.4 and 6.6 cases per 100,000 individuals. Similarly, in the United Kingdom, the incidence rose from 4 per 100,000 individuals in 2007 to 6.1 per 100,000 in 2012. A Canadian study highlighted an increase in NTM-PD prevalence from 29.3 cases per 100,000 individuals between 1998 and 2002 to 41.3 cases per 100,000 individuals from 2006 to 2010 [2].

Several factors contribute to the rising incidence of NTM-PD:

- NTM Evolution: Genetic mutations have enhanced the virulence of NTM species.
- Environmental and Climatic Changes: Expanding human-made infrastructure has altered environments conducive to NTM growth.
- Vulnerable Populations: The growing number of immunocompromised individuals and patients with chronic lung conditions has increased susceptibility.
- Declining TB Burden: Reduced herd immunity associated with lower tuberculosis prevalence may indirectly contribute.
- Improved Diagnostics: Advances in CT imaging, laboratory infrastructure, and heightened awareness have led to increased detection rates.

These factors underscore the need for heightened surveillance, research, and reporting to better understand and address the evolving burden of NTM disease globally [2].

14.5 Diagnosis

14.5.1 Microbiologic Diagnosis of Non-Tuberculous Mycobacteria (NTM) Infections

Non-tuberculous mycobacteria (NTM) are ubiquitous in the environment, commonly found in soil and water, including municipal and residential water systems. Vigilance is crucial during sample collection to prevent environmental contamination of biological specimens, which could result in false-positive findings. Diagnostic specimens may be obtained from any tissue or organ suspected to harbor the infection [4].

For pulmonary NTM infections, the diagnostic criteria established by the American Thoracic Society (ATS) and the Infectious Disease Society of America (IDSA) include:

- Positive sputum cultures on two separate occasions, or.
- A single positive culture from a lower respiratory tract sample, such as bronchial lavage or washing.

When clinical suspicion is high but initial tests are inconclusive, additional sputum samples should be collected. For patients unable to produce sputum, induction or bronchoscopy may be necessary. While the optimal interval between sample collections remains uncertain, a minimum 1-week gap is suggested to minimize diagnostic confusion caused by transient environmental contamination. Though rarely required, lung biopsy may provide valuable histopathological evidence, such as granuloma formation, to support a diagnosis beyond positive cultures or stains.

In non-pulmonary NTM diseases, the diagnostic approach varies based on the site of infection:

- Lymphadenitis**:** Excisional biopsy or fine needle aspiration for microscopy and mycobacterial culture.
- Disseminated NTM Disease**:** Mycobacterial blood cultures are essential, with bone marrow or liver biopsy indicated in cases of cytopenia.
- Skin Infections: Deep tissue biopsies are more reliable than superficial swabs, which may only detect environmental exposure rather than active disease.

A thorough and systematic approach to microbiologic diagnosis is critical for confirming NTM infections and guiding effective management strategies [4].

14.6 Antimicrobial Susceptibility Testing

Antimicrobial Susceptibility Testing (AST) in Non-Tuberculous Mycobacteria (NTM). The Clinical and Laboratory Standards Institute (CLSI) and the American Thoracic Society (ATS)/Infectious Diseases Society of America (IDSA) have established guidelines for performing antimicrobial susceptibility testing (AST) in non-tuberculous mycobacteria (NTM). The definitive method for assessing antimicrobial sensitivity is **broth microdilution**. AST is typically reserved for isolates deemed clinically significant, as testing low-pathogenicity species such as *Mycobacterium gordonae*, *M. mucogenicum*, and *M. terrae* is not recommended by CLSI [4]

Key Considerations in AST for NTM

1. Clinical Correlation:
   - The relationship between in vitro susceptibility and clinical response is not universally established for all NTM species or antimycobacterial drugs.
   - Exceptions include specific correlations for *Mycobacterium avium* complex (MAC) and *Mycobacterium kansasii*.
2. AST for *M. avium* Complex (MAC):
   - Susceptibility testing is recommended only for clarithromycin and amikacin, as these are the only drugs where minimum inhibitory concentration (MIC) results correlate with clinical outcomes.
   - Testing for other drugs is not routinely necessary since clinical responses do not align with MIC results.
3. AST for *M. kansasii*:
   - Rifampin susceptibility testing is critical, as treatment failure is often linked to rifampin resistance.
   - MIC values for ethambutol (EMB) and isoniazid (INH) are not reliable indicators of clinical response.
   - When rifampin resistance is detected, testing for alternative drugs should be conducted to guide treatment decisions.

4. Rapidly Growing Mycobacteria:
   - For species like *M. abscessus*, AST is recommended across a broader range of antimicrobials.
   - The goal is to provide guidance for potential treatment options, as MIC thresholds for most drugs in these cases have not been established.

AST should be used judiciously to inform treatment decisions for NTM infections. The decision to perform susceptibility testing should be guided by clinical significance, species involved, and the availability of drugs with proven in vitro and in vivo efficacy [4].

14.7 Radiological Imaging

Radiological imaging is crucial in cases when there is suspicion of non-tuberculous mycobacteria (NTM) lung disease, characterized by diverse arrays of abnormalities including bronchiectasis, nodular lesions, cavitary lesions, and parenchymal consolidation. The appearance of the disease can be categorized into two main forms, namely, fibrocavitary and nodular bronchiectatic. The fibrocavitary variant bears resemblance to pulmonary TB and primarily affects older males with preexisting lung conditions. It is distinguished by the presence of cavities with regions of heightened opacity, typically found in the upper lobes. Frequent occurrences include pleural thickening and volume reduction due to fibrosis, accompanied by traction bronchiectasis. Cavitation is the predominant radiological characteristic observed in cases with pulmonary TB. In contrast, NTM lung disease typically leads to the formation of thin-walled cavities, frequently affecting the pleura without the presence of lymph node calcification or atelectasis. The disease also has a slower progression compared to pulmonary TB [5].

The nodular bronchiectatic type of non-tuberculous mycobacterial (NTM) lung disease is characterized by bilateral, multilobar bronchiectasis, most commonly affecting the middle and lower lung lobes. High-resolution computed tomography (HRCT) and chest radiography reveal hallmark features, including small nodules and bronchiectatic changes [5].

This condition is predominantly observed in older, non-smoking women without pre-existing lung diseases, particularly those with a slender body build. Emerging evidence suggests a bidirectional relationship between bronchiectasis and NTM infection:

- NTM infection may contribute to the development of bronchiectasis by causing chronic inflammation and structural lung damage.
- Conversely, bronchiectasis may precede NTM infection, creating a favorable environment for mycobacterial colonization and infection.

A recent meta-analysis reported that the prevalence of NTM infection among patients with bronchiectasis is approximately 9.3%, underscoring the importance of vigilance in these cases.

Due to the significant overlap in HRCT findings, differentiating between various NTM species based solely on radiological patterns remains challenging. Clinicians should maintain a high index of suspicion for NTM lung disease in patients with bronchiectasis and use microbiological confirmation to guide diagnosis and management [5].

14.8 Clinical Manifestation

Although pulmonary disease is the most common presentation, non-tuberculous mycobacteria (NTM) can also cause localized infections in the skin, bones, and soft tissues. In patients with significant immune suppression, disseminated infections may occur [4].

The clinical manifestations of NTM infections are diverse and often nonspecific. Pulmonary NTM disease typically presents with a persistent or recurrent cough, with or without sputum production. Constitutional symptoms such as fever, fatigue, weight loss, and night sweats may also occur, along with chest pain or shortness of breath, particularly in advanced stages of the disease. Diagnosing NTM infections can be especially challenging in patients with underlying lung conditions such as bronchiectasis or chronic obstructive pulmonary disease (COPD), as the symptoms overlap [4].

Infections involving the skin, soft tissues, and musculoskeletal system may present as skin nodules, ulcers, wound drainage, or abscesses, often accompanied by systemic symptoms. Musculoskeletal involvement may cause joint pain, stiffness, swelling, muscle atrophy, and draining sinuses. Mycobacterial lymphadenitis usually presents as painless, swollen lymph nodes. Disseminated NTM infections may appear as scattered skin lesions or systemic illness, such as disseminated Mycobacterium avium complex (MAC) infection in advanced HIV patients, which manifests as a febrile disease with abdominal pain and diarrhea [4].

Physical signs of NTM infections vary depending on the affected system and may include erythema, warmth, localized pain, swelling, ulceration, or abscess formation in cutaneous and soft tissue infections. Cosmetic procedures are a recognized risk factor for NTM infections in the skin and soft tissues. NTM lymphadenitis often presents as a hard, painless mass with visible skin changes, which can be easily identified on physical examination. In disseminated MAC disease, hepatosplenomegaly is a frequent finding during physical examination [4].

This broad range of presentations underscores the need for clinicians to maintain a high index of suspicion for NTM infections, particularly in at-risk populations or patients with underlying conditions [4].

14.9 Management

The management of *M. abscessus* lung disease remains a significant challenge due to poor treatment outcomes and limited efficacy of available therapies, underscoring the need for further clinical trials. Current guidelines advocate a combination therapy involving an oral macrolide alongside two parenteral agents for several months to help control symptoms and slow disease progression [6].

The most effective parenteral agents include [1, 6]:

- Amikacin: 10–15 mg/kg/day or 15–25 mg/kg administered three times per week.
- Cefoxitin: 200 mg/kg/day (up to a maximum of 12 g/day in divided doses).
- Imipenem: 500–1000 mg administered two to four times daily.
- Tigecycline: 50 mg once or twice daily.

The exact role of inhaled amikacin in treatment remains unclear. Studies indicate that slightly more than 50% of *M. abscessus* isolates exhibit moderate susceptibility to moxifloxacin, though the results are inconsistent, and neither amikacin nor moxifloxacin demonstrates robust bactericidal activity [6].

Due to concerns about toxicity and the inconvenience associated with prolonged parenteral treatment, it is recommended to administer intensive parenteral therapy for 2–4 months. This is followed by a step-down approach involving macrolide therapy combined with oral agents such as:

- Fluoroquinolone
- Linezolid
- Clofazimine
- Inhaled amikacin

This approach balances the need for effective therapy with considerations of patient safety and treatment tolerability. Further studies are essential to optimize treatment regimens and improve clinical outcomes [6].

The presence of inducible resistance may elucidate the unsatisfactory treatment outcomes observed with macrolide-based regimens for *M. abscessus* lung disease. Given the lack of consistently successful medication treatment, it is advisable to consider surgical removal, particularly in cases where the disease is localized [6].

14.10 Surgical

Managing non-tuberculous mycobacterial (NTM) lung disease solely with antimicrobial therapy, except *M. kansasii*, is challenging. Although the exact impact of supplementary surgical methods is uncertain, surgery can be efficacious in instances of substantial medication resistance or the ineffectiveness of medical intervention. For individuals with NTM lung disease, surgical treatment for isolated lesions could significantly enhance the possibility of successful treatment outcomes. In selected patients, debulking surgery on the most severely affected part of the damaged lung may be recommended to slow down the progression of the disease. Furthermore, surgery is beneficial for managing symptoms such as excessive hemoptysis [6].

Adjuvant surgical resection can lead to successful treatment results with sputum conversion in 81–100% of patients. Although the treatment success rate was positive, there were still a significant number of postoperative problems. Recent data showed that morbidity rates ranged from 7 to 25% and fatality rates ranged from 0 to 3%. It is important for physicians to meticulously select patients for surgery following deliberation in a multidisciplinary environment, and a thorough preoperative assessment is essential. Furthermore, the use of surgery, without the addition of combination antimicrobial therapy may not yield satisfactory outcomes. Continuing perioperative antibiotic medication during the postoperative period is crucial. The ideal length of antimicrobial medication before and following surgery remains a subject of discussion. However, patients are considered to have experienced treatment failure when there is no response within 6 months of receiving proper medical care, or when sputum does not convert within 12 months. Medical practitioners should consider the possible association of surgical intervention in these instances. In cases with localized disease, a rigorous medical treatment lasting a minimum of 2 months is recommended before considering surgery. Current guidelines advise that medical treatment should be maintained until the patient consistently tests negative for sputum cultures for a duration of 12 months, while also receiving surgical interventions [1, 6].

14.11 Prognosis

Patients infected with non-tuberculous mycobacteria (NTM) had a significantly worse prognosis compared to those with tuberculosis (TB) or the general population, particularly in cases of TB coinfection. NTM mortality correlated with specific demographic variables, but prolonged use of macrolides may offer advantages in terms of survival [6].

Key Points

Complicated lung infection due to *M. Abscessus* is difficult to treat, as conservative treatment does not provide favorable outcome. Surgical resection is the recommended option in this condition.

Question

1. The following are factors contributing to increased NTM incidence except:
   (a) NTM resulting in elevated virulence, as well as environmental and climatic changes due to increased human-manufactured infrastructure
   (b) Immunocompromised patient
   (c) Decreasing herd immunity due to declining TB burden
   (d) Widespread availability of CT scanning and laboratory infrastructure for NTM diagnosis
   (e) Lack of awareness about NTM
2. The following are the most common symptoms of pulmonary NTM except:
   (a) Shortness of breath
   (b) Chest pain

(c) Night sweats
(d) Fatigue
(e) Recurring cough with or without sputum production

3. Which of the following is TRUE about Hyper Immunoglobulin E Syndrome?
   (a) Patients with Hyper Immunoglobulin E Syndrome are predisposed to infections with nontuberculous mycobacteria (NTM) as bronchiectasis develops
   (b) Autosomal recessive signal transducer and activator of transcription 3 (STAT3) deficiency (hyper immunoglobulin E, HIES or Job's) patients develop recurrent pyogenic respiratory infections
   (c) NTM infections are detected in HIES patients who do not have preexisting airway abnormalities
   (d) The primary causes of mortality in HIES are predominantly associated with bronchial infections
   (e) Nontuberculous mycobacteria (NTM) are commonly isolated from patients with patent airway clearance
4. The most active oral macrolide to improve and slow down the disease progression for *M. abscessus* lung disease is:
   (a) Cefoxitin (20 mg/kg/day up to 12 g/day in divided doses)
   (b) Imipenem (500–750 mg up to four times daily)
   (c) Amikacin (10–15 mg/kg/day or 15–25 mg/kg thrice weekly)
   (d) Tigecycline (50 mg once or four times daily)
   (e) Amikacin (10–15 mg/kg/day or 15–25 mg/kg twice weekly)
5. Below are radiological patterns seen in NTM lung disease, except:
   (a) Bronchiectasis
   (b) Infiltrate
   (c) Nodular lesions
   (d) Cavitary lesions
   (e) Parenchymal consolidation

Answer keys

1. E
2. E
3. A
4. C
5. B

Acknowledgments Cipta Mahendra MD, Department of Internal Medicine, Respirology and Critical Illness Division, Universitas Indonesia, Dr. Cipto Mangunkusumo General Central National Hospital, Jakarta, Indonesia.

Ersananda Arlisa Putri MD, Department of Internal Medicine, Respirology and Critical Illness Division, Universitas Indonesia, Dr. Cipto Mangunkusumo General Central National Hospital, Jakarta, Indonesia.

Cleopas Martin Rumende MD DM PhD, Department of Internal Medicine, Respirology and Critical Illness Division, Universitas Indonesia, Dr. Cipto Mangunkusumo General Central National Hospital, Jakarta, Indonesia.

References

1. Haworth CS, Banks J, Capstick T, et al. British thoracic society guideline for the management of non-tuberculous mycobacterial pulmonary disease (NTM-PD). BMJ Open Respir Res. 2017;4:e000242.
2. Sharma SK, Upadhyay V. Epidemiology, diagnosis & treatment of non-tuberculous mycobacterial diseases. Indian J Med Res. 2020;152:185–226.
3. Melia E. Pulmonary nontuberculous mycobacterial infections in hyper-IgE syndrome. J Allergy Clin Immunol. 2009;124(3):617–8.
4. Pennington KM, Vu A, Challener D, Rivera CG, Shweta FNU, Zeuli JD, Temesgen Z. Approach to the diagnosis and treatment of non-tuberculous mycobacterial disease. J Clin Tuberc Mycobact Dis. 2021;24:100244. https://doi.org/10.1016/j.jctube.2021.10024.
5. Ryu YJ, Koh WJ, Daley CL. Diagnosis and treatment of nontuberculous mycobacterial lung disease: clinicians' perspectives. Tuberc Respir Seoul. 2016;79:74–84.
6. Lee H, Myung W, Lee EM, Kim H, Jhun BW. Mortality and prognostic factors of nontuberculous mycobacterial infection in Korea: a population-based comparative study. Clin Infect Dis. 2021;72:e610–9.

Non-Resolving Lymphadenitis Tuberculosis

15

15.1 Case Report

A 24-year-old female presented at the hospital with a complaint of continuous fluid secretion from an orifice located on the right side of her neck, which appeared exudative and yellow-whitish. A year ago, the patient had been admitted to another hospital with a bulging neck (Fig. 15.1) and frequently experienced fever and body aches. An interferon-gamma release assay (IGRA) was ordered and yielded a positive result, leading to a suspicion of tuberculosis (TB). The patient was subsequently treated for 1 year with first-line anti-TB medication, including rifampicin, isoniazid, pyrazinamide, ethambutol, and RHZE.

Despite nearly completing the 11-month RHZE treatment regimen, the neck bulging worsened instead of improving. A lymph node biopsy of the neck showed the presence of *Mycobacterium tuberculosis*, establishing a diagnosis of tuberculosis lymphadenitis (TL). This condition necessitated surgery to reduce the bulging and evacuate the pus from the infected lymph nodes, which was performed a week after TL diagnosis. Although the surgery was completed, pus continued to flow from the surgical wound, as shown in Fig. 15.2. A few days later, the wound developed necrosis, and debridement were performed to clear the necrotic debris. However, no significant clinical improvement was observed, making the treating physician refer the patient to this hospital for further evaluation.

An initial observation showed an open surgical wound approximately 1 cm wide, with no tenderness or erythema, similar in appearance to Fig. 15.2. The patient had no previous history of TB, even though her mother and brother had contracted the infection 7 years ago. The managing physician discontinued the patient's anti-TB medication after the 1-year treatment period had elapsed.

A week later, pus was still present, and mupirocin ointment and azithromycin were administered after rinsing to dry the wound. The patient began to complain about the pain felt at the wound site. A month after, pus was still observed, even

G. Singh, *Challenging Cases in Respirology and Critical Care*,
https://doi.org/10.1007/978-981-96-5002-6_15

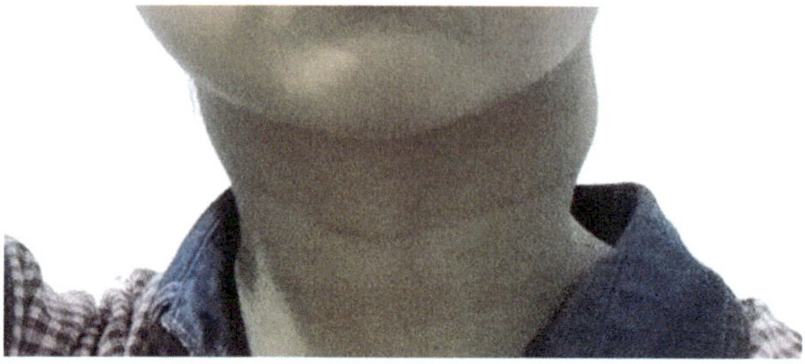

Fig. 15.1 The patient's neck was seen bulging on both the right and left sides

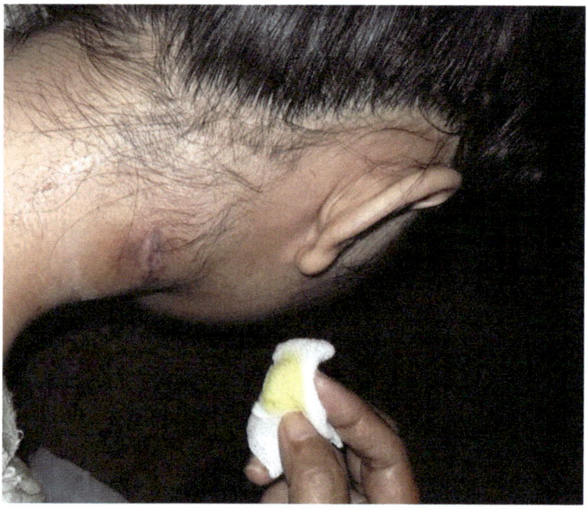

Fig. 15.2 After about 3 weeks since the surgery, pus was still flowing out from the resulting wound. The exudate was rinsed and cleaned out from the surgical wound using gauze

though the quantity had reduced. Therefore, cetirizine was prescribed, along with multivitamins, L-carnitine, and L-cystine to improve wound healing.

The following month, the wound continued to secrete yellow-whitish fluids, even though they were slightly thinner in consistency compared to the initial observation. The treating physician then decided to administer streptomycin monotherapy injections in accordance with the management guidelines for resistant TB and did not readminister the RHZE regimen. The injection regimen was planned for three times a week, totaling 56 injections over 5 months. Furthermore, chloramphenicol ointment was applied after each pus cleaning and gauze replacement during control visits.

Several days after initiating streptomycin injections, significant improvements were observed in the wound. The fluid secretion was markedly decreased, and the consistency was thinned. Moreover, significant wound healing was evident, with minimal cicatrix formation and the fistula drying out completely (Fig. 15.3).

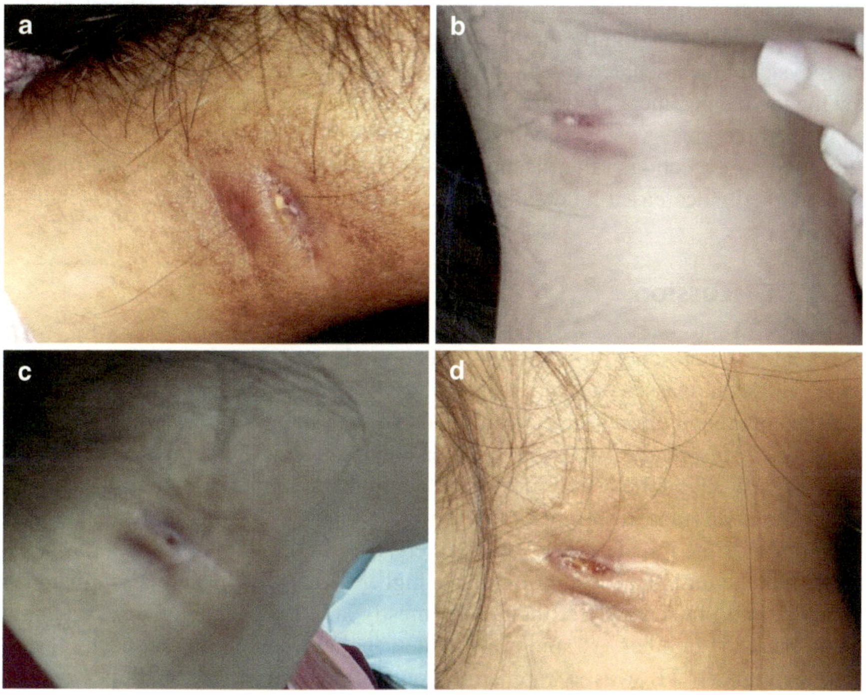

Fig. 15.3 The wound conditions after successive streptomycin injections. The photos were taken at 2 weeks (**a**), 4 months (**b**), 5 months (**c**), and 6 months (**d**) after the first injection

Granulation tissue began to form toward the conclusion of the streptomycin injection treatment period, as shown in the figure. Tinnitus began to appear in the middle of the treatment period but faded by its conclusion.

15.2 What Is the Patient's Problem Focus?

A 24-year-old female presented to this hospital with a complaint of continuous fluid secretion from an orifice located on the right side of her neck, which appeared exudative and yellow-whitish. The patient was diagnosed with TL based on an IGRA test result and a biopsy. She was then treated for 1 year with first-line anti-TB medication, particularly rifampicin, isoniazid, pyrazinamide, ethambutol, and RHZE, followed by surgery. Despite the surgery, pus continued to flow from the surgical wound.

The patient was repeatedly admitted to the hospital, and mupirocin ointment and azithromycin were administered after rinsing the pus to dry the wound. The patient began to complain of pain at the wound site, and a month after, pus was still present, even though the quantity had reduced. Cetirizine was then prescribed, along with multivitamins, L-carnitine, and L-cystine to improve wound healing. Despite antibiotics and supplements, the wound continued to secrete yellow-whitish fluids, with the consistency slightly thinner compared to the initial observation. The treating physician then decided to administer streptomycin monotherapy injections following the management guidelines for resistant TB. The injections were planned to be given three times a week, totaling 56 injections. A few days after the initiation of streptomycin injections, significant improvements were observed in the wound, with markedly decreased fluid and thinned consistency.

15.3 Discussion

Tuberculosis represented a persistent infection characterized by the formation of small, inflamed masses caused primarily by *Mycobacterium tuberculosis*. It could also be contracted through the consumption of unpasteurized cow's milk contaminated with *Mycobacterium bovis* or other uncommon types of mycobacteria. TB was a significant public health problem, affecting approximately eight million individuals annually and resulting in three million deaths due to complications. The prevalence of the infection was rapidly increasing in developing nations, possibly attributable to unsanitary conditions and a higher incidence of acquired immunodeficiency syndrome (AIDS). Although TB mostly affected the respiratory system, it could manifest in other extrapulmonary sites, including the head and neck region. Extrapulmonary TB was a rare condition, affecting only a small percentage (0.05–5%) of individuals with TB. Therefore, the condition was seldom considered a potential diagnosis for head and neck symptoms. This report presented the case of a pediatric patient diagnosed with submandibular TL, which was successfully treated with anti-TB medication, resulting in complete resolution [1].

Tuberculosis lymphadenitis was considered the predominant non-pulmonary symptom of TB. Although the general incidence of pulmonary TB was declining in certain nations, there has been an increase in extrapulmonary cases. In the United States, in 2012, out of the 9945 identified cases of TB, 846 (8.5%) were specifically lymphadenitis. Similarly, in 2011, Spain reported 6762 cases, with an incidence rate of 14.7 cases per 100,000 person-years. From these cases, a total of 1785 (26.4%) were classified as extrapulmonary TB. In non-endemic nations, the majority of TL patients were either nonnative inhabitants, primarily from Asia, or individuals with an immunosuppressive infection, such as HIV [2].

The diagnosis of TL could be challenging due to the non-specific clinical presentation, which might resemble symptoms of other viral and non-infectious disorders. Although culture remained the most reliable diagnostic method, it might take 3–4 weeks to obtain the results. A positive acid-fast bacilli (AFB) stain could suggest the presence of mycobacterial infection, even though the sensitivity was low compared to culture, ranging from 5% to 38% depending on the study. When AFB was not detected or cultures were negative, histological characteristics, such as granulomas with or without caseous necrosis, or nonspecific lymphadenitis, could support a probable diagnosis of TL [2].

15.4 Current Update

Aminoglycosides and capreomycin, which were second-line injectable medications, were primarily used to treat drug-resistant TB. These medications were effective against multidrug-resistant bacillus but were often associated with frequent side effects. In many countries with a high prevalence of multidrug-resistant tuberculosis (MDR-TB), treatment was administered through intramuscular injection [3].

World Health Organization (WHO) recommended an 8-month intensive phase for treatment, during which an injectable medication was provided.[3] The efficacy of aminoglycosides against *Mycobacterium TB* has been established for several decades, and resistance remained uncommon, even in cases of MDR-TB. However, aminoglycosides were known for their toxicity, specifically ototoxicity and nephrotoxicity, and prolonged parenteral administration was associated with numerous adverse effects [4].

Streptomycin was commonly used as a conventional treatment for TB due to the minimal side effects and strong ability to eradicate the tubercidin bacillus extracellular. Clinicians have extensively used streptomycin for TB treatment, primarily through the intramuscular administration. Moreover, the use of the medication might lead to the formation of localized solid masses near the injection site. Despite its clinical efficacy, streptomycin's utility was limited by the risk of adverse reactions and high rates of drug resistance. To mitigate these risks, streptomycin was administered through localized injection rather than systemic administration [5].

Streptomycin was particularly effective in eradicating the tubercidin bacillus extracellular and maintaining a high concentration in the lymph node tissues, facilitating rapid and complete elimination of the bacillus. When compared to isoniazid, rifamycin, and amikacin, streptomycin showed superior clinical efficacy. Geographically, the medication had a higher concentration than others, contributing to its significant therapeutic benefit. Although drug resistance might develop during treatment, it remained specific to streptomycin and did not diminish the therapeutic efficacy of other medications. Therefore, the use of streptomycin proved more effective than the administration of isoniazid and others [5].

Key Points
Apart from regular anti-TB medication and surgery, streptomycin can be an option to accelerate recovery in patient with TL.

Question

1. The following might support the diagnosis of probable TL:
   (a) AFB-negative and/or culture-negative cases
   (b) Histological features, such as granulomas with or without caseous necrosis
   (c) Specific cervical lymphadenitis
   (d) Present an immunosuppressive condition
   (e) Specific cervical lymphadenitis accompanied by fatigue

2. The most common extrapulmonary TB manifestation included one of the following:
   (a) Disseminated TB
   (b) Pot disease
   (c) Tuberculosis Lymphadenitis
   (d) Peritoneal tuberculosis
   (e) Adrenal tuberculosis
3. The efficacy of aminoglycosides on *Mycobacterium TB* has been known for many decades, but they could cause:
   (a) Hepatotoxic
   (b) Immunotoxicity
   (c) Neurotoxic
   (d) Pancreatoxic
   (e) Ototoxic
4. A second-line injectable anti-TB in the management of resistant TB. was one of the following:
   (a) Aminoglycosides
   (b) Fluoroquinolone
   (c) Sulfanomide
   (d) Penicillin
   (e) Cephalosporin
5. Which of the following was the drug action of streptomycin?
   (a) Eliminating tubercidin bacillus extracellular
   (b) Bacteriostatic activity by virtue of inhibition of arabinosyl transferase
   (c) Inhibit bacterial DNA-dependent RNA polymerase
   (d) Inhibit bacterial cell wall synthesis
   (e) Inhibits InhA, the enoyl reductase by forming a covalent adduct with the NAD cofactor.

Answer keys

1. B
2. C
3. E
4. A
5. A

Acknowledgments Cipta Mahendra MD, Department of Internal Medicine, Respirology and Critical Illness Division, Universitas Indonesia, Dr. Cipto Mangunkusumo General Central National Hospital, Jakarta, Indonesia.

Ersananda Arlisa Putri MD, Department of Internal Medicine, Respirology and Critical Illness Division, Universitas Indonesia, Dr. Cipto Mangunkusumo General Central National Hospital, Jakarta, Indonesia.

Adi Wijaya MD DM. Department of Internal Medicine. Gastroenterology and Hepatology division. Karya Bhakti Pratiwi Hospital, Bogor, Indonesia.

Hadian Setia MD. Department of Surgery. Karya Bhakti Pratiwi Hospital, Bogor, Indonesia.

References

1. Clin Infect Dis. 2011;53:555–62.
2. Salvador F, Los-Arcos I, Sánchez-Montalvá A, Tórtola T, Curran A, Villar A, Saborit N, Castellví J, Molina I. Epidemiology and diagnosis of tuberculous lymphadenitis in a tuberculosis low-burden country. Med Baltim. 2015;94:e509.
3. Quenard F, Fournier PE, Drancourt M, Brouqui P. Role of second-line injectable antituberculosis drugs in the treatment of MDR/XDR. Tuberc J Antimicrob Agents. 2017;50:252–4.
4. Cambau E, Viveiros M, Machado D, Raskine L. Revisiting susceptibility testing in MDR-TB by a standardized quantitative phenotypic assessment in a European multicentre study. J Antimicrob Chemother. 2015;70:686–96.
5. An H, Wang Z, Chen H, et al. Clinical efficacy of short-course chemotherapy combined with topical injection therapy in treatment of superficial lymph node tuberculosis. Oncotarget. 2017;8:109889–93.

Kartagener Syndrome: A Rare Autosomal Recessive Disorder

16

16.1 Case Report

A 38-year-old female complained of difficulty breathing for 1 week prior to hospital admission. The patient initially experienced breathlessness 4 months ago, which worsened with moderate and heavy physical activities. Gradually, she began experiencing difficulty breathing even during routine activities, finding relief in a semi-fowler position (45 degrees). The patient reported frequent leg swelling when urinating and complained of a persistent cough producing thick, yellow phlegm that was difficult to expel, but denied experiencing fever, weight loss, and night sweats. A previous CT thorax showed dextrocardia and raised suspicion of a lung infection.

Based on the physical examination, the patient appeared breathless and had hypotension (91/68), an increased pulse rate of 128 beats per minute, and SpO_2 desaturation at 59%. The pale conjunctiva was observed, along with minimal bilateral wet rhonchi upon lung auscultation and bilateral lower extremity pitting edema. The laboratory examination showed several abnormalities, including a high level of leukocytes at 39750, with blood gas analysis signifying pH of 7.52, $paCO_2$ of 32.7, paO_2 of 63.8, HCO3− of 27.4, and SaO_2 of 94.3%. Differential count results included basophils, eosinophils, neutrophils, lymphocytes, and monocytes at 0.4, 0, 81.5, 11.7, and 6.7, respectively. Additionally, CRP level was elevated at 83.1 mg/dl, procalcitonin at 0.21 ng/dl, prothrombin time (PT) at 14.5 sec, albumin at 2.9 g/dl, and phosphate at 5.5 mg/dl. The chest X-ray (Fig. 16.1) showed suspected situs inversus, cardiomegaly, and partially nodular infiltrates in both lung fields, with the largest nodule located in the lower left lung field. Furthermore, there was an upper field cavity in the right lung and fibrosis in the right upper lung field and left lower lung field.

CT Thorax examination conducted at the previous hospital showed cystic bronchiectasis in the inferior lobe bilaterally, suspected secondary pneumonia, dextrocardia, cardiomegaly with the liver in the left hemiabdomen, situs inversus view, and suspected KS, along with bilateral superior lobe fibrosis. Based on the initial

G. Singh, *Challenging Cases in Respirology and Critical Care*,
https://doi.org/10.1007/978-981-96-5002-6_16

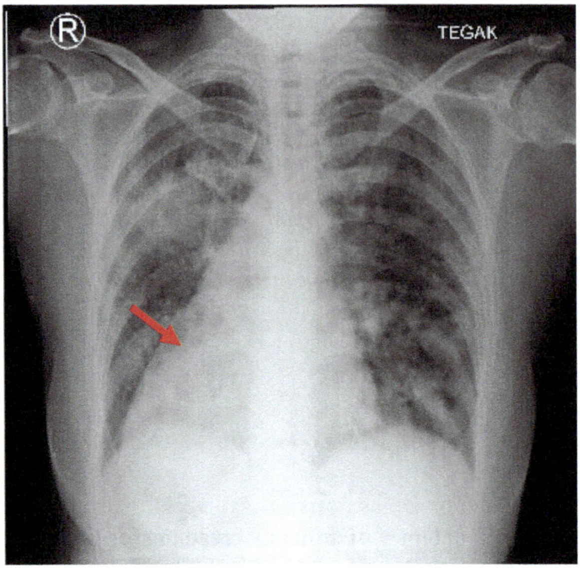

Fig. 16.1 Chest x-ray showed infiltrates partially nodular (honeycomb appearance), dextrocardia (red arrow), and cardiomegaly. (Figure courtesy: Trifonia Pingkan Siregar MD)

clinical and laboratory results, the patient received a diagnosis of Acute Decompensated Heart Failure Wet-Warm, Hospital Acquired Pneumonia (HAP) with a high-risk differential diagnosis of infected bronchiectasis, and KS. The patient was first administered oxygen at a rate of 12 lpm through a nonrebreathing mask (NRM), antibiotics, furosemide drip, and nebulization.

Following hospitalization as an inpatient, the patient was scheduled to experience another echocardiography. Additionally, several examination procedures were planned to establish potential causes of infection. The following day, the patient reported a reduction in complaints such as difficulty breathing and coughing but experienced a tendency to fall accidentally while moving. Based on the physical examination, the patient appeared moderately ill, with hypotension (94/65), oxygen saturation of 96% through the Nasal Cannula of 3 lpm, and a murmur detected upon heart auscultation. The laboratory examination showed several abnormalities, including a high level of hemoglobin at 17.4 mg/dl, hematocrit at 53.7 mg/dl, leukocytes at 26750 cells/mm^3, CRP at 98.7, and aprocalcitonin at 0.14. Subsequent follow-up chest X-ray examination (Fig. 16.2) aimed to monitor the patient's lung condition, showed consolidation and partially nodular infiltrates in the upper, middle, and lower fields of both lungs. Consolidation in the right mid-lung field indicated reduction, while the left side had an increase, raising suspicion of pneumonia. Moreover, an echocardiography examination showed decreased left ventricular systolic function (EF: 43.5%).

The following day, the patient was scheduled for CT Abdomen examination with contrast (Fig. 16.3), indicating situs inversus totalis, cystic bronchiectasis partially affected by infection, reticulonodular opacity in a part tree in bud, fibrosis, and

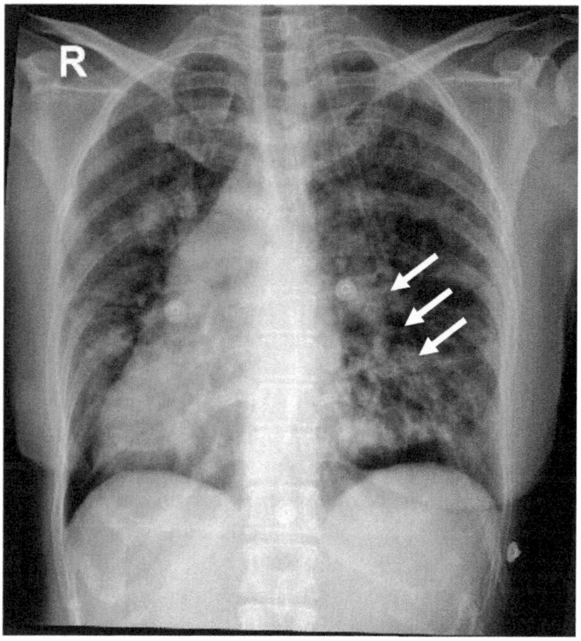

Fig. 16.2 Chest x-ray showed increased consolidation (white arrow) of the left lung. (Figure courtesy: Vally Wulani MD)

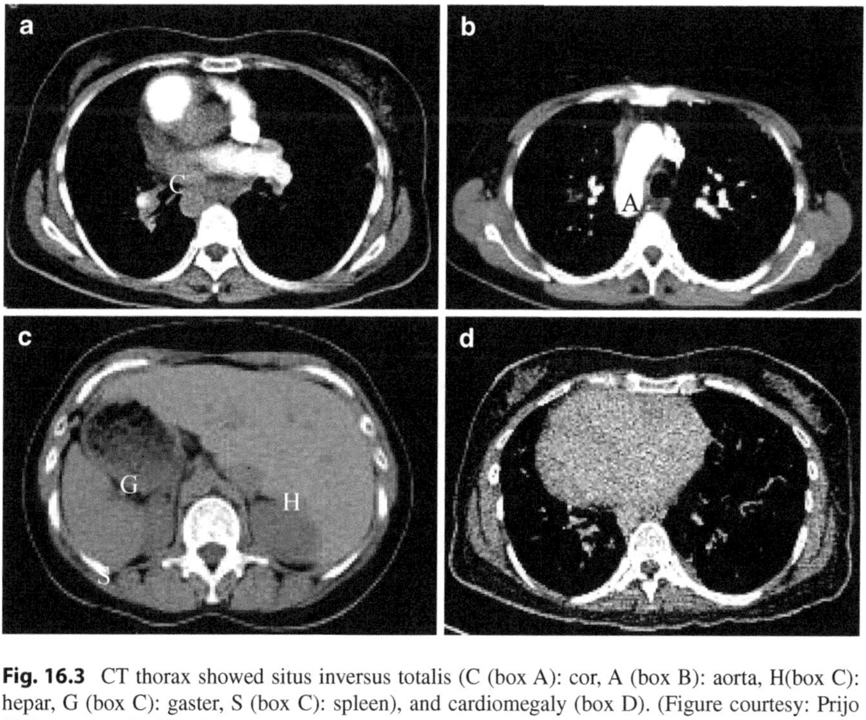

Fig. 16.3 CT thorax showed situs inversus totalis (C (box A): cor, A (box B): aorta, H(box C): hepar, G (box C): gaster, S (box C): spleen), and cardiomegaly (box D). (Figure courtesy: Prijo Sidipratomo MD DM PhD)

multiple consolidations, particularly in the superior lobes of both lungs and cardiomegaly with suspect pulmonary hypertension. The laboratory results showed negative galactomannan (0.6) and negative Aspergillus IgG. After several examinations and initial treatment to improve her clinical condition, the patient's breathing difficulties improved, even though desaturation persisted, possibly due to reduced lung function. Furthermore, a family meeting was held to discuss the provision of home oxygen and her restricted optimal condition, attributed to structural and congenital abnormalities. Plans were made for the patient's discharge and subsequent outpatient monitoring.

A week later, the patient returned to the hospital due to worsening breathing difficulties, with a saturation of only 50% at home. Based on physical examination, she appeared severely ill, with hypotension (76/53 mmHg) and high respiratory rates (111 times/minute). A thoracic inspection showed the use of auxiliary breathing muscles, and lung auscultation indicated bilateral coarse wet rhonchi. Moreover, bilateral pitting edema of the lower extremities was observed.

The laboratory examination showed several abnormalities, including a high level of leukocytes at 18870, with blood gas analysis signifying pH of 7.378, $paCO_2$ of 50, paO_2 of 68.7, HCO3− of 29.7, and SaO_2 of 92.4%. Differential count results included basophils, eosinophils, neutrophils, lymphocytes, and monocytes at 0.5, 2.7, 73.2, 19.7, and 3.9, respectively. Additionally, blood urea, potassium, chloride, procalcitonin, CRP, PT, and aPTT levels reached 30, 3.7, 103.2, 0.05, 3.8, 69.6, and 65.3, respectively. The chest X-ray examination showed consolidation and partial nodular infiltrates in both lungs, along with an increased impression and cardiomegaly.

Based on the clinical and laboratory results, the patient was diagnosed with cardiogenic shock and received initial oxygen treatment at 15 lpm through NRM, along with a 250 mg dobutamine drip in 50 ml water for injection. She was then admitted as an inpatient and scheduled for treatment in the High Care Unit (HCU) due to the need for high-pressure oxygen. Several interventions were planned to improve the patient's clinical condition and address the identified abnormalities (Table 16.1).

In the HCU, the patient continued to experience difficulty breathing, which worsened when she tried to move from one position to another. Routine blood gas analysis monitoring was conducted to address her complaints. Furthermore, the patient was tested for daily chest physiotherapy to improve her clinical condition.

The following day, a central venous catheter (CVC) was inserted to administer heparin. The gram staining of the sputum was negative, but Klebsiella pneumonia was identified in the culture. Additionally, the patient received antibiotic treatment based on the culture results, leading to clinical improvement (Table 16.1). Plans were made to transfer the patients from the HCU to outpatient care using CPAP or a simple mask.

Table 16.1 Initiatives medication

Intervention	Group/type	Drugs/fluids
Medicamentosa/fluids	Medical gas	Oxygen
	Blood products	Packed red cells
	Intravenous (IV) fluids	NaCl 0.9%
	Anticoagulant	Heparin
	Proton pump inhibitor	Omeprazole
	Antacids	Sucralfate
	Mucolytic	N-acetyl cysteine
	SSRIs	Sertraline
	Antifungal	Mycamine Nystatin drop
	Antibiotics	Meropenem Amikacin Azithromycin
Devices/tools	Tubes/catheters	Central venous catheter (CVC)

16.2 What Is the Patient's Problem Focus?

A 38-year-old female presented with difficulty breathing for 1 week before the hospital admission. The patient also reported leg swelling during urination and a productive cough. Following a thorough history, physical test, and laboratory examination, she was diagnosed with KS, Decompensated Heart Failure Wet-Warm, and HAP, with a differential diagnosis of bronchiectasis infection. Previous echocardiography, CT thorax, and CT abdomen with contrast showed dextrocardia and situs inversus.

The patient was initially admitted to the hospital and treated with 12 lpm oxygen through an NRM, antibiotics, a furosemide drip, and nebulization. The follow-up echocardiography examination showed decreased left ventricular systolic function (EF: 43.5%). Based on the second admission, the patient was further diagnosed with cardiogenic shock and received initial oxygen treatment at 15 lpm through NRM and a 250 mg dobutamine drip in 50 ml water for injection. She was planned for treatment in the HCU, requiring high-pressure oxygen, with several initiatives to improve her clinical condition and address laboratory abnormalities (Table 16.1). Subsequently, a central venous catheter (CVC) was inserted to administer heparin. Although the gram stain of the sputum was negative, klebsiella pneumonia was cultured. The patient also received targeted antibiotic treatment, resulting in clinical improvement.

16.3 Discussion

Kartagener syndrome is a rare genetic disorder inherited in an autosomal recessive manner, with an occurrence rate of approximately 1 in every 30,000 live births. This condition was characterized by the presence of situs inversus, chronic sinusitis, and bronchiectasis. The fundamental issue in KS arose from impaired ciliary motility, resulting in recurrent respiratory infections, symptoms affecting the ears, nose, and throat, as well as infertility [1, 2].

The lower respiratory tract was lined with ciliated epithelium, extending from the trachea to the respiratory bronchioles. Each ciliated cell generated around 200 cilia, which were 5 to 6 μm in length, decreasing in size as the airway narrowed. Individuals diagnosed with primary ciliary dyskinesia had various abnormalities in the structure and movement of their cilia, resulting in compromised ciliary beating and the ability to remove mucus effectively [3].

16.4 Diagnosis

The diagnostic criteria for KS included a history of chronic bronchial infection and rhinitis from early childhood, combined with one or more of the following features, (a) situs inversus or dextrocardia in the patient or a sibling, (b) immotile spermatozoa, (c) absent or impaired tracheobronchial clearance, and (d) cilia showing characteristic ultrastructural defects on electron microscopy [4].

The laboratory screening tests included the measurement of exhaled nasal nitric oxide levels and the saccharin test, which evaluated nasal epithelial mucociliary function. Additionally, confirmatory laboratory procedures consisted of high-speed video microscopy to examine ciliary beat frequency and pattern, transmission electron microscopy to detect ultrastructural ciliary defects, and genetic testing for DNAI1 and DNAH5 mutations. Abnormal laboratory results in KS showed a significant decrease in nasal nitric oxide levels (about 10% of the normal), prolonged saccharin clearance time (more than 1 hour), decreased ciliary beat frequency (less than 11 Hz/second), absence of ciliary ultrastructure (dynein arms), and mutations in DNAI1 and DNAH5 genes [4].

16.5 Management

The management of KS, a rare congenital condition, covered the use of antibiotics to treat infections in both the upper and lower airways. These antibiotics could be administered intravenously or orally and also be administered intermittently or continuously. The most prevalent pathogens were Hemophilus influenzae and Staphylococcus aureus. Children might require long-term administration of low-dose preventive antibiotics, and the treatment for obstructive lung disease and bronchiectasis includes the use of inhaled bronchodilators, mucolytics, and chest physiotherapy. Although the available information was primarily based on anecdotal reports, there was potential for the use of inhaled antibiotics, inhaled and oral corticosteroids, and recombinant DNAs. Therefore, the promotion of influenza and pneumococcal immunization was suggested [3].

In surgical care, tympanostomy tubes were used to mitigate the occurrence of repeated infections and conductive hearing loss, though multiple insertions might be necessary, and chronic otitis media could be a persistent issue. Endoscopic sinus surgery, along with the creation of a nasal antral window beneath the inferior turbinate, provided temporary relief for symptoms related to the upper and lower respiratory tracts [3].

Advanced surgical procedures, including lobectomy, lingulectomy, and anterior segmentectomy of the left upper lobe of the lungs, have been performed. In severe cases, lung and heart-lung transplantation have been attempted with varying degrees of success [5, 6].

16.6 Prognosis

The prognosis of KS depended on the extent of lung damage, and the annual decline in forced expiratory volume in the first second (FEV1) has been estimated to range from 0.8% to 3% of the expected value. The life expectancy of patients with KS was influenced by the quality of care received at specialized centers and the timeliness of diagnosis [4, 6].

Key Points

Kartagener syndrome is a very rare disease, but apparently still exists. It is often difficult to obtain a diagnosis due to the symptoms being similar to most respiratory infections. Awareness toward this syndrome should be raised to obtain an early diagnosis and administer proper treatment.

Questions

1. The inheritance pattern of Kartagener syndrome:
   (a) Autosomal dominant
   (b) X-linked recessive
   (c) X-linked dominant
   (d) Autosomal recessive
   (e) Fragile-X
2. A laboratory screening test that assesses nasal epithelial mucociliary function:
   (a) Exhaled nasal nitric oxide level determination and saccharin test
   (b) High-speed video microscopy for assessing ciliary beat frequency and pattern
   (c) Transmission electron microscopic for detecting an ultrastructural ciliary defect
   (d) Genetic testing for DNAI1 and DNAH5 mutations
   (e) Inhaled nasal nitric oxide level determination and saccharin test
3. Below are given on the management of Kartagener syndrome, except:
   (a) Antibiotic
   (b) Corticosteroid
   (c) Bronchodilator
   (d) Antiviral
   (e) Influenza vaccine

4. Below are the preferred surgical interventions for the management of Kartagener syndrome:
   (a) Lobectomy and lingulectomy
   (b) Anterior segmentectomy of the right upper lobe
   (c) Posterior segmentectomy of the right upper lobe
   (d) Anterior segmentectomy of the left lower lobe
   (e) Posterior segmentectomy of the left upper lobe
5. Below are the diagnostic criteria of Kartagener syndrome, except:
   (a) Situs inversus or dextrocardia in a patient or a sibling
   (b) Alive but immotile spermatozoa
   (c) Mesothelioma absent
   (d) Impaired tracheobronchial clearance
   (e) Cilia showing characteristic ultrastructural plenty on electron microscopy

Answer Keys
1. E
2. A
3. D
4. A
5. E

Acknowledgments **Cipta Mahendra MD**, Department of Internal Medicine, Respirology and Critical Illness Division, Universitas Indonesia, Dr. Cipto Mangunkusumo General Central National Hospital, Jakarta, Indonesia.
Ersananda Arlisa Putri MD, Department of Internal Medicine, Respirology and Critical Illness Division, Universitas Indonesia, Dr. Cipto Mangunkusumo General Central National Hospital, Jakarta, Indonesia.
Lie Khie Chen MD DM PhD, Department of Internal Medicine, Tropical Infectious Diseases Division, Universitas Indonesia, Dr. Cipto Mangunkusumo General Central National Hospital, Jakarta, Indonesia.
Resultanti MD DM, Department of Internal Medicine, Cardiovascular Division, Universitas Indonesia, Dr. Cipto Mangunkusumo General Central National Hospital, Jakarta, Indonesia.
Reza Prabowo MD, Department of Internal Medicine, Universitas Indonesia, Dr. Cipto Mangunkusumo General Central National Hospital, Jakarta, Indonesia.

References

1. Isabella C, Silva S, Nestor L, Müller M. The teaching files: chest. Elsevier Health Sciences; 2010.
2. Mishra M, Kumar N, Jaiswal A, Verma AK, Kant S. Kartagener's syndrome: a case series. Lung India. 2012;29:366–9.
3. Gupta S, Handa KK, Kasliwal RR, Bajpai P. A case of Kartagener's syndrome: importance of early diagnosis and treatment. Indian J Hum Genet. 2012;18:263–7.
4. Tadesse A, Alemu H, Silamsaw M. Kartagener's syndrome: a case report. J Med Case Rep. 2018; https://doi.org/10.1186/s13256-017-1538-2.

5. Otgün I, Karnak I, Tanyel FC, Senocak ME, Büyükpamukçu N. Surgical treatment of bronchiectasis in children. J Pediatr Surg. 2004;39:1532–6.
6. Alvarez A, Algar FJ, Santos F, Lama R, Baamonde C, Cerezo F. Pediatric lung transplantation. Transpl Proc. 2005;37:1519–22.

Transudative Pleural Effusion in Pleural Tuberculosis

17

17.1 Case Illustration

A 22-year-old male patient was admitted to the hospital with a chief complaint of shortness of breath, which had worsened 3 days before hospital admission. The complaint was affected by position, with the patient being more comfortable in a sitting position. Before the shortness of breath started, a fluctuating fever was felt in the previous month. The fever subsided when given paracetamol 500 mg, with the highest temperature being about 38 °C. Additionally, the patient occasionally had a wet cough, producing thick and white sputum accompanied by chest pain. There was also a reduction in weight by 6 kg and decreased appetite, but shortness of breath and a history of cold sweats at night were denied. Both the patient and other family members had no signs of active TB, while a history of hypertension, diabetes mellitus, asthma, heart, and kidney problems was denied.

On examination, the patient appeared short of breath with a respiratory rate of 25 per minute and a pulse rate of 119 times per minute. The oxygen saturation level was 99% with a nasal cannula delivering oxygen at 3 lpm. Examination of the lungs indicated decreased vesicular breath sound in the right lung up to ICS 2–3. Laboratory tests showed an increased erythrocyte sedimentation rate (ESR) of 88 mm/h, and a chest X-ray suggested a right pleural effusion.

A thoracocentesis procedure (Fig. 17.1) was carried out to remove the fluid and determine the etiology of pleural effusion. The fluid analysis results showed a transudate, negative for acid-fast bacilli (AFB), with Ca at 125 95.7 U/ml, as well as negative for malignant cells and microorganisms (sterile culture). The Sputum AFB was also negative, and then medical thoracoscopy was conducted for further diagnostic plan.

Pleural fluid obtained from medical thoracoscopy showed exudates, with cytological and histopathology features negative for malignant cells. Medical thoracoscopy was performed using a semirigid thoracoscope, while tissue extraction used forceps biopsy and cryobiopsy.

G. Singh, *Challenging Cases in Respirology and Critical Care*,
https://doi.org/10.1007/978-981-96-5002-6_17

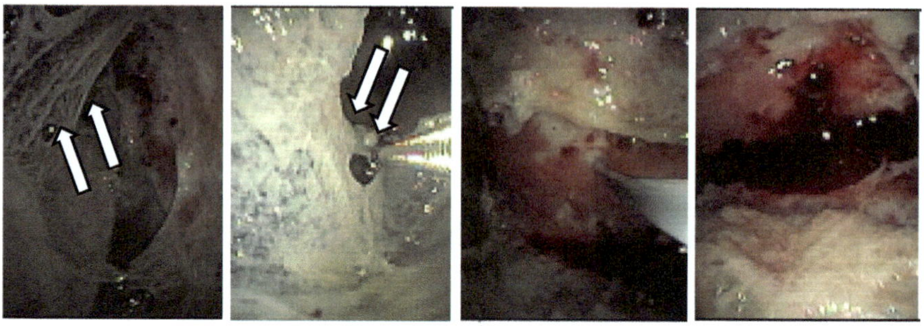

Fig. 17.1 Complex pleural effusion of the right lung postthoracoscopy with adhesiolysis suspected of chronic infection (white narrow). Fibrin deposition in pleural cavity. (Figure courtesy: Gumeet Singh MD DM PhD, Ray Bryan Charles Rattu MD)

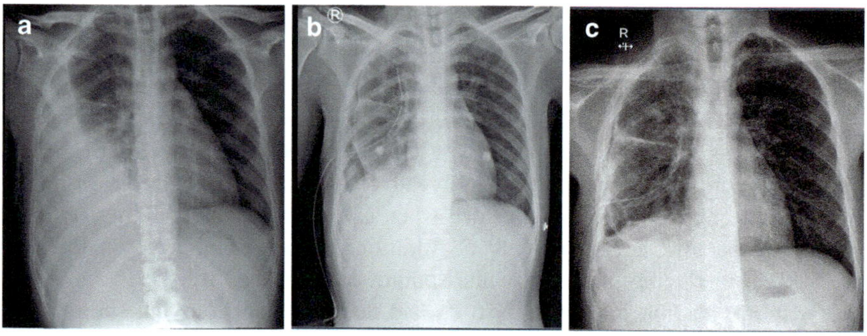

Fig. 17.2 (**a**) Patient's chest x-ray at initial hospital admission, (**b**) the chest x-ray after thoracoscopy, showed the opacity of the lung was decreased than before, (**c**) chest x-ray showed almost complete resolution after anti-TB drug treatment. (Figure courtesy: I Wayan Murna Yonathan MD DM, Damayanti Sekarsari MD DM, Sawitri Darmiati MD DM PhD)

Histological features showed chronic granulomatous inflammation, suggesting the possibility of tuberculosis (TB) infection. The cytology was composed of mesothelial cells, macrophages, and leukocytes with no feature indicative of malignancy. Molecular testing was positive for TB (sensitive rifampicin), while postmedical thoracoscopy chest X-ray (Fig. 17.2) showed right hydropneumothorax with thickening of the visceral pleura and opacity in the right lung, specifically at the base. The patient was placed under an anti-TB drug regimen for sensitive TB.

Two weeks after the drug consumption, pleural fluid production decreased gradually over time, from 800 ml/24 h until there was no fluid production remaining. The clinical symptoms, laboratory, and chest X-rays (Fig. 17.2) showed improvement, with a reduction in signs of effusion. The patient was discharged and advised for routine control in the outpatient department (OPD).

17.2 What Is the Patient's Problem Focus?

A 22-year-old male patient was admitted to the hospital with a chief complaint of shortness of breath, which had worsened 3 days before hospital admission. Additionally, fluctuating fever, wet cough, and decreased appetite were experienced. The condition was diagnosed as pleural effusion after a thorough history-taking, physical and laboratory examination, as well as a history of chest x-ray.

The patient was admitted to the hospital, and a thoracentesis procedure was carried out to remove the fluid and determine the etiology of the pleural effusion. The fluid analysis came as a transudate and was negative for malignant cells, while the Sputum AFB was negative. For further diagnosis, medical thoracoscopy was carried out, and pleural fluid obtained showed exudative effusion, negative for malignant cells based on cytological and histopathology features.

The features of the histology were indicative of chronic granulomatous inflammation, while molecular testing was positive for TB (sensitive rifampicin). The patient was placed under an anti-TB drug regimen for sensitive TB. Two weeks after the drug consumption, pleural fluid production decreased gradually over time. The patient was discharged and advised for routine control in the outpatient department (OPD).

17.3 Discussion

Pleural effusion is a common issue projected to affect more than 400 people out of every 100,000. It can be categorized into two distinct types, namely transudative and exudative, specifically, transudative pleural effusion occurs due to altered permeability of the lung capillaries. Meanwhile, exudative pleural effusion signifies the presence of a primary pleural ailment and requires inquiry into the underlying etiology [1].

Tuberculous pleural effusion (TPE) is the second most frequent manifestation of TB outside the lungs and the primary cause of pleural effusions in developing countries [1, 2]. It arises from an infection of the pleura by *Mycobacterium tuberculosis* and is distinguished by a persistent as well as severe buildup of fluid and inflammatory cells in the pleural cavity [3].

17.4 Epidemiology

In countries with a low prevalence of TB, there is a shift in the epidemiology and clinical manifestation of the disease. This includes a rise in the number of cases affecting organs outside the lungs (extrapulmonary) and a greater proportion of cases among individuals who are not native to the country. According to the European Union Statistical Agency, the number of immigrants who arrived in the

European Union (EU) in 2013 was 3.4 million. Among the nations that received immigrants, Spain was in the top five, with a total of over 280,000. Given the ongoing influx and the projected rise in rates in the future, TB will remain a significant health concern in the EU. Tuberculous lymphadenitis is followed by TPE as the most prevalent manifestation of TB beyond the lungs. TPE can manifest either as a secondary condition caused by a primary disease or a delayed consequence of infection spread several years after the initial onset [4].

17.5 Clinical Manifestation

Tuberculous pleural effusion is more common in men, with a male-to-female ratio of 2:1, and according to a study conducted in the United States, this condition is more prevalent than pulmonary TB among those over the age of 65. The average age of patients is 49 years, with approximately 50% being less than 45 years and 30% being older than 65 years. On the other hand, TPE primarily impacts younger individuals with an average age of 34 years in regions characterized by a high prevalence of TB. In these places, a significant portion of cases are caused by primary infection. TPE typically presents as a sudden and severe sickness, particularly in younger people with a stronger immune system [3].

The predominant symptoms include an unproductive cough and pleuritic chest discomfort. In cases where both cough and chest pain are present, the pain typically occurs before the cough. The majority of patients experience fever, while approximately 15% do not. Some patients may have dyspnea when the effusion is of significant size. Additional symptoms include nocturnal hyperhidrosis, reduction in body mass, and a general feeling of discomfort [3].

17.6 Diagnosis

The definitive diagnosis of TPE relies on the detection of *Mycobacterium tuberculosis* in samples of sputum, pleural fluid, or biopsy specimens. The preliminary diagnosis can also be confidently determined by observing the presence of granuloma in the parietal pleura and detecting high levels of adenosine deaminase (ADA), or interferon-γ in pleural fluid, given the appropriate clinical circumstances [3].

17.7 Adenosine Deaminase

Adenosine deaminase (ADA) is a primary enzyme found in T-lymphocytes that facilitates the transformation of adenosine and deoxyadenosine into inosine and deoxyinosine, respectively. Several studies have examined the efficacy of ADA in pleural effusion for the prompt identification of TPE, affirming that measuring ADA levels is a simple and cost-effective approach. Elevated levels can be observed in the pleural fluid of HIV patients, even in the presence of severely depleted CD4+ T cells. The vast majority of patients show pleural fluid ADA levels exceeding 40 U/L, which is the universally recognized threshold for diagnosing TPE. The presence of elevated levels can also be observed in pleural effusions caused by other factors. However, distinguishing TPE is not challenging because the clinical presentation and the composition of pleural fluid, which is predominantly composed of polymorphonuclear leukocytes, are significantly different in patients with parapneumonic effusions and empyemas compared to those with TPE. Currently, the measurement of pleural fluid ADA is commonly used in the diagnostic evaluation of pleural effusions in countries with a high burden of TB [3].

17.8 Carbohydrate Antigen 125

Pleural effusion may originate from pleural infections such as TB and neoplasia. In this context, Carbohydrate Antigen 125 (CA125) is a biomarker present on the outer layer of ovarian and other healthy cells, including pleural cells. Elevated levels have been observed in both the blood and pleural fluid of patients with pleural effusion caused by malignancy or TB. The mean concentration in TPE patients was elevated in comparison to other infections. According to a recent study, the concentration of CA125 in the pleural fluid of individuals having malignancies was markedly greater than those with tuberculous pleural fluid [5].

17.9 Xpert MTB/RIF

Tuberculous pleural effusion is the second most common type of TB that occurs beyond the lungs and is the leading cause of exudative pleural effusions in regions with a high prevalence of HIV infection. Individuals of all age groups show either unilateral or bilateral pleural effusion, characterized by a sudden to moderately rapid onset of chest discomfort, fever, loss of weight, shortness of breath, and cough. The diagnostic evaluation entails obtaining pleural fluid through aspiration and performing a pleural biopsy. Pleural fluid smear and culture tests are frequently uninformative due to the low presence of bacteria. The Xpert assay can be performed on pleural fluid samples, but it has limited sensitivity and is associated with a positive pleural fluid culture. In addition, there is evidence of a high specificity level. It is necessary to optimize the methods used to collect, store, and prepare pleural fluid samples to enhance the sensitivity of the Xpert assay on pleural fluid [6].

17.10 Thoracocenthesis Procedure

Thoracocentesis is recommended as the initial procedure in the evaluation of nearly all pleural effusions of uncertain etiology. It is recommended to consistently perform total and differential cell counts, as well as a biochemical study of total proteins, lactate dehydrogenase (LDH), glucose, and ADA on pleural fluid samples. LDH is valuable for identifying transudative effusions that show higher total proteins due to diuretic treatment. The measurement of pH in pleural fluid is widely acknowledged in algorithms for the treatment of parapneumonic pleural effusions, and it can also be beneficial in the management of malignancy. However, the true function of the entity must always be evaluated in relation to the specific clinical circumstances of the patient. Transudative effusions often have a pH within the range of 7.45–7.55, except for urinothorax, which presents an acidic pH, while most exudates have a pH ranging from 7.30 to 7.45. A pH level below 7.30 is associated with a limited range of diseases, including empyema, some acute tuberculous effusions, rheumatoid pleuritis, and highly aggressive malignant effusions. The concurrent presence of both low pH and glucose in malignant pleural effusions is associated with significant thickening and the hindrance of transfer between pleural space and systemic circulation [7].

17.11 Biopsy Pleura

An important critique of utilizing soluble biomarkers instead of culture or biopsy studies for diagnosing TPE is that none of the biomarkers offer a conclusive etiologic diagnosis. A conclusive diagnosis may only be made when *Mycobacterium tuberculosis* is detected in sputum or pleural samples, or when pleural biopsies show the presence of epithelioid cell granulomas or caseating granulomas [3].

17.12 Management

Patients who do not meet the criteria for nonsevere TB should receive the standard 6-month treatment regimen (2HRZE/4HR) (Table 17.1) or recommended treatment regimens for severe forms of extrapulmonary TB. These criteria include peripheral and intrathoracic lymph node TB without airway obstruction, as well as uncomplicated TB pleural effusion or paucibacillary, noncavitary disease, confined to one lobe of the lungs, and without a miliary pattern [8].

When resistance to isoniazid occurs but not to rifampin, a normal 6-month treatment regimen can still be effective by substituting isoniazid with a newer fluoroquinolone antibiotic such as levofloxacin or moxifloxacin. Furthermore, a 6-month treatment plan consisting of rifampin, moxifloxacin, pyrazinamide, and ethambutol for 2 months, followed by rifapentine and moxifloxacin for 4 months, has also demonstrated efficacy [8].

Table 17.1 Recommendation doses of first-line anti-TB drugs for adults

Drug	Dose (mg/kg body weight/daily)	Maximum (mg)
Isoniazid	5 (4–6)	300
Rifampicin	10 (8–12)	600
Pyrazinamide	25 (20–30)	–
Ethambutol	15 (15–20)	–

17.13 Therapeutical Thoracentesis

When the patient experiences difficulty breathing due to a significant accumulation of fluid in the pleural cavity, therapeutic thoracentesis is recommended. Meanwhile, completely removing pleural fluid using pigtail drainage, in combination with efficient anti-TB treatment, does not significantly reduce the occurrence of residual pleural thickening and other clinical symptoms [3].

17.14 Fibrinolytics

Following the completion of treatment for TB, about 25% of patients with TPE show persistent thickening of the pleura (1 cm). However, this gradually diminishes over time and has minimal impact on bodily functions. Administering fibrinolytics can reduce the extent of remaining pleural thickening in patients with localized TPE. The administration of fibrinolytics, together with anti-TB treatment, to patients with symptomatic loculated TB effusions can expedite the cure of pleural effusion and decrease the occurrence of persistent thickening [3].

17.15 Corticosteroids

The use of corticosteroids in the treatment of TPE is a subject of debate and disagreement. Two controlled investigations evaluating the efficacy of therapeutical thoracentesis yielded no discernible advantages. In another study where therapeutic thoracentesis was not conducted, there was a reduction in the duration of fever and the time needed for fluid resorption. A recent Cochrane review found that there was a lack of sufficient data to provide evidence-based recommendations on the use of additional corticosteroids in individuals with TPE. When the patient is experiencing symptoms beyond mild, a therapeutic thoracentesis is recommended. However, persistent and intense systemic symptoms such as fever, general discomfort, and chest pain during breathing occur following the thoracentesis procedure, it is advisable to administer 80 mg of prednisone every other day until the acute symptoms have subsided. The administration of steroids is gradually reduced at a fast pace [9].

17.16 Medical Thoracoscopy

Thoracoscopy can be used both for diagnostic and therapeutic objectives, with pleural effusion being the most common reason for performing a diagnostic thoracoscopy. This method can be used to determine the underlying cause of spontaneous pneumothorax. Meanwhile, pleurodesis, primarily chemical, is the most common reason for therapeutic thoracoscopy, aiming to avoid the reoccurrence of pleural effusion. The primary indication is the repeated occurrence of malignant pleural effusions. The majority of pleural exudates, a frequently encountered clinical issue, are malignant. Most of these individuals have progressed disease with an unfavorable prognosis, but a subset may experience a comparatively extended period of survival. Therefore, it is reasonable to pursue targeted treatment to alleviate symptoms. Only a small proportion of patients with malignant pleural effusions experience positive outcomes with appropriate systemic therapy. Pulmonologists are required to address these persistent pleural effusions promptly due to the tendency to reoccur quickly and cause significant disability for patients [7].

17.17 Prognosis

The prognosis of patients with TPE can be significantly affected when anti-TB medication is not administered promptly. The diagnosis relies on bacteria culture and histology, but the diagnostic sensitivity is restricted, and the process is time-consuming [10]. Patient prognosis is negatively impacted by the presence of significant effusions [11].

Key Points
In undiagnosed unilateral transudative pleural effusion, TB should be considered as one of the differential diagnoses. Medical thoracoscopy is also a precise method to confirm the etiology.

Questions

1. Which of the following statements is correct:
   (a) TPE predominates in women
   (b) TPE usually manifests as an acute illness
   (c) Chest pain can be present in some TPE patients when the effusion is large
   (d) TPE occurs significantly more often than pulmonary TB among persons <65 years old
   (e) TPE is the most common presentation of extrapulmonary TB
2. A definitive diagnosis of tuberculous pleural effusion is obtained through:
   (a) Pleural biopsy specimens
   (b) The average value of CA125
   (c) Interferon-γ in pleural fluid in the adequate clinical context
   (d) Elevated concentrations of adenosine deaminase (ADA)
   (e) Demonstrating granuloma in the parietal pleura
3. The following are clinical manifestations of TB-induced pleural effusion, except:
   (a) Dyspnea
   (b) Night sweats
   (c) Weight loss
   (d) Malaise
   (e) Chest pain
4. The most common indication for diagnostic thoracoscopy is:
   (a) Recurrent pleural effusion
   (b) Pneumothorax

   (c) Malignancy
   (d) Massive hemothorax
   (e) Pleuritis
5. Below are treatments given to tuberculous pleural effusion patients, except:
   (a) First-line anti-TB drugs
   (b) Corticosteroid
   (c) Medical thoracoscopy
   (d) Fibrinolytic
   (e) Diuretic

Answer Keys

1. B
2. A
3. E
4. A
5. E

Acknowledgments **Ersananda Arlisa Putri MD,** Department of Internal Medicine, Respirology and Critical Illness Division, Universitas Indonesia, Dr. Cipto Mangunkusumo General Central National Hospital, Jakarta, Indonesia.
Ray Bryan Charles Rattu MD, Department of Internal Medicine, Respirology and Critical Illness Division, Universitas Indonesia, Dr. Cipto Mangunkusumo General Central National Hospital, Jakarta, Indonesia.

References

1. Darooei R. Discriminating tuberculous pleural effusion from malignant pleural effusion based on routine pleural fluid biomarkers, using mathematical methods. Tanaffos. 2017;16:157–65.
2. Lo Cascio CM, Kaul V, Dhooria S, Agrawal A, Chaddha U. Diagnosis of tuberculous pleural effusions: a review. Respir Med. 2021;188:106607. https://doi.org/10.1016/j.rmed.2021.106607.
3. Zhai K. Tuberculous pleural effusion. J Thorac Dis. 2016;8:486–94.
4. Macias A. Epidemiology and diagnosis of pleural tuberculosis in a low incidence country with high rate of immigrant population: a retrospective study. Int J Infect Dis. 2019;78:34–8.
5. El-Hoshy M, Abdallah AA, Abd-Elhamid SM. Abd Elhamid, comparison of the diagnostic utility of ADA and CA125 in tuberculous effusion. Egypt J Chest Dis Tuberc. 2017;66:299–305.
6. Friedrich SO. Xpert MTB/RIF assay for diagnosis of pleural tuberculosis. J Clin Microbiol. 2011;49:4341–2.
7. Panadero FR, Janssen JP, Astoul P. Eur Respir J. 2006;28:409–22.
8. WHO. WHO consolidated guidelines on tuberculosis, module 4: treatment – drug- susceptible tuberculosis treatment in 2022.
9. Cohen LA, Light RW. Tuberculous pleural effusion. Turk Thorac J. 2015;16:1–9.
10. Wu S, Li S, Fang N. A scoring model for diagnosis of tuberculous pleural effusion. BMC Pulm Med. 2022;22:332.
11. Jiménez D, Díaz G, Gil D, Cicero A, Pérez-Rodríguez E, Sueiro A. Etiology and prognostic significance of massive pleural effusions. Respir Med. 2005;99:1183–7.

Disseminated Tuberculosis Infection (Pulmonary, Peritoneal, Colonic, and Adrenal)

18

18.1 Case Illustration

A 37-year-old female was admitted to the emergency room with a loss of consciousness for the past 4 h. According to the family, this incident occurred when the patient was preparing for hemodialysis. Initially, difficulty in communicating was observed 2 h before arrival at the hospital. There were no complaints of slurred speech, vomiting, or severe headaches, and the urinary output was <500 cc/24 h. One month before admission, fluctuating fever occurred but symptoms of coughing and shortness of breath were denied. The patient suffered from kidney failure, which started in 2018, and routine hemodialysis was initiated in January 2022 through double-lumen catheter tunneling every Tuesday and Friday. On initial hemodialysis, the HBsAg result was positive. In addition, there was a history of uncontrolled diabetes mellitus, which started in 2013, and a history of controlled hypertension, managed with amlodipine 5 mg, since 2018.

On physical examination, the patient appeared seriously ill with a Glasgow Coma Scale (GCS) score of E4M5V3. Hypertension (168/94 mmHg), pale conjunctiva, and edema in the lower extremities were also observed. Laboratory tests showed several abnormalities, including decreased hemoglobin level (8.6 g/dl), leukocytosis (34,620), decreased kidney function characterized by urea 96 mg/dl, creatinine 3.5 mg/dl, and eGFR 15.9 mL/min/1.73 m^2, as well as hyponatremia (128 mEq/l). Furthermore, chest X-ray (Fig. 18.1) indicated pulmonary interstitial edema infiltrates in both lung fields and left pleural effusion.

Based on clinical and initial laboratory results, the patient was diagnosed with impaired consciousness and aphasia, CKD stage V on HD, anemia, hypertension, type II DM, overweight, chronic hepatitis B, left pleural effusion, and hyponatremia. Oxygen therapy with 3 lpm and initial management was given to improve the condition, and a nasogastric tube was installed.

On the first day of admission, the patient appeared not to be fully conscious and could open the eyes but did not communicate. Physical examination showed pitting

G. Singh, *Challenging Cases in Respirology and Critical Care*,
https://doi.org/10.1007/978-981-96-5002-6_18

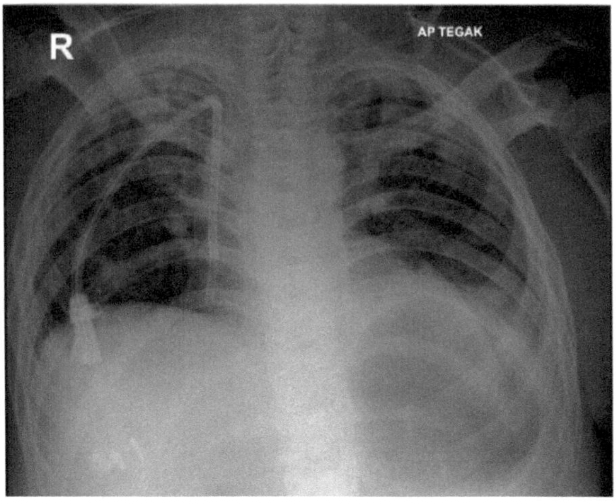

Fig. 18.1 Patient's chest x-ray shows pulmonary interstitial edema, infiltrates in both lung fields, and left pleural effusion. (Figure courtesy: Rahmad Mulyadi MD DM PhD)

edema on the right leg with a positive Homans sign. Subsequently, a noncontrast computed tomography (CT) scan of the head was scheduled to confirm the diagnosis. A follow-up examination of urea, blood culture, lactate, procalcitonin, CRP, APTT, and D-Dimer was also carried out. CT scan results showed a lacunar infarction in the subcortical left frontal lobe, and no bleeding or SOL was observed. Laboratory test results were as follows: urea (128 mg/dl), blood culture (sterile), lactate (1.8 mg/dl), procalcitonin (18.34 μg/L), CRP (147 mg/L), APTT (50), and D-Dimer (4550). The patient was suspected to have Suprainguinal Deep Vein Thrombosis. Hypoglycemia (blood glucose 64 mg/dl) was observed, and treatment was carried out using bolus D40% 2 flacons and IVFD D10% 500 ml/24 h. After therapy, the blood glucose increased to 100 mg/dl, and the current fluid balance reached +300 ml/24 h.

The following day, the patient experienced a fluctuating fever, with the highest temperature being 38.1 °C. Based on the examination results, the state of consciousness was reduced, and contact was inadequate, culminating in the transfer to the High Care Unit (HCU) room for monitoring. The blood pressure tended to decrease, leading to the administration of a titrated norepinephrine drip 0.05 mcg/kg body weight/min. Laboratory examination showed decreased hemoglobin level (8.2 g/dl; SI (25), TIBC (64), % transferrin (68%)), leukocyte count (21,840 μl), total bilirubin (3.81 mg/dl), direct bilirubin (3.02 mg/dl), indirect bilirubin (0.78 mg/dl), and APTT (60). AST to Platelet Ratio Index (APRI) and Fibrosis-4 (FIB-4) examinations were also carried out to evaluate the degree of liver cirrhosis in chronic hepatitis B. Based on the results, the APRI score was 4.7 and FIB-4 was 1.17.

The second day after moving to the HCU room, the patient was conscious, but the contact was inadequate. Complaints of coughing became increasingly frequent, and there was a shortness of breath. On physical examination, the temperature was elevated, and there were crackles in the lungs. An ultrasound of the chest showed no effusion, and the IVC was 1.8 cm, within normal limits. Based on the complaints and the investigation results, the diagnosis was septic shock, possibly due to Intravascular catheter-related bloodstream infection (CRBSI) with a differential diagnosis of Community-acquired pneumonia (CAP) and a pneumonia severity index (PSI) score in risk class V (PSI-V).

On the third day in HCU, the cough worsened and the fever persisted; hence, Ventolin inhalation was given, and suction was carried out according to indications. The patient was scheduled for an abdominal CT examination and repeat X-rays. The abdominal CT (Fig. 18.2) showed massive ascites with stinging of the peritoneal wall and multiple hypodense calcified central lymphadenopathy suspicious of peritonitis and tuberculous lymphadenitis. There was also extensive in-bud opacity in the lung bases visualized with bilateral pleural effusion, suggesting pulmonary TB. Furthermore, circumferential symmetrical thickening of the long segment in the terminal ileum and cecum that stings with water-target contrast type accompanied by the fat stranding of the surrounding mesenteric fat suggested ileocolitis

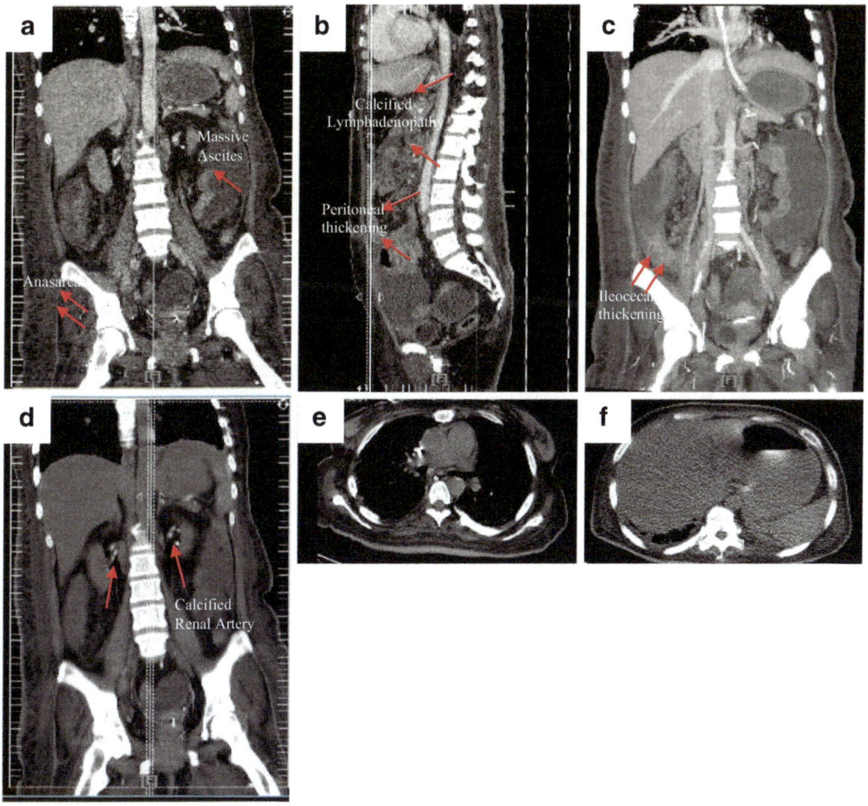

Fig. 18.2 (a-e) Patient's CT abdomen suspected of disseminated TB (pulmonary, peritoneal, colonic). Figure courtesy: Jacub Pandelaki MD DM PhD.

TB. Computed tomography angiography (CTA) of the abdomen did not show occlusion or significant stenosis. Abdominal Computed tomography venography (CTV) was within the limits, with no visualized intraluminal thrombus in the venous system. Additional findings included a Central Venous Catheter (CVC) in the right inguinal region, anasarca edema, a dislocated IUD in the cervical region, and bilateral calcified atrophy of the kidneys indicative of chronic parenchymal kidney disease.

Based on the results of X-rays, the opacity in both lung fields appeared to increase, and there was a left pleural effusion (Fig. 18.3). The patient was suspected of disseminated TB (pulmonary, peritoneal, and colonic).

From day 4 to 8 in HCU, the patient was conscious, but contact remained inadequate, and the focus was easily diverted. Several examinations were subsequently scheduled, including CT angiography, echocardiography, and sputum culture. Based on the echocardiography results, there was segmental hypokinetic, LV concentric remodeling, decreased left ventricular systolic function, and grade I diastolic dysfunction without increased left atrial pressure (LAP). The acid-fast sputum culture was negative, and hypoglycemia (blood glucose 64 mg/dl) occurred, but the condition improved to 100 mg dl after administering D40% 2 flacons. The supporting examination of the CDL tip culture was sterile. Furthermore, the patient had femoral central venous catheters connected to Bfluid 500 ml/24 h with a fluid balance of +1230 cc/24 h. A recent chest X-ray showed heterogeneous opacity over both lung fields, suggesting pneumonia. The CRP level increased (249.1), and the arterial blood gas (ABG) was indicative of respiratory alkalosis (pH: 7.56, pCO2: 31.4, pO2: 165, HCO3: 28.4). A lumbar puncture was scheduled for the next day to identify the etiology of decreased consciousness, including the possibility of tuberculous meningitis. Furthermore, cerebrospinal fluid (CSF) analysis showed colorless and clear fluid with cytoalbumin dissociation (cerebrospinal fluid protein (55),

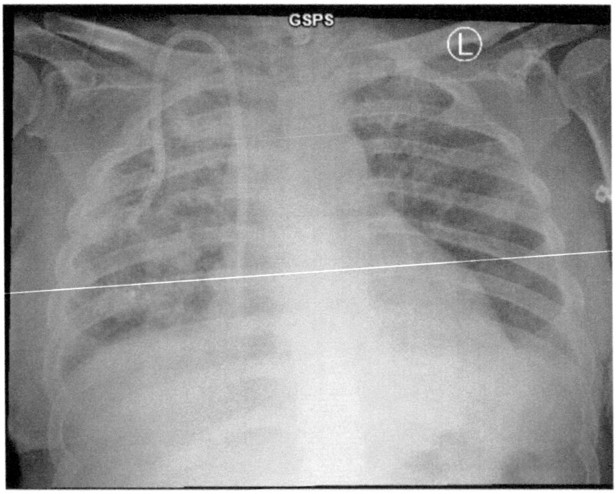

Fig. 18.3 The opacity in both lung fields increased. (Figure courtesy: Sahat Matondang MD DM)

cerebrospinal fluid glucose (30), serum glucose (94.2), and chloride (22)). Cerebrospinal fluid was negative for India ink, Gram stain, and smear, also, an anti-HIV screening test showed negative results.

On day 10, Xpert MTB/RIF Assay examination with sputum samples showed positive MTB and negative rifampicin resistance. Based on the clinical condition and supporting examinations, the patient was diagnosed with disseminated TB, confirmed by a molecular test. Consequently, the intensive phase of the anti-TB regimen was initiated by adjusting renal doses <50 kg. The OAT regimen consisted of rifampicin 1 × 400 mg, Isoniazid 1 × 300 mg, and pyrazinamide 750 mg taken orally three times a week. In addition, an antiviral was scheduled due to the reactive HBeAg test results.

The following day, the clinical condition had improved, and a lower gastrointestinal endoscopy was scheduled due to suspected intestinal TB but was not carried out because there was an underlying muscle injury in the lower back region. As the patient experienced desaturation, the condition worsened, the consciousness decreased to coma, and blood pressure decreased from 90/47 mmHg to 73/34 mmHg. After day 17 of treatment at HCU, at 02.00 pm, bradycardia and desaturation occurred, and consciousness decreased to a coma. As a DNR (Do Not Resuscitate) patient, at 02.05 pm, the pulse was not palpable, and the EKG showed true asystole, leading to death.

18.2 Discussion

Disseminated tuberculosis (TB) is a severe illness caused by the spread of *Mycobacterium tuberculosis* through the bloodstream. The diagnosis is difficult due to the modest and vague clinical presentation, which typically indicates the affected organ. Disseminated TB is characterized by the existence of two or more separate locations attributed to either the initial infection progressing, reactivation of a dormant infection followed by spreading, or in rare cases, due to medical intervention [1].

18.3 Epidemiology

The precise worldwide prevalence of disseminated TB remains uncertain, but in immunocompetent people, it constitutes less than 2% of all TB cases and up to 20% of all extrapulmonary TB cases [1]. The condition is recognized as a significant contributor to diseases and death in poor nations, particularly among youngsters aged 15 and below. However, the prevalence has increased in technologically advanced nations and across various age demographics due to multiple risk factors. These factors include human immunodeficiency virus (HIV) infection/acquired immunodeficiency syndrome (AIDS), as well as other causes of weakened immune system function such as the utilization of biologicals and immunosuppressive medications for the management of various medical conditions, the growing occurrence of organ transplantation, alcoholism, chronic liver disease, chronic hemodialysis, diabetes mellitus, malignancies, and silicosis [1].

18.4 Clinical Manifestation

Tuberculosis spreads in the body and can impact several anatomical regions. The manifestation of symptoms is contingent on the specific regions of the body impacted. The predominant initial symptoms included fever, cough, loss of appetite, weight loss, and nocturnal perspiration [1, 2]. Patients diagnosed with disseminated TB often had a higher prevalence of smoking and were more commonly impacted by chronic liver failure or cirrhosis, attributed to either alcohol consumption or HCV infection. Additionally, these patients experienced immunosuppression due to co-infection with HIV or immunosuppressive treatment [3].

The length of time between the onset of symptoms and the diagnosis can vary, ranging from over a period of days to weeks to several months in some cases. Therefore, identifying this ailment is typically challenging, and a majority of patients tend to postpone getting medical assistance for a duration exceeding 1 month. Diagnosing children is challenging due to the ambiguous nature of clinical presentations, often leading to missed diagnoses. The clinical manifestation of disseminated TB in adults and children differs. In adults, symptoms and signs such as anorexia, fatigue, difficulty breathing, excessive sweating at night, fever, abdominal pain, coughing up blood, headache, changes in mental state, accumulation of fluid in the chest cavity, accumulation of fluid in the abdomen, and swelling of the lymph nodes are more frequently observed compared to children. On the other hand, children are more likely to experience symptoms including diarrhea, vomiting, seizures, enlargement of the liver and the spleen, yellowing of the skin and eyes, and stiffness of the neck [1].

18.5 Diagnosis

To verify the diagnosis in individuals with suspected disseminated TB, it is necessary to obtain a variety of suitable samples for acid-fast bacilli (AFB) smear, polymerase chain reaction (PCR), mycobacterial culture, and histology [1].

18.6 Microbiological Studies of Specimens

Acid-Fast Bacilli smear and culture of specimens remain a valuable method for detecting disseminated TB. Although AFB smear is a quick, cost-effective, and highly accurate method for detecting TB, the ability may vary and be limited among various samples. It cannot also identify strains of TB that are resistant to drugs. Culture is often regarded as the benchmark for diagnosis, but traditional mycobacterial culture can take up to 4–6 weeks to produce results. Similarly, the liquid culture method requires a minimum of 2 weeks, which is still rather lengthy and has the potential to raise mortality and morbidity rates. Attempts have been made to use new quick diagnostic technologies such as PCR and certain biomarkers [1].

18.7 Polymerase Chain Reaction Study on Specimens

Nucleic acid amplification (NAA) assays using PCR have recently emerged as a swift diagnostic method for TB capable of directly detecting *M. tuberculosis* complex (MTBC) from patient samples in 2 h. This process comprises DNA extraction, amplification, and detection. PCR amplification target sequence is IS6110, a distinct gene segment found exclusively in MTBC and not observed in other mycobacterial species [1].

Xpert MTB/RIF is an example of an NAA test that has received approval from the Food and Drug Administration (FDA) for directly detecting MTBC from respiratory specimens. It also has the advantage of offering insights into potential resistance to rifampin. This is achieved by identifying mutations in an 81-base pair segment of the rpoB gene, which is responsible for conferring approximately 96% of rifampin resistance in MTBC. However, the diagnostic accuracy varies in different studies due to the lack of consistency in the approach used to handle the material, amplify the target of *M. tuberculosis*, and identify the amplified DNA. Physicians must be aware that negative results may not rule out the presence of TB due to limited sensitivity. Consequently, samples should be cultured to promote the growth of mycobacteria and avoid obtaining incorrect negative results when using NAA testing. This is crucial for identifying nontuberculous mycobacteria species and conducting antibiotic susceptibility testing [1].

18.8 Biomarker

Recently, several quick and noninvasive tests that use different types of samples other than sputum have been utilized for diagnosing TB. Biomarkers, such as adenosine deaminase (ADA) and IFN-γ, have been used to diagnose TB by measuring the levels in the supernatant of fluid specimens, including pleural, ascites, pericardial, and cerebrospinal fluid (CSF). Despite the abundance of studies on these biomarkers, the validation and confirmatory role remains equivocal [1].

18.9 Histologic Study of Specimens

Histopathology remains a crucial method for diagnosing TB, and histopathologic examination of a tissue sample typically shows the presence of caseating and noncaseating granulomas, which may or may not be positive for the AFB test [4].

18.10 Imaging in Tuberculosis

Pulmonary TB is commonly diagnosed with conventional chest X-rays, but other imaging methods such as CT, PET-CT, and MRI are valuable for evaluating both pulmonary and extrapulmonary TB. The use of imaging techniques in TB has shown significant and rapid expansion, mirroring the progress observed in many areas of medicine. An imaging study is generally the initial indication of the potential presence of TB, specifically in locations that are difficult to access.

Imaging is frequently needed in a confirmed case of TB to determine the scope of the disease, assess the effectiveness of treatment, or identify any remaining infection following the completion of therapy. Furthermore, imaging is crucial in directing aspirations and biopsies, as well as providing advice for the therapeutic drainage of abnormal fluid collections [5].

18.11 Chest Radiograph

Chest radiography is typically the primary and most economical modality used in the early detection of disseminated TB. The classic military pattern is observed in around 85%–90% of instances. These discoveries are not exclusive to disseminated TB but can be imitated by histoplasmosis, sarcoidosis, pneumoconiosis, metastasis, bronchoalveolar carcinoma, and pulmonary siderosis. Infrequent observations on chest X-rays include consolidation, cavities, calcification, granulomas, and pleural effusion [5].

18.12 High-Resolution Computed Tomography (CT)

High-resolution CT can identify abnormalities that are not detectable on chest X-rays, such as miliary nodules, ground-glass opacities, and thickening of the interlobular septa [5].

18.13 Abdominal Ultrasonography

Abdominal Ultrasonography imaging method can detect disseminated liver disease, localized abnormalities or enlargement of the liver and spleen, thickening of the peritoneum, many thin partitions, and various types of debris inside ascitic fluid. Other discoveries consist of para-aortic, mesenteric, or omental nodes. However, these irregularities lack specificity and can be imitated by various nontuberculous disorders [5].

18.14 Abdominal Computed Tomography (CT)

An abdominal CT scan can detect the presence of para-aortic lymph nodes, enlargement of the liver and spleen, thickness of the peritoneum, the presence of free or localized fluid in the abdomen (ascites), thickening of the mesentery or omentum, the presence of strands in the mesentery or omentum, and the presence of nodes in the mesentery or omentum. The nodes are typically clustered, characterized by slight fat infiltration and a centrally hypoattenuating area, with or without calcification [5].

18.15 Magnetic Resonance Imaging of Abdomen

Magnetic resonance imaging (MRI) is an effective method for detecting miliary lesions in hidden extrapulmonary locations due to its exceptional ability to visualize soft tissues and acquire images from several angles. Ultrasonography and MRI are the preferred imaging modalities for pregnant patients [5].

18.16 Brain Computed Tomography (CT) Scanning with Contrast or Magnetic Resonance Imaging

Brain Computed Tomography (CT) Scanning with Contrast or Magnetic Resonance Imaging can be used to evaluate suspected TB lesions, including meningeal enlargement, tuberculoma, tuberculous abscess, and cerebritis [5].

18.17 Echocardiography

Echocardiography is beneficial for identifying tuberculous lesions, such as pericardial effusion and heart masses [5].

18.18 Positron Emission Tomographic-Computed Tomography (PET-CT)

18F-FDG has recently been used for the identification of extrapulmonary TB. PET-CT can identify peripheral uptake and central hypometabolism, which depends on the extent of caseation. This information helps in identifying the most appropriate organ or site for biopsy [5].

18.19 Diagnostic Criteria

Disseminated TB should be clinically confirmed through the use of bacteriological methods such as AFB smear and culture in both liquid and solid media, as well as PCR or histological evidence. The disease is confirmed when a patient meets any of the following criteria: isolation of *M. tuberculosis*, positive PCR test, or histological evidence of caseating granulomatous inflammation from bone marrow, blood, or liver biopsy specimen, or from at least two separate organs, with or without miliary lung lesions [1, 6].

18.20 Management

The length of treatment for disseminated TB is typically equivalent to that of pulmonary TB. However, it may be necessary to customize the treatment plan for each case. Patients with a high level of microorganisms, delayed improvement in condition, weakened immune system, or central nervous system infection, as well as those with bone and joint problems who require a longer treatment period, may need additional therapy. The treatment for disseminated TB in susceptible organisms entails the administration of a "four-drug regimen" consisting of rifampicin, isoniazid (INH), pyrazinamide, and ethambutol/streptomycin. This treatment is given daily for the first 2 months and is divided into two phases. Subsequently, the regimen includes the administration of rifampicin and isoniazid for an additional duration of 4 months, which may be prolonged to 7 months in certain instances. The efficacy of first-line anti-TB medicines is well-documented in numerous reports. To effectively treat multidrug-resistant TB, it is necessary to administer a minimum of one injectable medicine that is susceptible to the bacteria, along with a minimum of three other susceptible drugs. This combination is crucial to avoid the development of further resistance [1].

The effect of corticosteroids on treatment outcomes remains uncertain due to limited evidence from randomized controlled trials focused on TB infection rather than specifically on individuals with disseminated TB. Adjunct corticosteroid treatment is typically administered in cases of disseminated TB accompanied by meningitis, pericarditis, adrenal insufficiency, and refractory hypoxemia [1].

18.21 Prognosis

Although there have been improvements in the treatment and care of individuals with disseminated TB, the death rate remains significant, ranging from 25 to 30%. Several factors can predict death, including meningismus, liver cirrhosis, leukopenia, leukocytosis, advancing age, presence of underlying disease, impaired mental status, and night sweats [1]. The mortality rate is greater among patients with disseminated TB as compared to those with locoregional TB [3].

Key Points

Disseminated TB is rare in patients without HIV and who are immunocompromised. Prognosis is worse in these patients compared to those with locoregional TB.

Questions

1. The exact global incidence of disseminated TB is:
   (a) Accounts for <2% of all cases of TB and up to 20% of all pulmonary TB cases
   (b) Accounts for <2% of all cases of TB and up to 20% of all extrapulmonary TB cases
   (c) Accounts for >2% of all cases of TB and up to 20% of all pulmonary TB cases
   (d) Accounts for >2% of all cases of TB and up to 20% of all extrapulmonary TB cases
   (e) Accounts for >2% of all cases of TB and up to 10% of all extrapulmonary TB cases
2. Below are common symptoms of disseminated TB, except:
   (a) Fever
   (b) Cough
   (c) Anorexia
   (d) Weight loss
   (e) Muscle Pain
3. To confirm the diagnosis in patients with suspected disseminated TB, a selection of appropriate specimens is needed, except:
   (a) AFB smear
   (b) Adenosine deaminase
   (c) Mycobacterial culture
   (d) Polymerase chain reaction (PCR)
4. In general, adjunct corticosteroid treatment can be given in disseminated TB with:
   (a) Meningitis
   (b) Encephalitis
   (c) Pot Disease
   (d) Pleuritis
   (e) Disseminated TB with Alkalosis
5. These mortality predictors are associated with disseminated TB, except?
   (a) Meningismus
   (b) Liver cirrhosis
   (c) Neutrophilia
   (d) Leukocytosis
   (e) Altered mental status

Answer Keys

1. B
2. E
3. B
4. A
5. C

Acknowledgments Ersananda Arlisa Putri MD, Department of Internal Medicine, Respirology and Critical Illness Division, Universitas Indonesia, Dr. Cipto Mangunkusumo General Central National Hospital, Jakarta, Indonesia.

Kemal Fariz Kalista MD DM PhD, Department of Internal Medicine, Hepatobilliary Division, Universitas Indonesia, Dr. Cipto Mangunkusumo General Central National Hospital., Jakarta, Indonesia.

Hasan Maulahela MD DM PhD, Department of Internal Medicine, Gastroenterology Division, Pancreatobilliary and Digestive Endoscopy, Universitas Indonesia, Dr. Cipto Mangunkusumo General Central National Hospital, Jakarta, Indonesia.

References

1. Khan FY. Review of literature on disseminated tuberculosis with emphasis on the focused diagnostic workup. J Fam Community Med. 2019;26:83–91.
2. Ellner JJ, Jacobson KR. Tuberculosis. 26th ed. Philadelphia: Elsevier; 2020.
3. Meira L. Predictors and outcomes of disseminated tuberculosis in an intermediate burden setting. Pulmonology. 2019;25:320. https://doi.org/10.1016/j.pulmoe.2018.11.001.
4. Gupta M, Lobo FD, Adiga DS, Gupta A. A histomorphological pattern analysis of pulmonary tuberculosis in lung autopsy and surgically resected specimens. Pathol Res Int. 2016;2016:8132741.
5. Bomanji JB. Imaging in tuberculosis. Cold Spring Harb Perspect Med. 2015;5(6):a017814.
6. Ribeiro S, Trabulo D, Cardoso C, Oliveira A, Cremers I. Disseminated tuberculosis in an immunocompetent patient: the answer is in the liver. GE – Port J Gastroenterol. 2016;23:208–13.

19 Benign Lung Mass: Necrosis Fibrinoid

19.1 Case Illustration

A 52-year-old male presented to the internist with a chief complaint of continuous coughing, which was productive in nature. The patient also reported occasional episodes of hemoptysis, along with symptoms of fluctuating fever and shortness of breath, which were not affected by changes in position. The results of chest X-rays showed no abnormalities in the heart and lungs (Fig. 19.1). Subsequently, the patient was given medication to take home and later reported improvement in the condition.

At the beginning of 2020, the complaints reappeared, and the coughing and tightness worsened. Consequently, the patient was taken to the nearby hospital and appeared breathless, with an increased respiratory rate of 28 times per minute and a body temperature of 38.2 °C. The patient was hospitalized and underwent a chest X-ray and computed tomography (CT) scan examination. Chest X-ray results showed an impression of atelectasis in the midfield and lower left lung accompanied by pneumonia (Fig. 19.2). Meanwhile, a CT scan suspected a mass in the left lung with a differential diagnosis of malignancy (Fig. 19.3). The patient was then advised to go to another hospital for a biopsy.

Following referral to another hospital, the patient underwent several examinations and tissue biopsies. Chest X-ray results showed lung mass and atelectasis, while the echocardiogram was normal. *Subsequent* bronchoscopy biopsy (Fig. 19.4) *did not show any malignant cells*, and the histopathological results of lung tissue were consistent with necrotic tissue.

To seek a second opinion, the patient was evaluated at another hospital and underwent a bronchoscopy procedure (Fig. 19.5). The results showed a mass in the left lung, raising suspicion of malignancy.

In June 2020, the symptoms reappeared, leading to a visit to the outpatient department of Cipto Mangunkusumo Hospital with complaints of left chest pain since October 2019, specifically when coughing and inhaling. The patient also reported experiencing episodes of hemoptysis since the same period, which had

G. Singh, *Challenging Cases in Respirology and Critical Care*,
https://doi.org/10.1007/978-981-96-5002-6_19

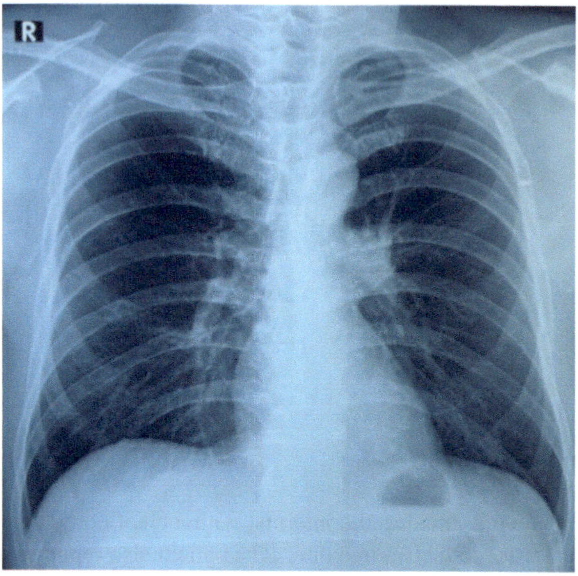

Fig. 19.1 Patient's chest x-ray. (Figure courtesy: Kahar Kusumawidjaja MD)

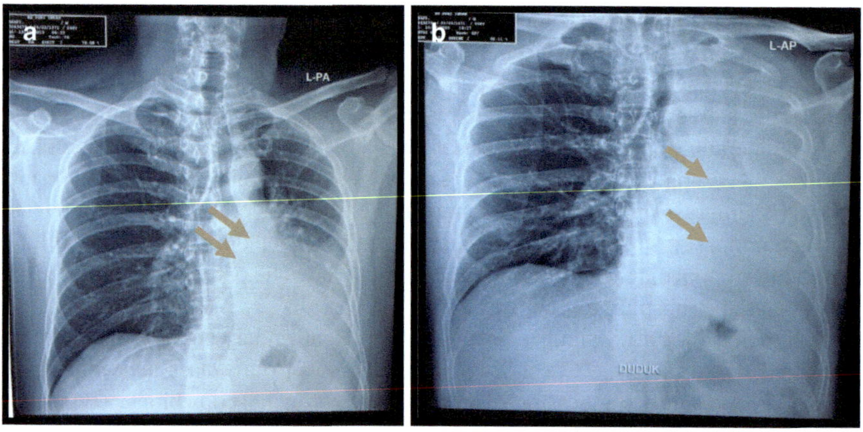

Fig. 19.2 Patient's chest x-ray showed opacity homogenous in the upper, middle, and lower left lung (**a**) PA position; (**b**) erect position. (Figure courtesy: Annisa Safitriana MD)

resided but reappeared. In addition, a lump was observed in the neck, along with hoarseness, a month ago. An ultrasound examination was carried out, showing a mass appearing on the left side of the lung (Fig. 19.6).

The patient was later hospitalized for a bronchoscopy procedure, and the results showed a malignant necrotic mass in the left bronchus and a nodular lesion of the left vocal cords (Fig. 19.7). The biopsy results from the bronchoscopy revealed lung tissue with inflammation accompanied by fibrinoid necrosis, with no signs of malignancy.

Immunoserological examination (ANA, C3 Complement, C4 Complement, Anti-dsDNA-NcX) was performed, with the result being negative. Subsequently,

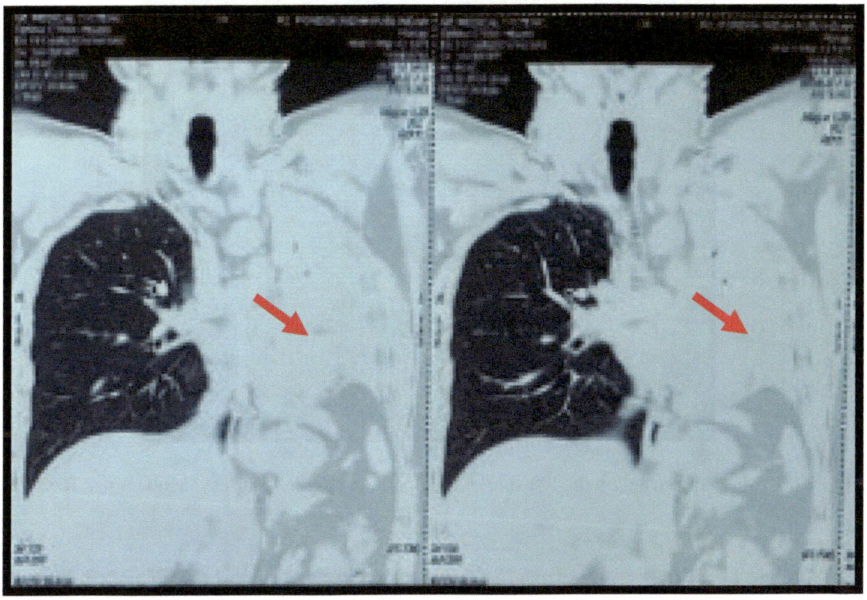

Fig. 19.3 The patient's CT scan showed a mass in the left lung. (Figure courtesy: Andi Darwis MD)

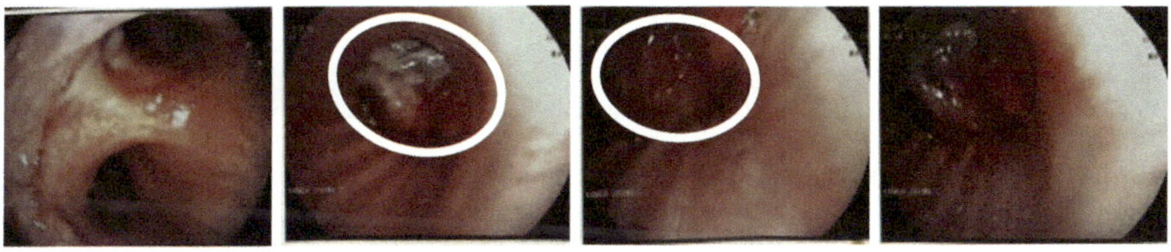

Fig. 19.4 Patient's bronchoscopy showed a necrotic mass in the left bronchus. (Figure courtesy: Eddy Suratman MD)

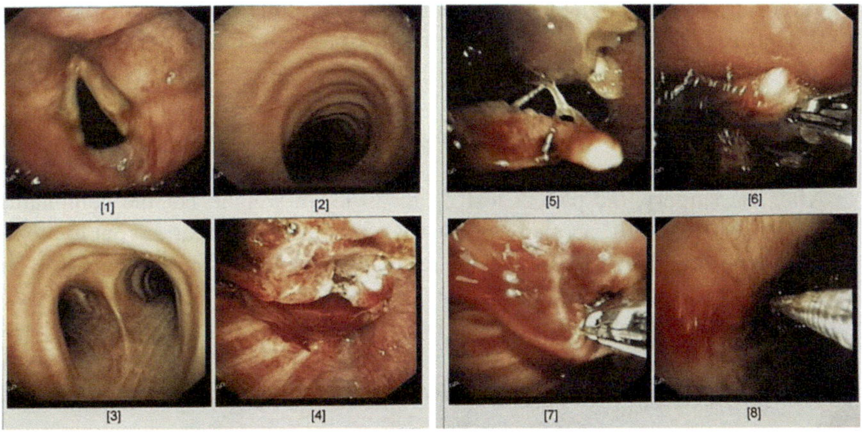

Fig. 19.5 The Patient's bronchoscopy showed a mass in the left lung. (1) Plica vocalis, (2) Trachea, (3) RMB and RLB, (4) Necrotic mass, (5) (6) (7) (8) Forceps biopsy of the necrotic mass. (Figure courtesy: Paulus Embran MD)

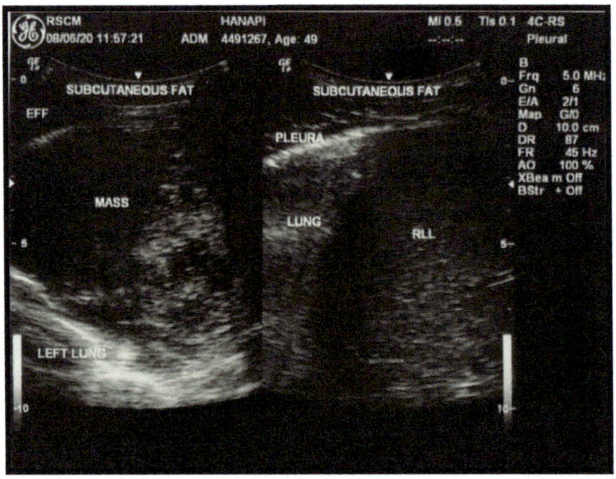

Fig. 19.6 Mass appearing on the left side of lung patient. (Figure courtesy: Mohammad Reynalzi Yugo MD)

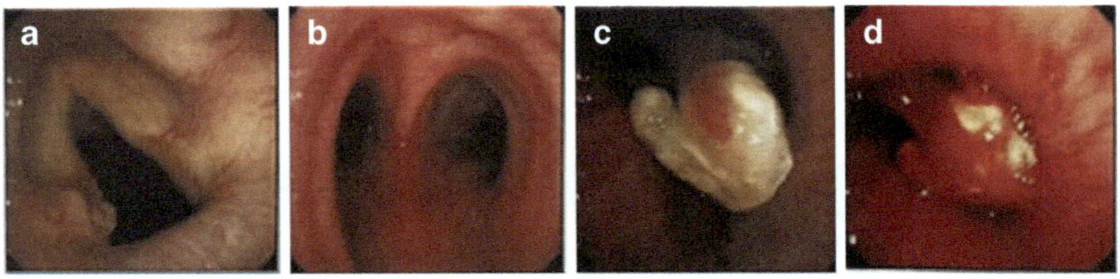

Fig. 19.7 Patient's bronchoscopy. (**a**) A nodular lesion of the left vocal cords (black arrow). (**b**) Main bronchus. (**c**) Malignant necrotic mass in the left bronchus. (**d**) Malignant necrotic mass in the left bronchus. (Figure courtesy: Gurmeet Singh MD DM PhD)

the patient consulted a thoracic surgeon and was advised to undergo lobectomy surgery, comprising the removal of the lower lobe of the left lung. Chest CT examination was performed before the lobectomy, and the results showed a complex solid mass causing obliteration of the left lower lobe of the lung with a differential diagnosed mass in the left lower lobe and left pleural mass. An invasion of the left main bronchus was also observed, causing atelectasis of the left inferior lobe (Fig. 19.8).

The patient later underwent lobectomy, and the mass of the left lower lobe was successfully removed (Fig. 19.9).

After the surgery, the patient lost up to 20 kg in weight, but the complaints improved. Subsequently, another chest X-ray examination was carried out to monitor lung condition (Fig. 19.10), with the result showing the absence of lung opacity in the left field.

Following the completion of the surgery, extensive histological examination was conducted on all lung sections showing macroscopic abnormalities (approximately 60 slides). The histological analysis revealed only areas of necrosis and bleeding,

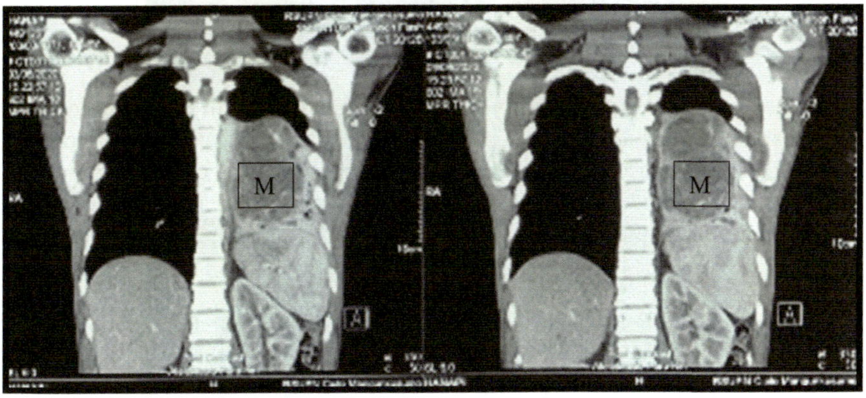

Fig. 19.8 Patient's CT scan prior to surgery. M, mass. (Figure courtesy: Taufik Agung MD)

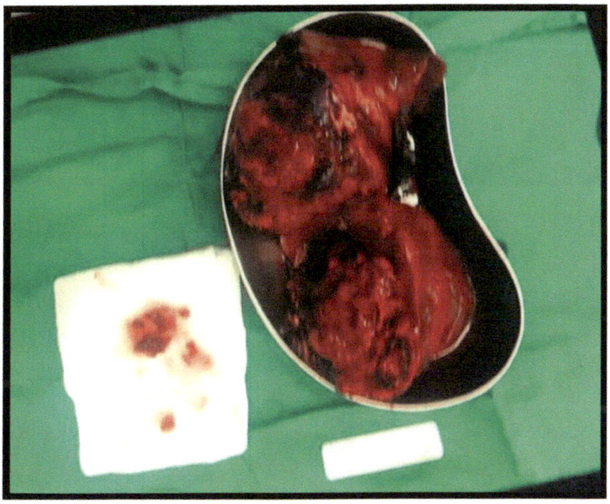

Fig. 19.9 Postoperative mass of the left lower lobe. (Figure courtesy: Muhammad Arza Putra MD DM PhD)

with several reactive atypical cells at the edges of the necrosis area. In addition, there was no sign of malignancy, as shown in Fig. 19.11.

After hospital discharge, the patient reported a return to normalcy in daily life. The surgical wound was described as tolerable, with no impediments to performing routine activities. Moreover, the patient expressed satisfaction with his overall well-being. In May 2023, during a follow-up visit, there were no complaints of coughing or shortness of breath. Physical examination showed weight gain, while ultrasonography revealed no evidence of pleural effusions. Consequently, the patient was deemed physically fit to undertake the Hajj pilgrimage.

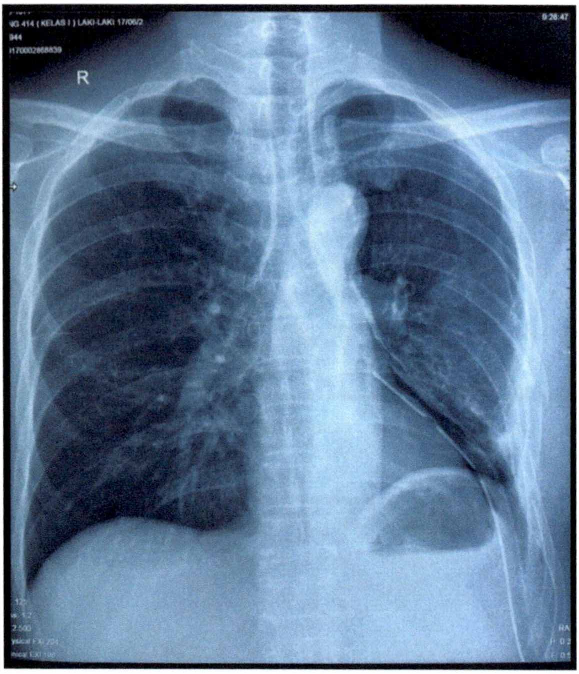

Fig. 19.10 Chest x-ray after surgery. (Figure courtesy: Reyhan Edy Yunus MD)

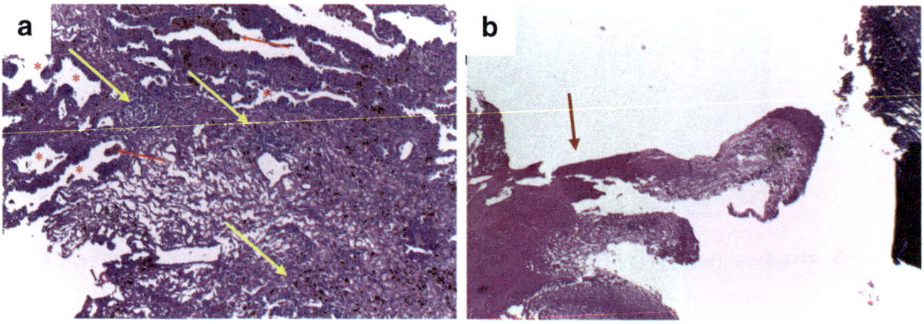

Fig. 19.11 Histology of completion surgery. (**a**) lung parenchyma with alveoli (*), alveolar macrophages (red arrow), and inflammatory cells (yellow arrow). (**b**) Areas of necrosis (red arrow). (`ure courtesy: Yayi Dwina Billianti Susanto MD)

19.2 Discussion

Pulmonary neoplasms are among the most prevalent tumors and can be classified into two categories, namely benign and malignant. However, benign lung tumors are significantly less common compared to malignant tumors. According to previous reports, benign neoplasms constitute less than 1% of pulmonary neoplasms and 8–18% of pulmonary solitary nodules. These tumors can be classified into five distinct categories, namely, epithelial, mesodermal, of uncertain origin or developmental, inflammatory, and pseudotumors or polypoid lesions. Building on this idea, the prevalence of noncancerous growths can differ based on factors such as the size and location of lung mass, the patient's age, the method used to discover the condition, and the accuracy of the final diagnosis. Patients affected by this condition typically fall in the age range of 17–77 years, with an average of 56.2 years. Tumors are considered benign in the presence of several factors, including (1) advanced nuclear organization, (2) well-differentiated cells, (3) low mitotic rate, (4) no local invasion, and (5) no distant metastasis [1, 2].

Fibrinoid necrosis is a distinct form of cell death that is irreversible and uncontrolled. This condition often occurs when complexes formed by antigens and antibodies are deposited. The occurrence of fibrinoid necrosis in lung tissue is typically associated with autoimmune diseases and can be classified as either of unknown origin or due to developing malignancies [1, 3, 4].

19.3 Clinical Manifestation

Benign lung tumors typically exhibit no symptoms due to their nonspecificity and can only be detected through radiography. Therefore, histological examination is necessary to diagnose these tumors and select the most suitable therapy approach. Respiratory symptoms typically arise from the blockage of the trachea and subsequent development of pneumonitis. In this context, the symptomatic lesions are primarily located in the central region and can function as a one-way valve depending on their size and ability to move. The phenomenon permits the intake of air into the lungs during inhalation, but hinders the passage of air through the airways during expiration, leading to the development of lobar or segmental emphysema. Partial blockage can lead to noticeable wheezing and impaired clearance of secretions, which causes pneumonia, recurring bronchitis, bronchiectasis, and the formation of abscesses. Advancement toward total blockage of the bronchus typically leads to atelectasis and necrosis of lung tissue. Hemoptysis is infrequent, with a documented incidence of 3%. Tracheal lesions commonly cause symptoms such as coughing, difficulty breathing, and wheezing [1].

19.4 Diagnosis

19.4.1 Computed Tomography (CT)

The complete extent of the influence of CT scan on the assessment and management of patients with intrathoracic anomalies has not yet been fully understood. The application of this approach in detecting numerous pulmonary lesions that are not visible using normal radiologic methods is widely recognized due to the capability to accurately document the progression of malignancy in the mediastinum. Despite the potential, the extent to which it can assist in distinguishing between stage I lung malignancies and benign pulmonary tumors remains unclear. CT scan has enhanced sensitivity in identifying calcium in peripheral pulmonary nodules, while the significance of this level of calcification remains undetermined. In certain cases, it may be feasible to accurately identify the lobulated shape and popcorn calcification of a typical hamartoma, allowing for safe nonoperative surveillance. Building on this idea, it is plausible that certain benign lesions, such as lipomas and homogenous pseudotumors, can exhibit a distinct density pattern when observed using a CT scan. The efficacy of the applications has not been confirmed, and further investigation is needed to determine the accuracy of CT scan in distinguishing between benign and malignant isolated peripheral pulmonary lesions [2].

Necrotic pulmonary lesions appear as areas of relatively low density on contrast-enhanced CT. However, distinguishing between malignant and benign necrotic pulmonary lesions by CT scan is challenging due to their comparable peripheral enhancement. To overcome the challenges, several studies have proposed the use of dual-energy spectral CT (DESCT) [5].

19.5 Percutaneous Needle Biopsy

According to previous reports, there is considerable confidence about the efficacy of percutaneous needle biopsy and aspiration biopsy in accurately diagnosing up to 91% of malignant pulmonary lesions and a significant proportion of localized inflammatory lesions. When the radiographic appearance indicates either benign or malignant tumors, needle biopsy offers limited extra information that can impact patient treatment decisions. The diagnostic accuracy for identifying benign lesions has varied between 10 and 50%, depending on the proportion of tumors in the dataset. Several studies have reported that if three consecutive needle biopsies do not indicate the presence of tumors, it is medically advisable to monitor the patient without resorting to surgery. However, the use of the approach must be restricted to high-risk patients, considering the associated time, effort, expense, and morbidity. These factors need to be contrasted with those of a prompt limited thoracotomy and removal of lesions [2].

19.6 Fiberoptic Bronchoscopy

The diagnostic efficacy of fiberoptic bronchoscopy, either alone or in combination with percutaneous needle biopsy, has been assessed for peripheral pulmonary lesions. The diagnosis accuracy for benign tumors, primarily inflammatory masses, was shown to be 38%. In this context, the diagnostic accuracy was found to be lowest in lesions with a diameter of less than 2 cm. Therefore, fiberoptic bronchoscopy is particularly beneficial for individuals at high risk or those with multiple pulmonary lesions [2].

19.7 Management

Complete removal of lesions is the preferred treatment due to the possibility of malignancy in certain lesions and their associated morbidity. Each patient is carefully assigned a specific surgery technique, with the scope of the procedure defined intraoperatively in all instances. For peripheral lesions, wedge resection is typically the preferred method. In addition, sleeve-type resection and reanastomosis can be used to preserve lung tissues in case of big bronchial tumors. This surgical approach comprises removing and reconnecting the area behind tumors while leaving the growth untouched. In the presence of pneumonia or atelectasis, the extent of lung damage hinders the preservation of lung tissues. The required procedure in this scenario is either segmentectomy or lobectomy [1].

The outcomes of surgical intervention are typically outstanding in cases of benign lung tumors, with no reported fatalities following the procedure and a 2% occurrence of postoperative problems. The advantages of this method for patients with nonmalignant conditions were found to include prompt preoperative assessment, short hospital stay, reduced expenses, and high patient satisfaction due to the confirmation of a conclusive diagnosis leading to a permanent remedy. The results show the ongoing significance of surgical excision in the treatment of individuals with nonmalignant tumors of the lung and bronchus [2].

19.8 Prognosis

Surgical treatment for patients with benign lung tumors is typically highly effective, with no report of death after the surgery. Subsequent evaluation was conducted using a standard chest radiograph, revealing no instance of recurrence after the surgical procedure [1, 2].

Key Points

Tissue biopsy is an essential diagnostic procedure in suspected cases of thoracic malignancy. Immunologic disorders are considered one of the possible etiologies in the development of lung mass.

Questions

1. The following is TRUE about lung tumors:
   (a) Benign lung tumors are very rare compared to malignant lung tumors.
   (b) 20% of pulmonary solitary nodules are comprised of benign neoplasms.
   (c) Fibrinoid necrosis pattern of lung tissue usually occurs as manifestation malignancy.
   (d) The patients are in the age range of 35–77 years with an average age of 56.2 years.
   (e) They are categorized into four groups: epithelial, mesodermal, inflammatory, pseudo tumors or polypoid lesions.

2. Impaired removal of secretions in benign lung tumors can lead to these conditions, except:
   (a) Pneumonia
   (b) Recurrent bronchitis
   (c) Bronchiectasis
   (d) Abscess formation
   (e) Wheezing
3. What is the best method to diagnose lung tumor?
   (a) Computed Tomography
   (b) Percutaneous Needle Biopsy
   (c) Fiberoptic Bronchoscopy
   (d) Thoracoscopy
   (e) Magnetic Resonance Imaging
4. The best management of lung tumor with pneumonia or atelectasis:
   (a) Lobectomy
   (b) Pneumonectomy
   (c) Bilobectomy
   (d) Radiation
   (e) Tyrosine kinase inhibitors
5. The accuracy of percutaneous needle biopsy is:
   (a) 50%
   (b) 38%
   (c) 91%
   (d) 28%
   (e) 40%

Answer Keys

1. A
2. E
3. B
4. A
5. C

Acknowledgments Ersananda Arlisa Putri MD, Department of Internal Medicine, Respirology and Critical Illness Division, Universitas Indonesia, Dr. Cipto Mangunkusumo General Central National Hospital, Jakarta, Indonesia.

Muhammad Arza Putra MD DM PhD, Department of Cardiovascular and Thoracic Surgery, Universitas Indonesia, Dr. Cipto Mangunkusumo General Central National Hospital, Jakarta, Indonesia.

References

1. Bagheri R. Evaluation of the results of surgery treatment in patients with benign lung tumors. Lung India Off Organ Indian Chest Soc. 2015;32:29–33.
2. Oldham HN. Benign tumors of the lung and bronchus. Surg Clin North Am. 1980;60:825–34.
3. Gao L-Y. Clinicopathologic characteristics of Weneger's granulomatosis: a report of three cases. Exp Ther Med. 2016;11:1340–4.
4. Kumar V, Abbas AK, Aster JC, Perkins JA. Robbins and Cotran pathologic basis of disease. 9th ed. Philadelphia; 2014.
5. Li Q. Differentiating malignant and benign necrotic lung lesions using kVp-switching dual-energy spectral computed tomography. BMC Med Imaging. 2021;21:81.

Endobronchial Lipoma

20

20.1 Case Illustration

A 60-year-old male patient presented to the hospital with a chief complaint of a fever for 2 weeks, characterized by fluctuations, with the highest temperature being 38 °C. The fever improved temporarily with paracetamol administration but later recurred. In addition, the patient reported experiencing a persistent dry cough for more than a year, intermittently disappearing and reoccurring. Occasional shortness of breath was also experienced, but symptoms of coughing up blood, heavy coughing at night, cold sweats at night, and weight loss were denied. The patient had a history of type 2 diabetes mellitus (T2DM), hypertension, smoking, and lipomas, which were spread over the back, hands, and feet. The lipomas had been successfully removed 15 times at Cipto Mangunkusumo Hospital.

On physical examination, decreased vesicular breath sounds were observed in the left lung compared to the right lung, along with minimal rhonchi at the base of the right lung. The laboratory results showed that the leukocyte value increased by 19,100 μl (4.500–11.000 μl), ESR increased 22 mm/hour (<15), CRP increased 92.2 mg/L (<5.0), HbA1c increased 6.6% (<5.7), creatinine decreased 0.70 mg/dl (0.08–1.30), eGFR increased 102.6 ml/min/1.63 m^2 (66.00–96.00), Na decreased 134 mEq/L (136–145), and K decreased 3.1 Meq/L (3.5–5.1). In addition, chest X-ray revealed the presence of cardiomegaly with aortic elongation, infiltrates in the perihilar, and left pericardiac with a differential diagnosis of pneumonia. The results also showed right perihilar fibrosis, suggestive of a previous procedure. A high left hemidiaphragm position was observed with a differential diagnosis of subdiaphragmatic process, phrenic nerve palsy, diaphragmatic events, and thoracic scoliosis (Fig. 20.1). Given these findings, the patient was advised to undergo a chest computed tomography (CT) examination.

Based on clinical findings and initial laboratory results, the patient was admitted to the hospital with a temporary diagnosis *of Community-Acquired Pneumonia* (CAP). Subsequently, thoracic CT examination procedure with contrast was

G. Singh, *Challenging Cases in Respirology and Critical Care*,
https://doi.org/10.1007/978-981-96-5002-6_20

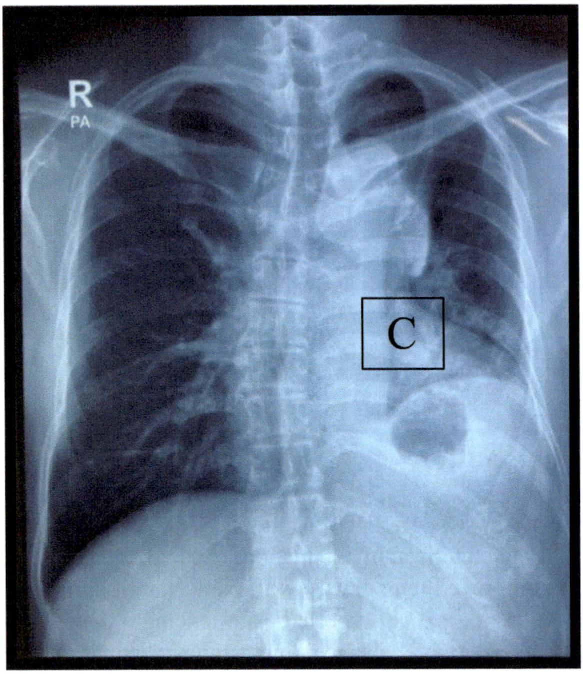

Fig. 20.1 Chest x-ray showed cardiomegaly with aortic elongation, infiltrates in the perihilar, and left pericardiac, right perihilar fibrosis. C, consolidation in the left lung. (Figure courtesy: Indrati Suroyo MD DM)

performed. The results showed a solid lesion with a fat component in the intralumen of the left main bronchus to the superior branch bronchus, which caused atelectasis of the superior lobe of the left lung. Consolidation with air bronchogram and ground glass was observed in segments 6, 7, and 8 of the left lung, with a differential diagnosis of pneumonia (Fig. 20.2).

After admission, the patient was subjected to bronchoscopy for diagnostic purposes, with the result showing a mass of the upper lobe and left bronchial lingula (Fig. 20.3).

Following the bronchoscopy, the biopsy results indicated no evidence of malignant tumor cells in the left bronchial brushing cytology. Histopathology results showed acute and chronic inflammation in the bronchial mucosa with no single feature that was indicative of malignancy. Based on the results of these examinations, the patient was diagnosed with CAP and endobronchial lipomas. Subsequently, the patient consulted a thoracic surgeon to remove the mass because bronchoscopy resection equipment was not available in the current facility. However, the patient declined the surgical intervention, leading to the administration of symptomatic therapy based on the complaints. The clinical condition improved, and the patient was advised to attend regular appointments to evaluate the size of the lipomas.

During a follow-up visit in March, the patient reported a significant reduction in coughing and shortness of breath. Subsequently, a thoracic CT examination was performed for lipomas evaluation. The results showed that there was still an

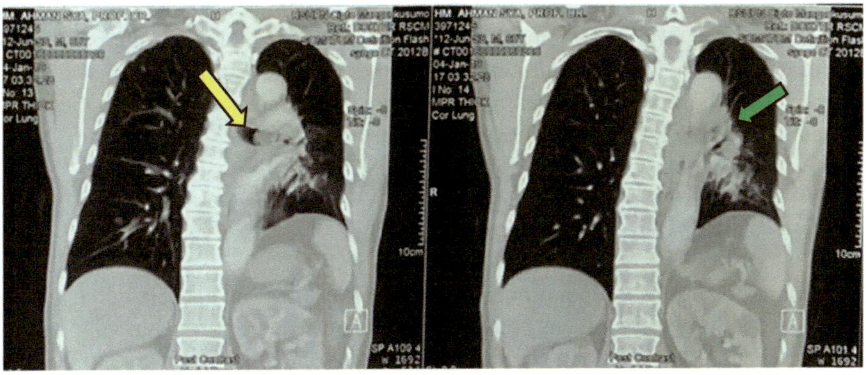

Fig. 20.2 Thoracic CT showed a solid lesion with a fat component in the intralumen of the left main bronchus to the superior branch bronchus (yellow arrow), postobstructive atelectasis is present (green arrow). (Figure courtesy: Indrati Suroyo MD DM)

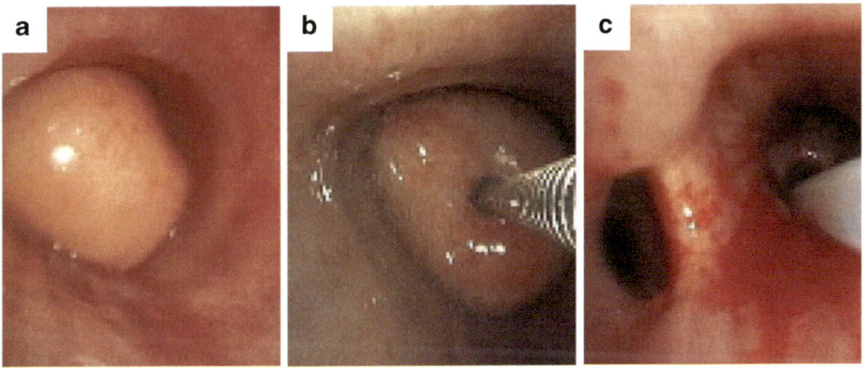

Fig. 20.3 Bronchoscopy results in the patient contained a mass of the upper lobe and left bronchial lingula. (**a**) Endobronchial lipoma in left main bronchus. (**b**) Forceps biopsy on endobronchial lipoma. (**c**) Brushing in the lower lobe of left bronchus. (Figure courtesy: Gurmeet Singh MD DM PhD)

irregular oval heterogeneous lesion in the intralumen of the left main bronchus and an extension to the superior branch bronchus, which caused atelectasis of the superior lobe of the left lung. However, the impression was reduced compared to the previous CT scan. Despite recommendations for surgical intervention, the patient declined and continued routine follow-ups without respiratory problems.

20.2 Discussion

Endobronchial lipomas are infrequent noncancerous growths in the lung that can lead to blockage of the bronchial tubes and damage to lung tissue. Although rare in origin, these conditions are frequently misdiagnosed due to the similarity in their clinical presentation to obstructive lung diseases, such as COPD and asthma. In addition, the occurrence rate ranges from 0.1% to 0.5% of all lung tumors. Several studies have shown that endobronchial lipomas are not harmful but can lead to blockage of the bronchial tubes and associated consequences, such as the early onset of difficulty breathing and wheezing [1].

20.3 Clinical Manifestation

Common indications of endobronchial lipomas consist of an enduring cough, thoracic discomfort, difficulty in breathing, recurring fever, and pneumonia. In this context, hemoptysis is a rare occurrence, but can sometimes occur due to postobstructive infection. However, none of these clinical characteristics can differentiate endobronchial lipomas from their malignant equivalents, such as bronchial carcinoid and mucoepidermoid carcinoma postobstructive alterations, such as atelectasis or pneumonia [2]. Clinically, distinguishing signs and symptoms of endobronchial neoplasms from those produced by other respiratory disorders is often. Therefore, imaging investigations play a crucial role in determining the diagnosis of endobronchial neoplasms. Identifying abnormalities on routine chest radiography can also be challenging, as it typically shows normal or vague postobstructive alterations, such as atelectasis or pneumonia [2].

20.4 Diagnosis

The diagnosis is often established using imaging techniques, primarily CT scan, followed by confirmation with a biopsy. The presence of endobronchial lipomas is typically identified using a CT scan, which reveals an intrabronchial mass with a density similar to that of fat and no enhancement after the administration of contrast material. Building on this idea, a CT scan is highly useful for precisely determining the location and size of tumors. Chest X-ray can reveal atelectasis or consolidation of lung beyond tumors. CT scan and chest X-ray are essential diagnostic instruments for detecting potential endobronchial abnormalities. A definitive diagnosis is typically achieved through either an incisional or excisional biopsy. For these noncancerous tumors, excisional biopsy is preferred as it provides a higher probability of confirming the diagnosis, compared to techniques such as brushing or lavage performed using a flexible bronchoscope, which may not capture abnormal cells effectively [3].

Endobronchial lipomas are noncancerous tumors composed of mature fat cells, which do not exhibit any abnormal cellular characteristics. These tumors often originate in the mucosa but can also develop in the spaces between cartilages. Several studies have reported their distinctive hourglass form and association with the bronchial walls. A lipomatous hamartoma is typically assigned to tumors that contain cartilage, bone, or smooth muscle. Therefore, prompt diagnosis is crucial to avert potential bronchial blockage or other problems [3].

20.5 Management

Endobronchial lipomas have been surgically treated due to the occurrence of post-obstructive alterations in lung tissue and the challenge of distinguishing the growth from cancerous tumors. However, surgical procedures, such as pneumonectomy, lobectomy, bilobectomy, and resection by bronchotomy, must only be performed under certain conditions. These include when there is a potential presence of malignant tumors, irreversible damage to lung tissue, an extension of the disease beyond the bronchial area or into the outer layer of the lung, and when there are anticipated challenges in using bronchoscopy due to multidirectional growth [4].

At present, bronchoscopy resection is recommended as the primary approach for treating endobronchial lipomas, as it serves both diagnostic and therapeutic purposes. In addition, both flexible and rigid bronchoscopy have proven to be effective in this regard [4, 5].

Various methodologies can also be used with the flexible bronchoscope to extract endobronchial malignancies. The most commonly used method comprises removing tumors, either partially or entirely in the event of a growth with a stalk, using an electrocautery snare. The excised tumors can be removed using either biopsy forceps or Dormia basket forceps. The technique can also be conducted using the rigid bronchoscope, where the barrel of the rigid scope is used to remove excess tissue mechanically, and the growth can be retrieved using stiff forceps. Endobronchial electrosurgery, a cost-effective and readily accessible treatment, has been reported as both affordable and reasonably simple to perform [6].

Despite the potential, the rigid bronchoscope remains the most important instrument for therapeutic airway procedures and provides excellent airway control, as shown in this case. In addition, a flexible bronchoscope can be introduced through the barrel of a rigid bronchoscope and appears to be the preferred mode for performing these therapeutic procedures. The complete elimination of harmless tumors in the bronchial tubes has been effectively accomplished by employing electrosurgical snaring with a fiberoptic scope inserted through the rigid bronchoscope. Excised tissue can be extracted using the instrument, and in instances of substantial tissue, it can be removed along with the rigid bronchoscope [7].

20.6 Prognosis

Several studies have shown that the recurrence rate of endobronchial lipomas is typically low. In two extensive studies where interventional bronchoscopy was used to treat endobronchial lipoma, none of the patients experienced a recurrence of tumors [4, 5].

Key Points

Endobronchial lipomas usually occur in patients with multiple superficial lipomas. Conservative treatment can be a possibility in cases where interventional pulmonology procedures are not available.

Questions

1. The incidence of endobronchial lipomas:
   (a) 0.1% of all lung tumors
   (b) 0.5% of all lung tumors
   (c) 0.2% of all lung tumors
   (d) 0.1 to 0.5% of all lung tumors
   (e) 0.1 to 0.2% of all lung tumors
2. Below are common symptoms of endobronchial lipoma, except:
   (a) Chest pain
   (b) Dyspnea
   (c) Loss weight
   (d) Persistent cough
   (e) Recurrent fever
3. A definitive diagnosis of endobronchial lipoma is obtained from:
   (a) MRI
   (b) CT scan
   (c) Bronchoscopy
   (d) Excisional biopsy
   (e) Medical thoracoscopy
4. Endobronchial lipomas are histologically benign tumors that consist of:
   (a) Cartilage
   (b) Bone
   (c) Smooth muscle
   (d) Cellular atypia
   (e) Mature adipose tissue
5. Indications of surgery in endobronchial lipoma include the following, except:
   (a) Possible coexistent malignant tumor
   (b) Distal irreversible parenchymal destructive changes
   (c) Proximal irreversible parenchymal destructive changes
   (d) Extra-bronchial extension or subpleural disease and
   (e) Expected technical difficulties during bronchoscopy resection

Answer Keys

1. D
2. C
3. D
4. E
5. C

Acknowledgments Ersananda Arlisa Putri MD, Department of Internal Medicine, Respirology and Critical Illness Division, Universitas Indonesia, Dr. Cipto Mangunkusumo General Central National Hospital, Jakarta, Indonesia.
Muhammad Arza Putra MD DM PhD, Department of Cardiovascular and Thoracic Surgery, Universitas Indonesia, Dr. Cipto Mangunkusumo General Central National Hospital, Jakarta, Indonesia.

References

1. Anbazhakan L. Endobronchial lipoma. Autopsy Case Rep. 2022;12:e2021377.
2. Cao D. Endobronchial lipoma: an unusual cause of bronchial obstruction. Case Rep Med. 2011;2011:939808.
3. Elsayed H, Traify R, McKeon D, Poullis M. An endobronchial lipoma. J Bronchol Interv Pulmonol. 2010;17:95–6.
4. Muraoka M, Oka T, Akamine S, Nagayasu T, Iseki M, Suyama N. Endobronchial lipoma: review of 64 cases reported in Japan. Chest. 2003;123(1):293–6.
5. Nassiri AH, Dutau H, Breen D, Colchen A, Quiot JJ, Nguyen B. A multicenter retrospective study investigating the role of interventional bronchoscopic techniques in the management of endobronchial lipomas. Respiration. 2008;75:79–84.
6. Huisman C, Kralingen KW, Postmus PE, Sutedja TG. Endobronchial lipoma: a series of three cases and the role of electrocautery. Respiration. 2000;67:689–92.
7. Gerasin VA, Shafirovsky BB. Endobronchial electrosurgery. Chest. 1988;93:270–4.

21 Multiple Primary Malignant Tumors (MPMTs): Lung, Thyroid, and Mammae Cancer

21.1 Case Illustration

A 39-year-old female patient presented with complaints of severe shortness of breath 2 days before admission. This condition was not affected by activity but aggravated with a supine position. Accompanying symptoms included sleeping using two to three pillows and a productive cough. Although experiencing no nausea and vomiting, there was no decreased appetite, with only a few mouthfuls consumed due to a sensation of fullness. Additionally, there was a complaint of heartburn, and the last defecation was 6 days ago, without weight loss. A post-total thyroidectomy of thyroid carcinoma was conducted 2 weeks ago, and the patient was referred from the previous hospital for the ablation plan. In the past 11 years, there was a complaint of a lump in the left neck, the size of a quail egg, and painless. The patient had a *fine needle* aspiration *biopsy* and an ultrasound of the neck before, but the result was a benign tumor, which did not require further action.

Two years before admission, the lump had increased in size and felt tight. Subsequently, chest X-ray and computed tomography (CT) scan were conducted, showing lung fluid taken 10 times without infection. After the thyroidectomy surgery, consultation with an oncologist led to the prescription for thyrax 1 × 50 mcg, sucralfate, paracetamol, lansoprazole, triacetate 2 × 15 ml, and redacid 250 1 × 1. However, the patient denied a history of hypertension, diabetes mellitus, hepatitis, pulmonary tuberculosis (TB), and autoimmune disease.

On physical examination, blood pressure was 159/90 mmHg, the left breast appeared larger than the right, no erythema was observed, and all the breasts were hard to feel, immobile, and tender. The thorax appeared asymmetrical, the left lung lagged during inspiration, the fremitus decreased in the left lung, and the left vesicular was reduced. Laboratory results showed various abnormalities, including a high level of leukocytes (12.200/μL), a high level of TSH sensitivity (61.407), and a low level of thyroglobulin (5.78). The histological of the left isthmolobectomy at the

G. Singh, *Challenging Cases in Respirology and Critical Care*,
https://doi.org/10.1007/978-981-96-5002-6_21

previous hospital showed encapsulated tumor pieces arranged in follicles and microfollicles consisting of proliferation of cells with clearing nuclei, ground glass, groves, arranged overlapping, and thin cytoplasm. The tumor did not penetrate the capsule, consistent with a diagnosis of *papillary thyroid carcinoma*, follicular variant. The pathological results of right thyroid completion surgery showed pieces of thyroid tissue comprising a proliferation of follicles of various sizes and shapes, covered by a single layer of cuboidal epithelium without nuclear atypia. After these evaluations, tumor cell infiltration was observed. The patient passed through chest X-ray (Fig. 21.1) and ultrasound of the neck, which showed a suspected massive left pleural effusion with an atelectasis component. However, there were no metastatic nodules visualized in the right lung.

The ultrasound of the neck (Fig. 21.2) showed heterogeneous lesions in bilateral thyroid beds, suspected postoperative inflammation, without visible structures suggesting thyroid tissue in bilateral thyroid beds, and lymphadenopathy.

A pleural ultrasound procedure was performed and continued with a pleural puncture, which showed 700 ccs of hemorrhagic fluid. The patient was hospitalized in the usual room, as TB was not suspected based on current complaints.

On the 2nd day of treatment, the patient reported a reduction in shortness of breath but experienced occasional coughing. Complaints were also accompanied by pain near the gut and left-side back pain (VAS 3), with the last defecation occurring 7 days ago. Physical examination showed blood pressure of 139/84 mmHg and decreased vesicular sounds on auscultation of the vesicular of the left thoracic, with a fluid balance of −250 ml/12 hours.

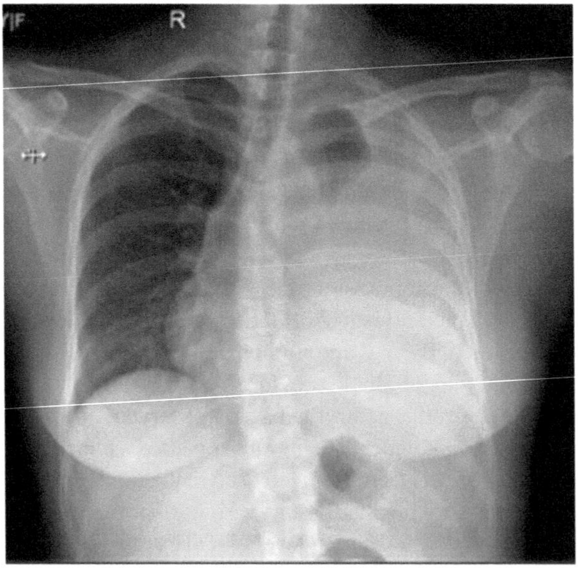

Fig. 21.1 Chest x-ray shows homogenous opacity in the left hemithorax, suggesting a pleural effusion or mass. (Figure courtesy: Vally Wulani MD DM)

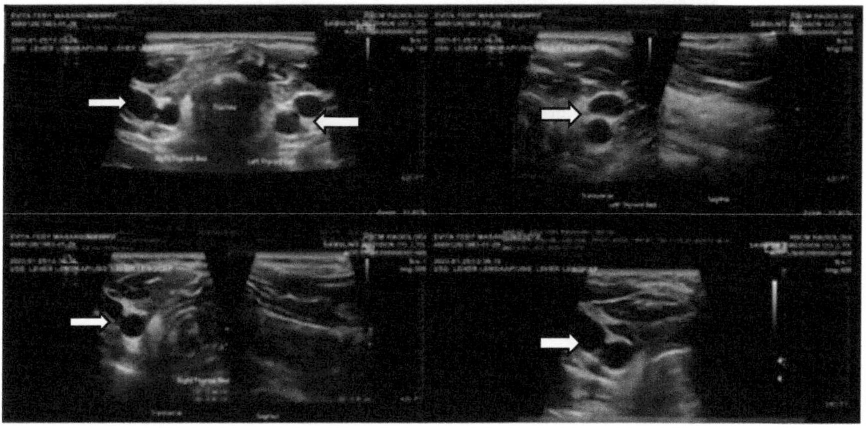

Fig. 21.2 Neck ultrasound showed heterogeneous lesions in bilateral thyroid beds (white arrows). (Figure courtesy: Vally Wulani MD DM)

On the 1st day of hospitalization at Cipto Mangunkusumo Hospital, the voice became hoarse with prolonged talking, and constipation was reported. Physical examination showed a blood pressure of 149/100 mmHg, with persistent decrease of vesicular sounds in the left thoracic on auscultation. Laboratory examination showed a high level of CRP (34.6), CA125 (167.2 U/ml), D-Dimer (950 ng/ml), and C3 complement (149). The analysis of pleural fluid showed an exudative and negative for acid-fast bacilli (AFB).

On the 2nd day in the hospital, the patient complained of heartburn, decreased appetite, and pain in the pleura puncture area. Physical examinations showed a blood pressure of 130/89 mmHg, with Daily Blood Glucose Curve at 05.00: 103 mg/dl; 11.30: 202 mg/dl; 16.00: 269 mg/dl.

The next days (around the 3rd–fifth day) in the hospital, laboratory examination showed high level of SGOT (64) and SGPT (121). The urine culture showed isolates of Klebsiella pneumonia (colonies >10,000) resistant to cefotaxime, ceftriaxone, ceftazidime, piptazo, cefosulbactam, cefepime, meropenem, imipenem, and levofloxacin. Chest X-ray showed pleural effusion with differential diagnosis of pleural thickening, with Daily Blood Glucose Curve at 05.00: 103 mg/dl; 12.00: 255 mg/dl; 18.00: 277 mg/dl. The patient was subjected to a chest X-ray (Fig. 21.3) to evaluate the lungs after a puncture. The results showed pleural effusion in the left hemithorax, with suspicion of an atelectasis component. Pleural effusion slightly increased, without visualized metastatic nodules in the right lung.

The patient was subjected to a thoracic ultrasound and medical thoracocentesis. Subsequently, pleural fluid was brought to the anatomical pathology department for pleural cytology examination.

On the 6th day in the hospital, the patient passed through an abdominal ultrasound examination (Fig. 21.4) in the Radiology room. The examination showed a left pleural effusion, but there was no accumulation of intraperitoneal fluid, signs of peritonitis, or abnormalities in the visualized intraabdominal organs.

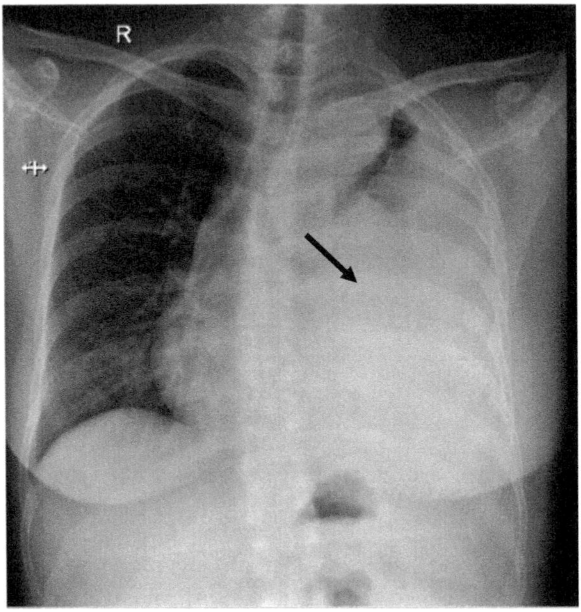

Fig. 21.3 Chest x-ray shows no visualized metastatic nodules in the right lung. Suspected left lung complicated pleural effusion. (Figure courtesy: Taufik Agung Wibowo MD DM)

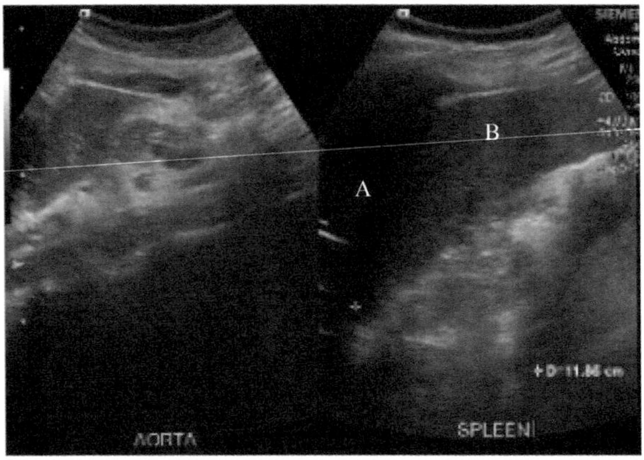

Fig. 21.4 The abdominal ultrasound shows a left pleural effusion. (**a**) Pleural effusion; (**b**) spleen. (Figure courtesy: Taufik Agung Wibowo MD DM)

The next days (around the 10th–16th day) in the hospital, the patient had a chest tube insertion procedure and was connected to a water-sealed drainage (WSD) system. Laboratory examination showed a high level of CRP (8.6), elevated D-Dimer (>32,000), and Adenosine Deaminase was non-TB (23.00). The second pleural fluid analysis showed an exudative fluid and tested negative for AFB as well as malignant cells. Furthermore, medical thoracoscopy was performed (Fig. 21.5).

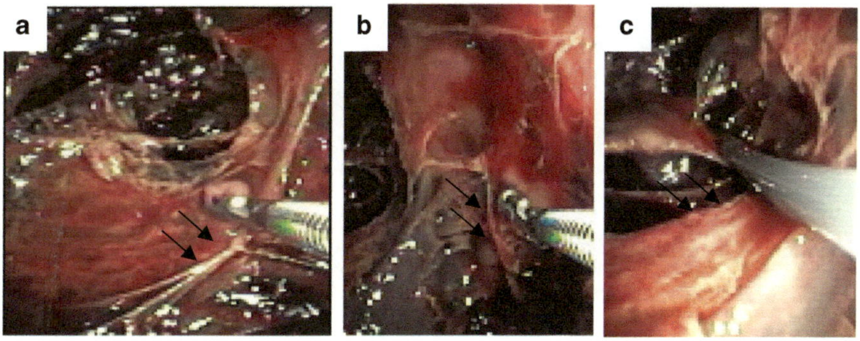

Fig. 21.5 (**a**–**c**) Thoracoscopy imaging shows hemorrhagic pleural fluid with multiple septal in pleural space. (Figure courtesy: Gurmeet Singh MD DM PhD, Ray Bryan Charles Rattu MD)

The histological of the tissue showed carcinoma but could not conclude the type and origin (Fig. 21.6). The immunohistochemical results *showed positive TTF1, positive CK7, focal P40, Ki67 30%, and positive Napsin A*. The histopathological and immunohistochemical staining support a nonsmall cell lung cancer of the adenocarcinoma type with eGFR mutation exon 21 L858R.

The patient received systemic chemotherapy and was planned to begin targeted treatment. Chest X-ray imaging (Fig. 21.7) showed left hydropneumothorax; the effusion component was reduced compared to the previous day, accompanied by an atelectatic component.

On the 19th–24th day of hospitalization, WSD production was gradually reduced. Laboratory examination showed a normal level of PCT (16.5) and CRP (57.6). The urination test showed clear yellow urine, leukocytes 2–3, erythrocytes 2–3, epithelium +1, amorphous crystals +2, BJ 1.010, pH 8.0, blood +1, Urobilinogen 3,2. Cylinders, bacteria, albumin, glucose, ketones, bilirubin, nitrites, and leukocyte esterase were negative. The patient fasted to receive an EGD examination procedure, with the results showing grade A left antrum reflux esophagitis and antrum gastritis.

On the 26th day in the hospital, laboratory examination showed a high level of TSH (41.657) and a low level of Thyroglobulin (0.53). The complaint had improved, but the patient was scheduled for control at the outpatient department while waiting for the ablation schedule.

Two days after discharge from the hospital, the patient returned and complained of persistent shortness of breath, particularly when changing positions. Additionally, there was a complaint of pain in the left side of the chest, lack of appetite, and general weakness. Physical examination showed a decreased vesicular on the left lung and a palpable lump in the left breast approximately 5 cm in diameter and hard in consistency. Chest X-ray examination showed there was left hydropneumothorax accompanied by passive atelectasis, with an increasing effusion component. Based on the results, chest tube reinsertion with a water-sealed drainage (WSD) system was planned to remove the fluid from the lungs. Subsequently, the patient was admitted for further management.

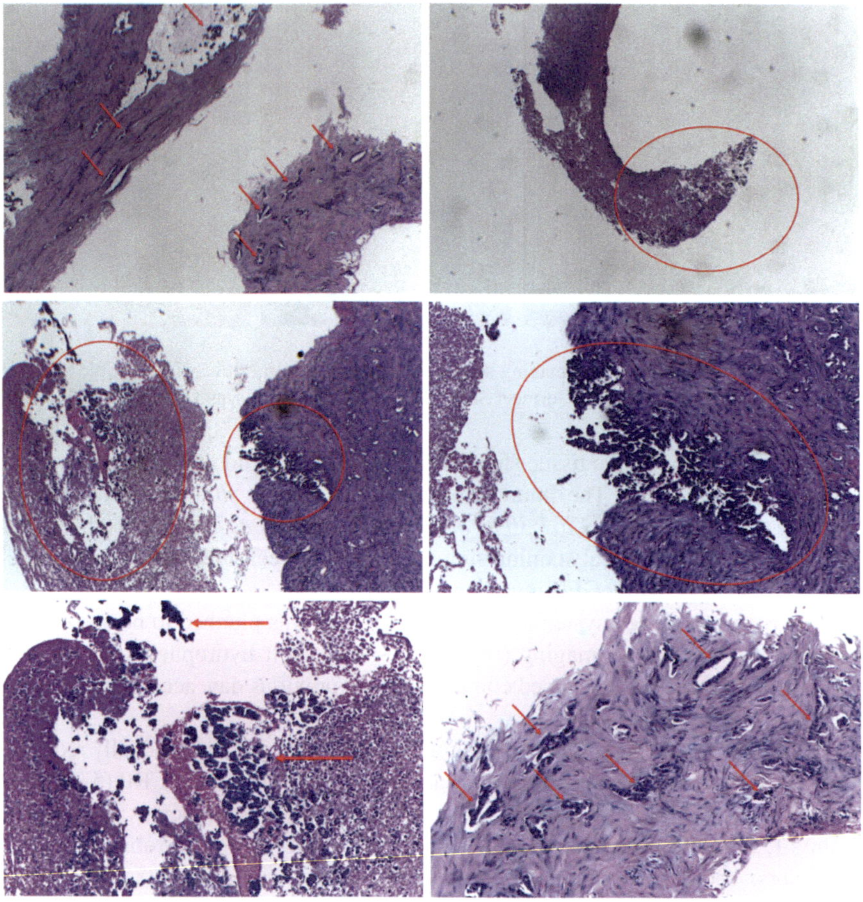

Fig. 21.6 The histological showed lung tissue with an infiltrative tumor mass (red arrow; red circle). (Figure courtesy: Yayi Dwina Billianti Susanto MD DM PhD)

On the next day, a whole-body scan examination (Fig. 21.8) was conducted, showing residual thyroid tissue in the thyroid bed bilaterally. The results also showed a faint pathological active process in the left coli projection with a differential diagnosis of lymph node metastases and minimal active pathological process in bilateral hemithorax or lung projections. However, there was no clear imaging of the distant metastases in other parts of the body.

Water-sealed drainage fluid production decreased gradually. Subsequently, a CT scan of the whole abdomen with contrast (Fig. 21.9) and an ultrasound of the breast were performed (Fig. 21.10). The results showed there was atelectasis in the lower lobe of the left lung with multiple nodules suggestive of metastases, left hydropneumothorax with WSD catheter, hepatomegaly, a simple leid-renal cyst (Bosniak I), and thoracolumbar vertebral column scoliosis.

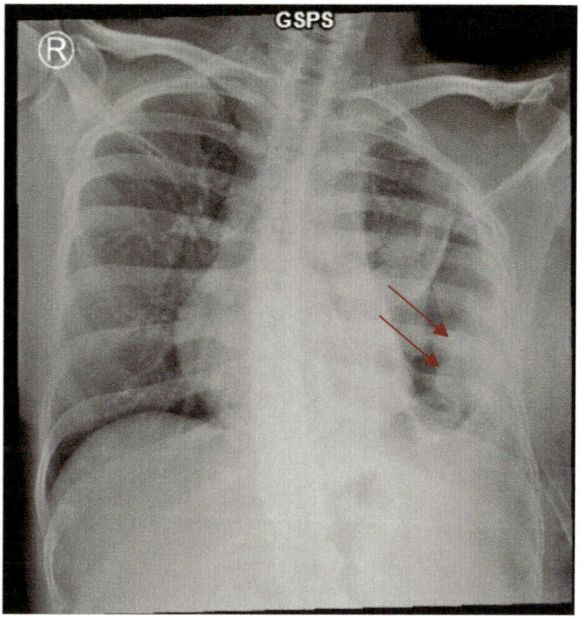

Fig. 21.7 Chest x-ray shows left hydropneumothorax, and the effusion component is reduced compared to the previous day. (Figure courtesy: Rahmad Mulyadi MD DM PhD)

Breast ultrasound showed a solid mass that filled the left mammary gland, compatible with BIRADS 5. A heterogeneous solid mass was observed in the right mammary gland, classified as BI-RADS 4b. Additionally, there was a cystic lesion on the left breast, compatible with BIRADS 2, and lymphadenopathy with malignant characteristics in the left axillary region (Fig. 21.10).

The patient received a fine needle aspiration biopsy procedure of the breast to obtain tissue samples. The *histology was positive* for malignant carcinoma leaning toward invasive carcinoma of "no special type" mammary dextra second degree (tubulus score 3, core score 2, mitotic score 1, and total score 6), with lymphovascular invasion (Fig. 21.11). Immunohistochemical examination showed molecular profile results consistent with triple-negative breast cancer.

Laboratory examination showed a low level of Albumin (2.2 g/dl), a normal level of FT4 (1.75 ng/dl), a low level of hemoglobin (9.2 g/dl), a normal level of Hematokrit (26.9%) and Trombosit (299 × 10^3/mL), a high level of Leukocytes (15.37 × 10^3/mL) and Urea (36.4 mg/dl), a normal level of Creatinine (1.0 mg/dl) and eGFR (70.6 ml/min/1.73m^2), as well as a low level of Sodium (Na) 129 meq/l, Potassium (K) 3.8 meq/l, and low level of Chloride (Cl) 84.8 meq/l. The patient planned to continue the chemotherapy after clinical improvement (Table 21.1).

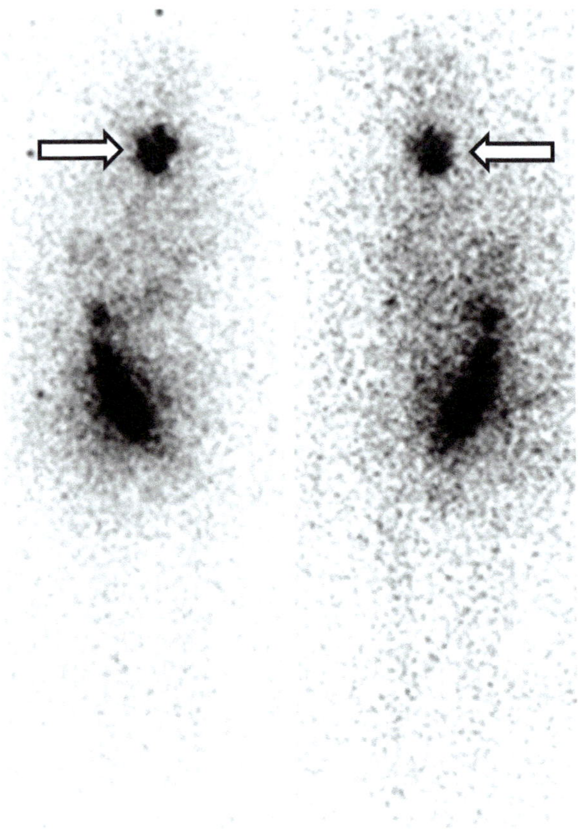

Fig. 21.8 A whole-body scan of the patient (white arrow) residual thyroid tissue in the thyroid bed bilaterally. (Figure courtesy: Alvita Dewi Siswoyo MD)

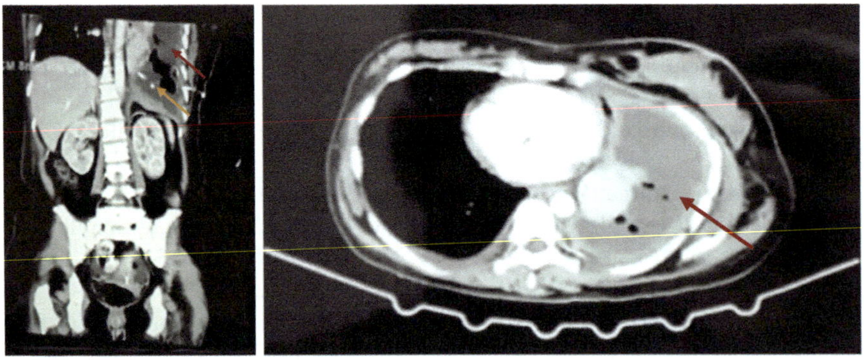

Fig. 21.9 CT scan of the whole abdomen with contrast results showed that there was atelectasis (red narrow) in the lower lobe of the left lung with multiple nodules (orange narrow) suggestive of metastases. (Figure courtesy: Vally Wulani MD DM)

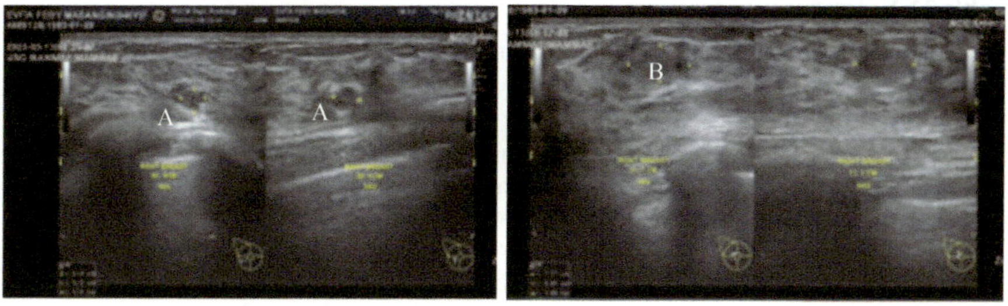

Fig. 21.10 Breast ultrasound of the patient. (**a**) Cystic lesion. (**b**) Solid mass that filled the left mammary gland. (Figure courtesy: Vally Wulani MD DM)

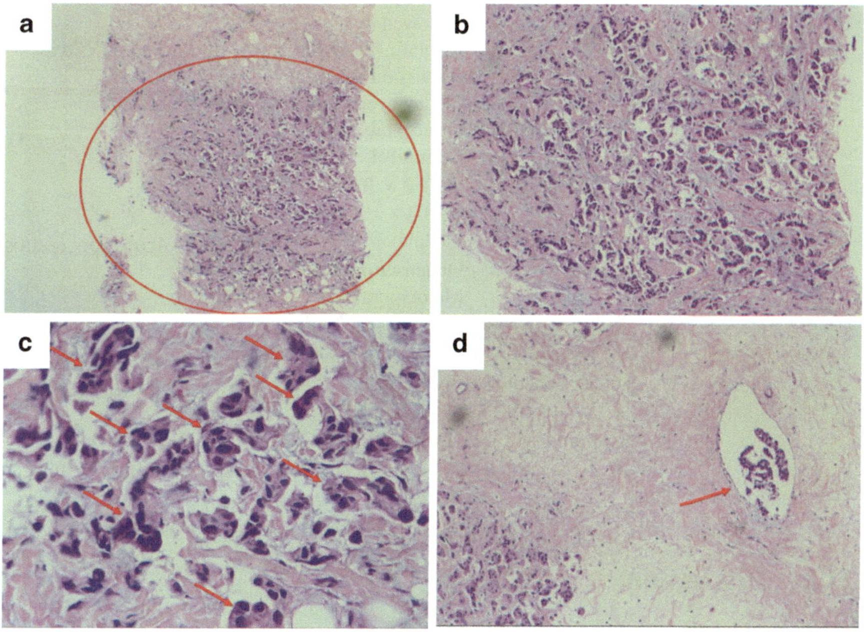

Fig. 21.11 The result of the biopsy procedure of the breast. (**a**) Tumor mass (red round); (**b**) tumor mass; (**c**) tumor cells (red arrow); (**d**) tumor cells in blood vessels (red arrow). (Figure courtesy: Yayi Dwina Billianti Susanto MD DM PhD)

Table 21.1 Treatment management

Intervention	Group/type	Drugs/fluids
Medicamentosa/ fluids	Medical gas	Oxygen
	Intravenous (IV) fluids	NaCl 0.9% Amino Acids and Glucose, Electrolytes and Vitamin B1 solution (Bfluid) Dextrose 40% Asering
	Chemotherapy agent	Docetaxel/cisplatin fourth cycle schedule June 28, 2023 if eligible (if eGFR<60 in cisplatin room replace carboplatin) BB 39 kg TB 160 cm BSA 1,35 m^2 Docetaxel 75 mg/m^2 = 101 mg = 100 mg IV over 60 minutes on day 1 Followed by Cisplatin 75 mg/m^2 = 101 mg = 100 mg IV over 2 hours on day 1 21-day cycle until disease progression or unacceptable toxicity Gefitinib 1 × 250 mg
	Cancer pain therapy	MST 2 × 30 mg orally MIR 4 × 10 mg orally Lactulax 3 × 15 ml orally
	CNIV therapy	Ondansetron 3 × 8 mg orally. Metoclopramide 3 × 10 mg orally. Omeprazole 2 × 20 mg orally.
	Thyroid therapy	Euthyrox 1 × 200 mcg orally
	Psychopharmaceutic	Fluoxetine 1 × 20 mg orally Clobazam 2 × 5 mg orally
	Hyponatremia therapy	Nacl 1000 mg × 3 orally
Devices/tools	Drain	Water-sealed drainage

21.2 Discussion

Multiple primary malignant tumors (MPMTs) refer to the occurrence of two or more separate malignant tumors in an individual that are not caused by recurrence, metastasis, or local spread. The most common tumor associations were found between genital–skin–breast, skin–skin–skin, digestive–genital–breast, and genital–breast–lung cancer [1].

21.3 Incidence

The incidence of second primary malignancies has increased in recent decades due to the expanding and aging population of individuals who have survived their first disease. The rising occurrence of numerous primary cancers can be attributed to several factors, including advancements in diagnostic testing, the development of more advanced and effective treatments, and enhanced screening and monitoring of cancer patients [2]. Moreover, the discovery of individuals with several primary malignant tumors has become a widespread phenomenon. In early 1921, research showed that among 3000 cases of malignancy, 4.7% had multiple growths. The prevalence of numerous primary cases in epidemiological research was typically reported to be between 2% and 17% [2].

21.4 Classification

Multiple primary malignant tumors (MPMTs) can be diagnosed either synchronously, within six months of detecting the first primary cancer, or metachronously, when diagnosed more than six months after the first primary cancer. Moertel proposed an alternative classification for MPMTs and multicentric malignancies in 1977, categorizing them into three main groups:

- *Group I*: Cancers occurring in organs with the same histology. This group is further divided into three subgroups:
  - *Subgroup A*: Cancer arising in the same tissue and organ.
  - *Subgroup B*: Cancer originating from the same tissue but in different organs.
  - *Subgroup C*: Cancer occurring in bilateral organs.
- *Group II*: Cancers originating from different tissues.
- *Group III*: Cancers from different tissues and organs coexisting with Group I cancers, resulting in three or more distinct primary cancers [3].

21.5 Diagnosis

The diverse clinical characteristics and rarity of multiple primary malignant tumors (MPMTs) often result in a lack of familiarity among practitioners in diagnosing and managing this condition. MPMTs are frequently mistaken for recurrences or metastases of the initial cancer, leading to inappropriate treatment strategies. The diagnostic criteria for MPMTs include: (1) each tumor must exhibit distinct malignant histological features; (2) each tumor must represent a separate pathological subtype; and (3) the possibility of the second cancer being a metastasis from the initial primary cancer must be excluded [4].

21.6 Management

The therapeutic approach to multiple primary malignant tumors (MPMTs) is guided by the stage and pathological type of each tumor, as well as the patient's overall physical condition. After confirmation through pathological examination, each tumor must be assessed and classified individually [1].

When a new lesion is detected in a patient with stage IV cancer, rebiopsy or multiple biopsies should be considered under the following circumstances:

1. The patient is in good physical condition with no contraindications for biopsy.
2. Tumor marker elevations are inconsistent with the expected cancer type (e.g., elevated AFP levels with new liver lesions in a patient with lung cancer).
3. Imaging reveals lesions in uncommon sites for metastasis.

A preliminary PET-CT scan can aid in identifying multiple tumors and guide treatment planning in certain cases. Patient financial capacity and willingness also play a significant role in shaping treatment strategies and outcomes. Multidisciplinary team (MDT) discussions are crucial for addressing complex cases. Treatment should prioritize the tumor that poses the greatest threat to the patient's survival or quality of life [1].

For patients eligible for surgery, resection of both tumors is ideal and can be supplemented with additional therapies such as chemoradiotherapy, endocrine therapy, or other modalities. Preoperative risk assessment and postoperative monitoring are critical, particularly for patients undergoing major organ resections. Postoperative care generally follows National Comprehensive Cancer Network (NCCN) guidelines tailored to the pathological stage of each tumor [1].

When a single chemotherapy regimen is unsuitable for all MPMTs, priority should be given to an effective regimen targeting tumors with higher malignancy or more advanced stages. A subset of patients with MPMTs may decline surgery, chemotherapy, or radiotherapy due to various factors, necessitating a personalized and patient-centered approach [1].

21.7 Prognosis

Patients with three tumors occurring at the same time had a mortality risk 6.5 times greater than those with tumors occurring at different dates. Additionally, patients who had one metachronous tumor and two synchronous tumors showed a mortality risk three times greater compared to the metachronous group. Being male and aged above 50 at the initial diagnosis of the main tumor was also correlated with an increased chance of death [5].

Key Points
Occurrence of triple primary malignant tumors is rare, but is still possible. Prognosis of three synchronous tumors is significantly worse compared to metachronous tumors.

Questions

1. The following is True about multiple primary malignant tumors (MPMTs):
   (a) The reported frequency of multiple primary tumors ranges from 2% to 17%.
   (b) The most common tumor associations are between digestive, skin, and breast cancers.
   (c) A contributing factor to the increased frequency of MPMTs is the lack of diagnostic tests.

   (d) The concept of MPMTs is not new, with one report documenting 300 cases.
   (e) MPMTs are defined as the presence of three or more histologically distinct malignant tumors.
2. The classification of MPMTs:
   (a) Group III includes multiple primary cancers originating from different tissues.
   (b) Group I includes multiple primary cancers occurring in organs with the same histology.
   (c) Metachronous tumors are diagnosed within six months of the first primary cancer.
   (d) Synchronous tumors are diagnosed more than six months after the first primary cancer.
   (e) Group II consists of cancers arising from different tissues and organs, occurring alongside group I cancers.
3. Which of the following is a diagnostic criteria of MPMTs:
   (a) Each tumor must exhibit definite malignant histopathological changes.
   (b) At least one malignancy must have an independent pathological type.
   (c) At least one malignancy must show definitive malignant histopathological changes.
   (d) The possibility of the second cancer being an invasion of the first must be excluded.
   (e) The possibility of the second cancer being a metastasis of the first must be excluded.
4. If a new stage IV lesion is detected, rebiopsy can be done in the following conditions, except:
   (a) The patient is in good physical condition.
   (b) There are no contraindications for biopsy.
   (c) Imaging findings suggest lesions in rare metastatic sites.
   (d) Elevated tumor markers align with the suspected tumor type.
   (e) Elevated tumor markers do not align with the expected tumor type.
5. Which one of the following statements regarding the prognosis of MPMTs is true?
   (a) Patients with three synchronous tumors have a 5.5-fold higher mortality risk compared to metachronous cases.
   (b) Patients with two metachronous and one synchronous tumor have a three-fold higher mortality risk compared to metachronous cases.
   (c) Male gender and being over 50 years old at the first tumor diagnosis are associated with higher mortality risk.
   (d) Female gender and being over 50 years old at the first tumor diagnosis are associated with higher mortality risk.
   (e) Male gender and being under 50 years old at the first tumor diagnosis are associated with higher mortality risk.

Answer Keys

1. A
2. B
3. A
4. D
5. C

Acknowledgments Ersananda Arlisa Putri MD, Department of Internal Medicine, Respirology and Critical Illness Division, Universitas Indonesia, Dr. Cipto Mangunkusumo General Central National Hospital, Jakarta, Indonesia.

Ray Bryan Charles Rattu MD DM, Department of Internal Medicine, Respirology and Critical Illness Division, Universitas Indonesia, Dr. Cipto Mangunkusumo General Central National Hospital, Jakarta, Indonesia.

Ardhi Rahman Ahani MD DM, Department of Internal Medicine, Medical Hematology and Oncology Division, Dr. Cipto Mangunkusumo General Central National Hospital, Jakarta, Indonesia.

References

1. Zhai C. Multiple primary malignant tumors – a clinical analysis of 15,321 patients with malignancies at a single Center in China. J Cancer. 2018;9:2795–801.
2. Vogt A. Multiple primary tumours: challenges and approaches, a review. ESMO Open. 2017;2:e000172.
3. Jena A. Multiple primary cancers: an enigma. South Asian J Cancer. 2016;5:29–32.
4. Yang X-B. High incidence combination of multiple primary malignant tumors of the digestive system. World J Gastroenterol. 2022;28:5982–92.
5. Almasan I, Piciu D. Triple primary malignancies: tumor associations, survival, and Clinicopathological analysis: a 25-year single-institution experience. Healthc Basel Switz. 2023;11:738.

Lung Hamartoma 22

22.1 Case Illustration

A 50-year-old female patient presented for a bronchoscopy, reporting a persistent dry cough that had been felt particularly at night for the past 1 year. Shortness of breath was felt continuously but did not interfere with daily activities. The patient denied fever and frequent night sweats, but there was a weight loss of approximately 10 kg in the past 1 year. Despite repeated visits to the public health center and administration of various cough medications, there was absolutely no improvement. However, no history of pulmonary tuberculosis (TB) was reported. After referral to the nearest hospital, chest X-ray was examined, suggesting Adenosine Deaminase (ADA) test and scheduled examinations of thoracic computed tomography (CT). ADA examination found normal results, while CT chest examination (Fig. 22.1) showed that there was a lung mass with calcification in the perihilar of the right lung accompanied by lung collapse and right pleural effusion.

The patient was advised to seek further treatment at the Cipto Mangunkusumo Hospital (RSCM). After arriving at RSCM, a bronchoscopy for tissue sampling was recommended. Complaints of swelling face and upper arms were experienced in the past month. Additionally, there was no personal or family history of malignancy, hypertension, diabetes mellitus, heart disease, and pulmonary TB. The patient has not smoked, although both husband and son engaged in smoking. As a vegetable seller in the market, these complaints did not interfere with daily activities, whether at work or house, which had adequate lighting and ventilation. Physical examination showed that the patient appeared moderately ill, with blood pressure 110/78 mmHg, breathing 22 times per minute, pulse 88 times per minute, temperature 36.8 degrees Celsius, height 155 cm, and weight 45 kg with BMI 18.7 kg/m^2. The conjunctiva was not pale or icteric, but there were distended neck veins, with chest wall showing widened veins. From the examination, palpation of vocal fremitus decreased in the right lung. Percussion showed that there was reddening in the right lung at the level of thoracic VI. Based on auscultation, the right breath sounds

G. Singh, *Challenging Cases in Respirology and Critical Care*,
https://doi.org/10.1007/978-981-96-5002-6_22

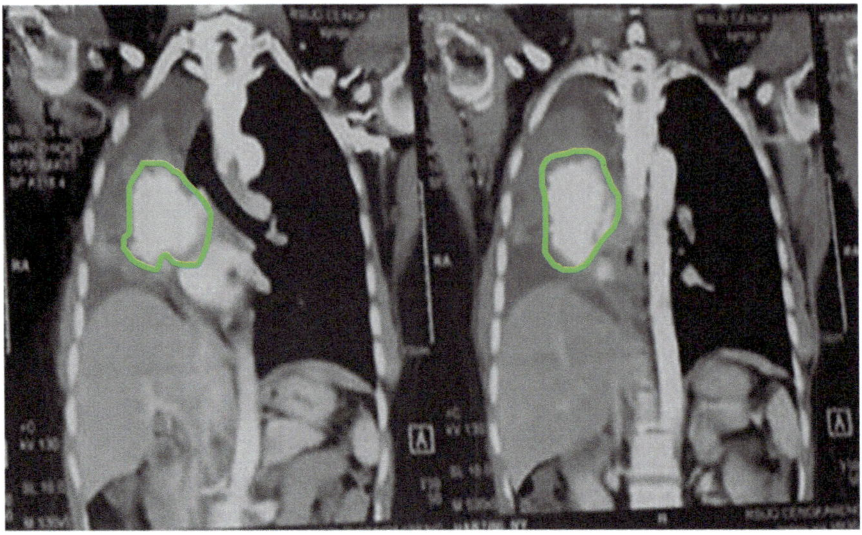

Fig. 22.1 Thoracic CT from the previous hospital showed lung mass with calcification in the perihilar of the right lung (green circle). (Figure courtesy: Mohammad Reynalzi Yugo MD)

decreased compared to the left without crackles and wheezing. Cardiac examination showed no palpable enlargement, regular heart sounds without murmurs and gallops. In the abdomen, bowel sounds were heard 3 times per minute, while liver and spleen were not enlarged on palpation. Examination of the extremities showed warm acral and *capillary refill time* <2 sec. Laboratory examination on initial admission showed Hb of 11.6 gr/dL, leukocytes 7120/uL, and platelets 312,000/uL. The results of the specific count showed basophils 0.3%, eosinophils 2.1%, neutrophils 66.8%, lymphocytes 24.3%, and monocytes 6.5%. Prothrombin time (PT) and activated partial thromboplastin time (APTT) were normal. Liver function tests showed normal SGOT and SGPT levels of 19 U/L and 14 U/L, respectively. Kidney function was normal with urea, creatinine, and eGFR 25.3 mg/dL, 0.60 mg/dL, and 106.6 mL/min/1.73m^2, respectively. Procalcitonin was normal, which was 0.04 ng/mL and CRP increased to 8.8 mg/L. Electrolytes were in normal ranges, namely sodium 138 mEq/L, Potassium 3.6 mEq/L, 102.2 mEq/L. Chest X-ray examination showed a perihilar mass with atelectasis of the right hemithorax, indicating a pleural effusion component. The patient was administered codeine 3 times 10 mg for the dry cough. The problem was considered a right lung mass suspected of malignancy with right pleural effusion. Additionally, physical examination showed that the possibility of superior vena cava syndrome could not be ruled out. Consequently, the patient planned for action endobronchial ultrasound-guided transbronchial lung biopsy (EBUS+TBLB) for diagnosis.

On the 3rd day of treatment, the EBUS + TBLB procedure was planned due to total stenosis of the right main bronchus. Subsequently, an examination of resistance to Microorganisms (MOR), gram, and acid-fast bacilli (AFB) was carried out. The results were negative from the slight smearing of gram-negative rods and moderate gram-positive cocci. The MOR examination identified >100,000 germs/mL of staphylococcus epidermidis and alpha-hemolytic streptococcus >100,000 germs/mL which were sensitive to ampicillin sulbactam. Therefore, the patient was given ampicillin sulbactam 3 times 1.5 grams intravenously for 7 days. On the 5th day of treatment, a diagnostic procedure medical thoracoscopy was planned. The results (Fig. 22.2) showed that the right lung collapsed, and nodular lesions were observed in the parietal pleura, visceral pleura, and diaphragm, without visible intrathoracic mass. Multiple biopsies were performed on nodular lesions and parietal pleura for further analysis.

Chest tube was inserted to drain the pleural fluid, which was examined for gram smear, AFB, and MOR, with results showing negative and sterile. After medical thoracoscopy, the face and arms were increasingly swollen, and the voice turned hoarse, leading to diagnosis of superior vena cava syndrome. Dexamethasone 2 × 10 mg intravenously was administered and there was a consultation with the radiation oncology department. The patient was given radiation 3 times 3Gy for 3 consecutive days, followed by the administration of prophylactic heparin of 1000 IU per 24 hours. Histology showed moderate–severe chronic inflammatory tissue (Fig. 22.3). Pleural fluid cytology and lung washings contained mesothelial cells, macrophages, and leukocytes, without malignant tumor cells.

Considering the inconclusive biopsy results, another option for diagnosis procedure was considered. The patient was consulted by the Thoracic and Cardiovascular Surgery department which decided on another bronchoscopy with a previous thoracic CT. This was due to the concerns that after radiation biopsy would be more difficult. Chest CT results (Fig. 22.4) showed a solid mass with a calcified component and malignant characteristics in the right lung. Additionally, there was intermittent thrombus in the intra lumen of the superior vena cava and bilateral brachiocephalic vein, with multiple left lung nodules.

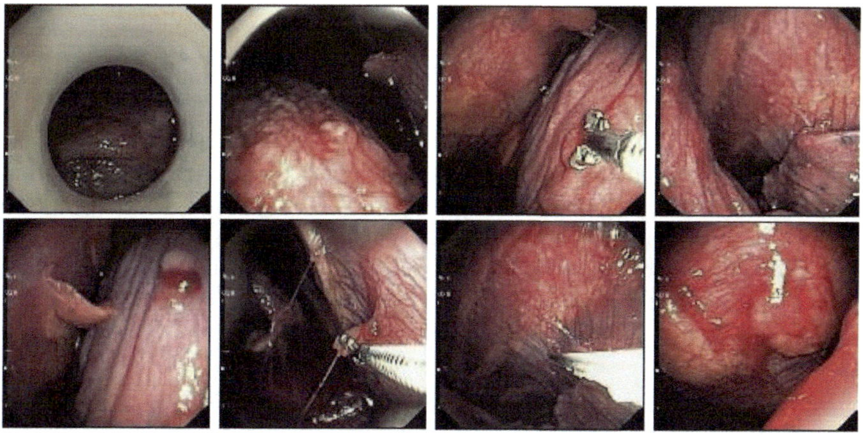

Fig. 22.2 Thoracoscopy showed collapse of the right lung and multiple nodular lesions. (Figure courtesy: Gurmeet Singh MD DM PhD)

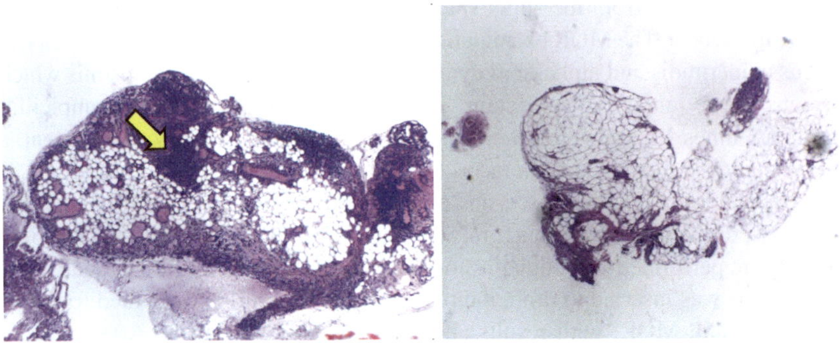

Fig. 22.3 Moderate severe–chronic inflammation, (yellow arrow) aggregates lymphoid. (Figure courtesy: Yayi Dwina Billianti Susanto MD DM PhD)

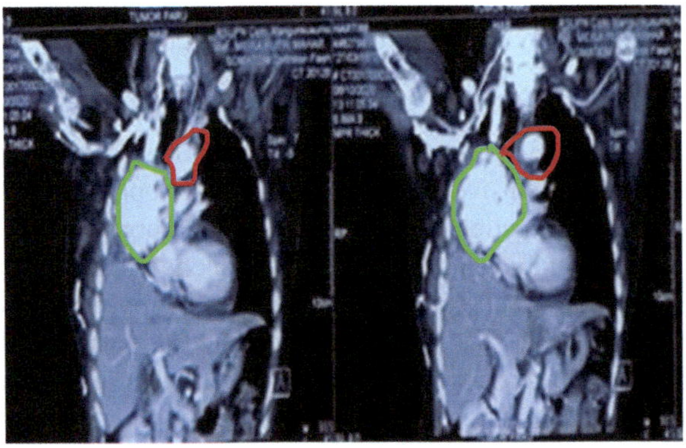

Fig. 22.4 Thoracic CT showed a solid mass with a calcified component with malignant characteristics in the right lung (green circle), and multiple left lung nodules (red circle). (Figure courtesy: Mohammad Reynalzi Yugo MD)

The histology from the right lung biopsy is suggestive of tumor necrosis with atypic cells (Fig. 22.5).

An abdominal CT scan was performed to rule out primary malignancy from other organs, showing only adenomyosis. Among the tumor markers, CA-125 was slightly increased, suggesting inconclusive results. Therefore, the patient was advised for an open biopsy and decided to undergo Video Assisted Thoracic Surgery (VATS). The results of the biopsy showed (Fig. 22.6) an appearance consisting of pieces of connective tissue containing reactive fibroblasts and moderate amounts of chronic inflammatory cells, and partially mineralized bone trabecular tissue, as well as bone marrow.

Histological analysis suggested fibrotic lung tissue accompanied by calcification, possibly part of pulmonary hamartoma (PH). After the procedure, the patient was transferred to the ICU.

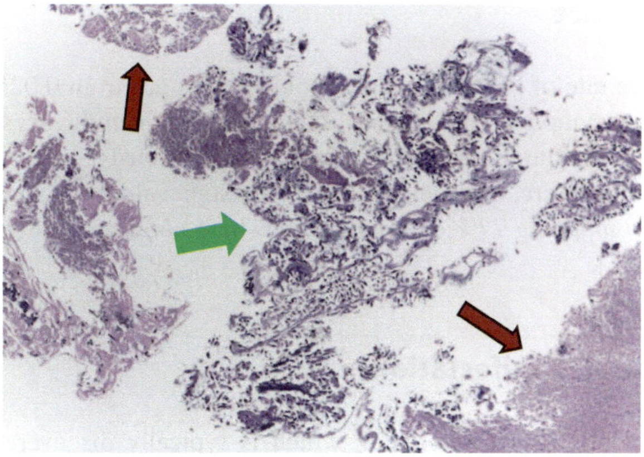

Fig. 22.5 Tumor necrosis (red arrow), atypic cells (green arrow). (Figure courtesy: Yayi Dwina Billianti Susanto MD DM PhD)

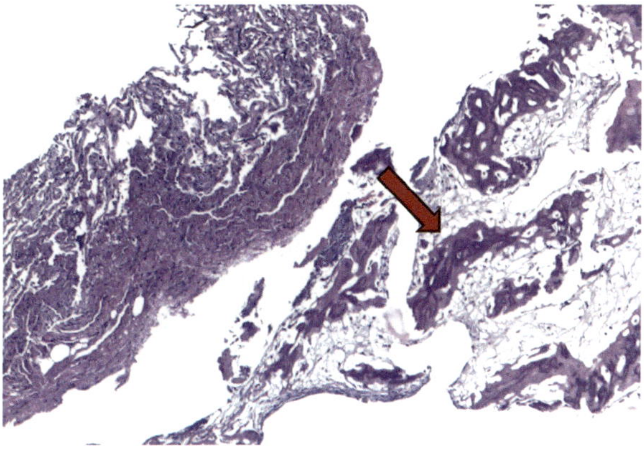

Fig. 22.6 Partially mineralized bone trabecular tissue (red arrow). (Figure courtesy: Yayi Dwina Billianti Susanto MD DM PhD)

22.2 Discussion

PH is the most frequent but uncommon noncancerous growths resembling tumors that develop in the lung from residual embryonic tissue. These growths are more prevalent in males and older individuals. PH consists of an atypical combination of tissue components, including cartilage, epithelium, fat, or muscle. However, the normal structure of the lung is not maintained in these cases [1]. Pulmonary neoplasms are the most often occurring noncancerous growths in the lungs of humans, but less prevalent in children. Typically, these abnormalities are found at the outside part of the tissue and rarely observed in the middle of chest wall. Lesions show a comparable rate of growth similar to the adjacent tissue [2].

22.3 Incidence

The occurrence rate of PH in the adult population ranges from 0.025% to 0.032%. Typically, these symptoms manifest in individuals between the ages of 40 and 59, with males being four times more likely to be affected compared to females. Although relatively rare, these lesions are the most prevalent noncancerous growths in the lungs, comprising 77% of noncancerous lung nodules and 8% of single lung abnormalities [3].

22.4 Clinical Manifestation

Most PH in adults is asymptomatic, which is typically discovered incidentally. However, depending on the position and extent of the lesion, patients can experience various symptoms, such as continuous coughing or wheezing, difficulty breathing, coughing up blood, abnormal breath sounds, increased risk of pneumonia, partial lung collapse, or even a collapsed lung. Endobronchial masses also present the risk of airway obstruction [1].

22.5 Evaluation

Hamartomas are frequently discovered incidentally during imaging tests and can resemble lung cancer. After discovery, or at the instance of an asymptomatic hamartoma, many diagnostic methods can be used to ascertain the characteristics of the abnormal growth. Imaging methods such as chest X-ray or CT scan show masses that appear as circular and solitary structures, with clearly defined boundaries, usually measuring less than 4 cm in diameter. Calcification is observed in approximately 25% to 30% of patients, often characterized by a popcorn or comma-shaped pattern, which is diagnostic of hamartomas. Although CT imaging is considered the most reliable method, further procedures may be required. FDG-PET scan is valuable for assessing the metabolic rate of lesions with an uncertain risk of malignancy by measuring the rate of FDG uptake. Biopsy is essential to exclude the presence of cancer, particularly in cases where there is no fatty component or a distinctive calcification pattern in the lesions. Bronchoscopy with fine needle aspiration (FNA) is often the preferred method but the aspirations can be limited due to the compactness of the lesions. Masses showing the characteristic appearance of a coin and meeting the CT criteria for hamartomas (size less than 4 cm, well-defined borders, presence of visible calcification or fatty component) should continue to be monitored conservatively through regular observation. However, surgical resection is only recommended for rapidly growing, symptomatic tumors, or cases where the potential for cancer cannot be ruled out [1].

Video-assisted thoracoscopic surgery (VATS) has significantly transformed the method and treatment of pulmonary as well as cardiac disorders in the last

20 years. The pleura was inspected thoracoscopically by Swedish physician Jacobeaus, with the patient under local anesthesia. This treatment was commonly conducted to assess and manage pleural effusions in individuals afflicted with pulmonary TB. Before implementation, the conventional method for addressing a thoracic pathology included performing a thoracotomy. The introduction of fiber-optic light was a significant technological achievement that led to advancements in all types of limited-access surgery. The quantity of VATS applications has increased throughout the decades due to technological developments, which enhanced the safety operations for old and weak patients. VATS has several benefits compared to standard thoracotomy, such as decreased postoperative pain, shorter hospital stays, faster recovery of respiratory function (particularly in patients with chronic obstructive pulmonary disease and the elderly), and lower total expenses [4].

VATS has been conducted using a uniportal or biportal method, based on the surgeon's discretion. During the procedure, the nodule enucleation method was used in peripheral cases that had a high degree of calcification based on palpation findings. The diagnosis was definitively confirmed using the frozen section method during surgery in cases when there was a strong suspicion of cancer. When the lesion was located centrally, a punch biopsy was performed to retrieve frozen examination material [4].

Recently, VATS has gradually supplanted open thoracotomies in the majority of thoracic surgery centers worldwide. This is due to favorable safety profile in geriatric patients, superior pain management, increased recovery periods, and enhanced hemostatic control. Results show that VATS reduces the duration of hospitalization in comparison to open thoracotomy due to the reduced time of chest tube placement. This was shown by previous studies which reported removal rates of 54% on day 1 for the VATS group, compared to 21% for open thoracotomies.

Surgery is the definitive curative treatment for PH to preserve functional lung tissue. Enucleation and wedge resections are the most preferred surgical options, while more extensive procedures such as lobectomy or total pneumonectomy are reserved for specific cases. These include deeply situated lesions, several lesions that cannot be removed through wedge resection, or lesions strongly attached to the hilum of the lung. Moreover, it is often advisable to obtain intraoperative frozen sections to prevent the possibility of missing any underlying malignant potential [5].

22.6 Prognosis

The overall prognosis for individuals diagnosed with lung hamartoma is typically favorable. These lesions show a slow rate of growth and in cases where symptoms are both apparent and enduring, surgical intervention is capable of providing a complete cure. The incidence of malignant transformation or future cancer is uncommon. However, when patients follow a conservative observation plan, recognition can be made at an early stage [5].

Key Points

Surgical intervention should be considered in cases of thoracic masses of unknown etiology before administration of chemotherapy and other oncologic therapies.

Questions

1. Pulmonary hamartoma is benign malformation of the lung and includes an abnormal mixture of:
   (a) Cartilage, epithelium, fat
   (b) Cartilage, fat, complex immune
   (c) Epithelium, fat, complex immune
   (d) Cartilage, muscle, complex immune
   (e) Cartilage, epithelium, complex immune
2. The incidence of pulmonary hamartoma:
   (a) They usually present in the fourth and fifth decade of life
   (b) Females being four times more likely to be affected than males
   (c) Males being two times more likely to be affected than females
   (d) These lesions are the most common benign pulmonary neoplasm
   (e) Pulmonary hamartoma occurs with an incidence of 0.25% to 0.32% within the adult population.
3. Clinical manifestation of hamartoma are as follows, except:
   (a) Wheezing
   (b) Atelectasis
   (c) Hemoptysis
   (d) Pneumothorax
   (e) Pleural effusion
4. The pathognomonic sign of hamartoma:
   (a) Parenchymal loos
   (b) Eggshell calcification
   (c) The popcorn shaped
   (d) Ground glass opacities
   (e) Loss of the regular vascular branching pattern
5. Below are curative methods to treat hamartoma, expect:
   (a) Enucleation
   (b) Segmentectomy
   (c) Wedge Resections
   (d) Radical Lobectomy
   (e) Total Pneumonectomy

Answer Keys

1. A
2. D
3. E
4. C
5. B

Acknowledgments Ersananda Arlisa Putri MD, Department of Internal Medicine, Respirology and Critical Illness Division, Universitas Indonesia, Dr. Cipto Mangunkusumo General Central National Hospital, Jakarta, Indonesia.
David Hutagaol MD DM PhD, Department of Cardiovascular and Thoracic Surgery, Vascular and Endovascular Surgery Division, Universitas Indonesia, Dr. Cipto Mangunkusumo General Central National Hospital, Jakarta, Indonesia.
Meisa Putri Maharani MD, Department of Internal Medicine, Universitas Indonesia, Dr. Cipto Mangunkusumo General Central National Hospital, Jakarta, Indonesia.

References

1. Lundeen KS, Raj MS, Rajasurya V Pulmonary hamartoma. In: StatPearls Internet. 2023. https://www.ncbi.nlm.nih.gov/books/NBK539806/
2. Umashankar T. Pulmonary hamartoma: cytological study of a case and literature review. J Cytol. 2012;29:261–3.
3. Saadi MM. Large multicystic pulmonary chondroid hamartoma in a child presenting as pneumothorax. Saudi Med J. 2015;36:487–9.
4. Erdogu V. Does pulmonary hamartoma increase the risk of lung cancer? Outcomes of 38 pulmonary hamartoma cases. Sisli Etfal Hastan Tip Bul. 2021;55:344–8.
5. Guo W. Surgical treatment and outcome of pulmonary hamartoma: a retrospective study of 20-year experience. J Exp Clin Cancer Res CR. 2008;27:8.

Pneumothorax Due to Fungal Infection 23

23.1 Case Illustration

A 20-year-old male presented to the emergency room with complaints of shortness of breath and chest pain one week before hospitalization, unaffected by position. The patient had been to the hospital and was diagnosed with a pneumothorax. At the previous hospital, a water sheil drainage (WSD) was installed, and surgery was planned. Due to the desire to use social security agency health, the patient was referred to Cipto Mangunkusumo Hospital. Additionally, there was a history of psoriasis 4 years ago, with methotrexate treatment. To prepare for further surgery, the methotrexate treatment was temporarily postponed and an additional dose of methylprednisolone was administered.

Physical examination showed decreased vesicular sound of the right hemithorax, while laboratory results indicated a high level of leukocytes (13.730). The result of thoracic CT at the previous hospital (Fig. 23.1) showed a prominent right pneumothorax attached to the distal end of the WSD in the right upper hemithorax. Additionally, there was prominent bullae originating from the superior lobe of the right lung with a wall defect in the posterolateral segment, potentially contributing to pneumothorax. A partial infiltrate was observed with consolidation of the posterior segment of the superior lobe and inferior media of the right lung.

A thoracocentesis procedure was performed to expel air from the patient's lungs, followed by the insertion of a chest tube to decompress the chest wall and connect to the WSD system. Evaluation was carried out by chest X-ray examination, showing a right pneumothorax with a chest tube extending the 3rd posterior intercostal space. However, no radiological abnormalities were observed in the heart, including pneumomediastinum or subcutaneous emphysema (Fig. 23.2). Based on clinical findings and initial laboratory results, the patient was diagnosed with spontaneous tension pneumothorax et causa bulla rupture.

The patient was admitted for a thoracotomy bullectomy action plan. Despite reporting intermittent chest pain, physical examination showed decreased vesicular

G. Singh, *Challenging Cases in Respirology and Critical Care*,
https://doi.org/10.1007/978-981-96-5002-6_23

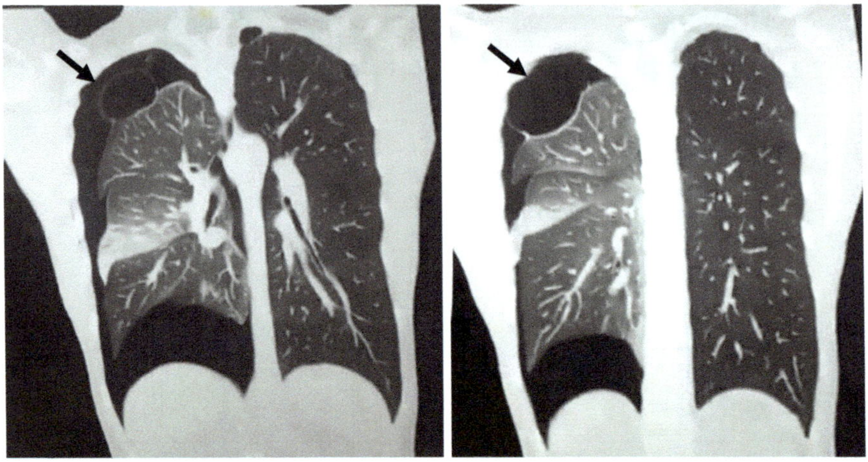

Fig. 23.1 Prominent bullae originating from the superior lobe of the right lung with a wall defect (pointed by arrows). (Image courtesy: Mohammad Reynalzi Yugo MD)

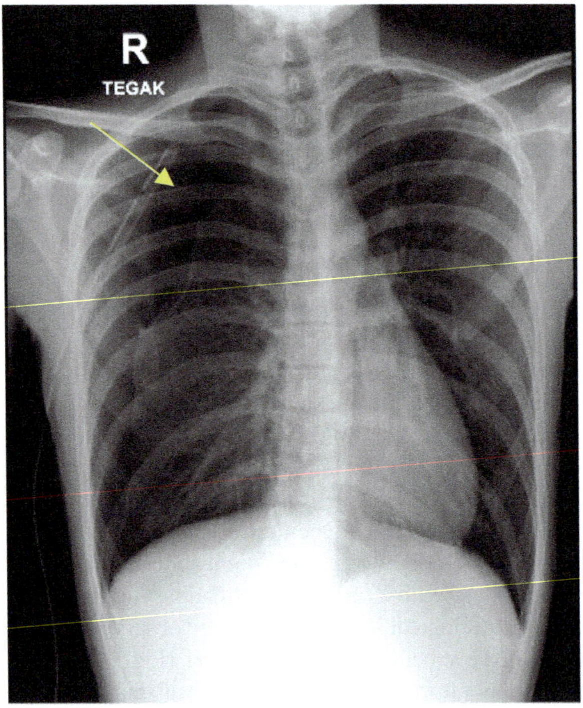

Fig. 23.2 Chest X-ray showed a right pneumothorax (pointed by arrow). (Image courtesy: Rahmi Afifi MD DM)

sound of the right hemithorax. The results of the histological image from thoracostomy showed lung parenchyma with atelectasis and fibrosis accompanied by fungal colonies that lead to aspergillosis. The blood gas analysis showed Ph 7.581, pCO_2 34.20, pO_2 121.60, and HCO3 32.40. The fluid production of WSD was reduced gradually, from 40 cc/8 hours to 30 cc/24 hours. Subsequently, the patient was subjected to the thoracotomy bullectomy procedure (Fig. 23.3) and had a parasitological examination of the operated tissue to confirm the diagnosis of fungal infection according to histological findings.

The patient was transferred to the ICU room and was subjected to laboratory evaluation as well as postoperative chest X-rays. Laboratory results showed an increase in leukocytes (19650), PT increased 1 times the normal value, and aPTT rose 1.2x from normal. Postoperative chest X-ray (Fig. 23.4) showed reduced right pneumothorax, right chest wall subcutaneous emphysema appeared, and there was no pneumomediastinum.

After surgery, the patient complained of pain at the postoperative site using a visual analog scale (2). However, there were no complaints of tightness, chest pain, and fever. WSD production decreased by 30 cc/24 hours, characterized as serohemorrhagic with positive undulation and negative bubbles. Consequently, an air–fluid

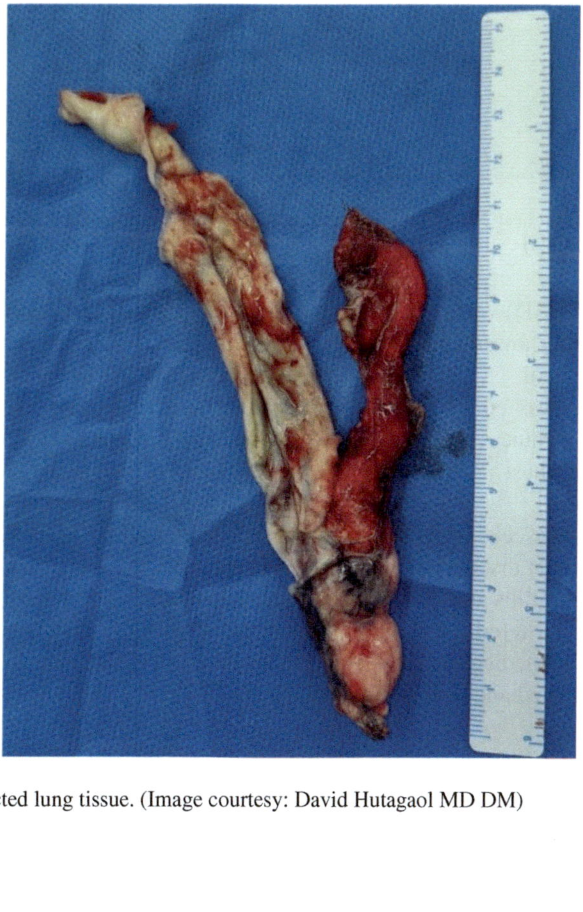

Fig. 23.3 Infected lung tissue. (Image courtesy: David Hutagaol MD DM)

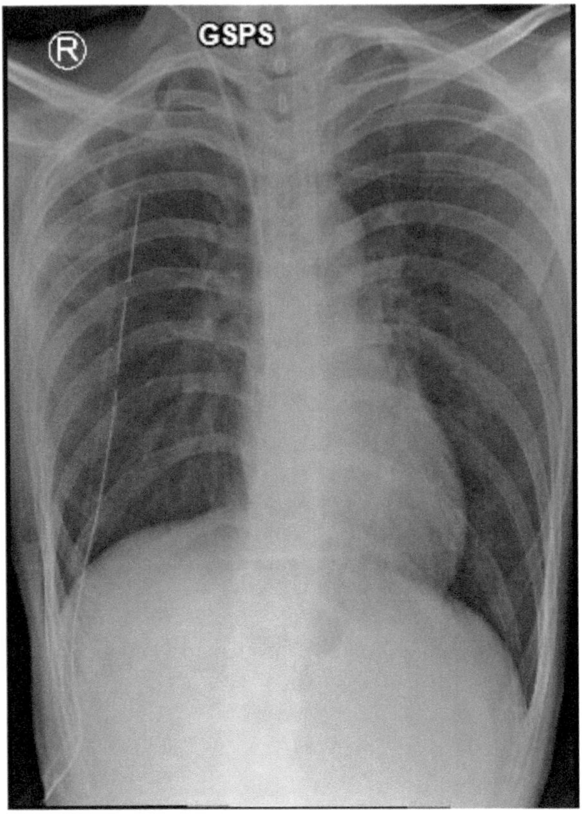

Fig. 23.4 Another chest X-ray showed reduced right pneumothorax. (Image courtesy: Reyhan Eddy Yunus MD PhD)

exchange (aff WSD) was performed on the patient. After being treated for several days, the patient showed significant improvement, leading to the plans for discharge and routine control.

The patient was controlled to the outpatient department (OPD), reporting no complaints of tightness and chest pain. CD4 and CD8 immunology showed normal results, while chest X-ray (Fig. 23.5) examination indicated the absence of pneumothorax.

After several weeks, the patient came back to the OPD for evaluation, with a complaint of chest discomfort. The results of parasitology found branched hyphae, leading to Aspergillus and wide hyphae, causing Mucorales. Subsequently, voriconazole was administered for 10 days and continued with itraconazole for 12 weeks. After taking the medication, the patient returned to the OPD, and respiratory complaints were denied and declared cured.

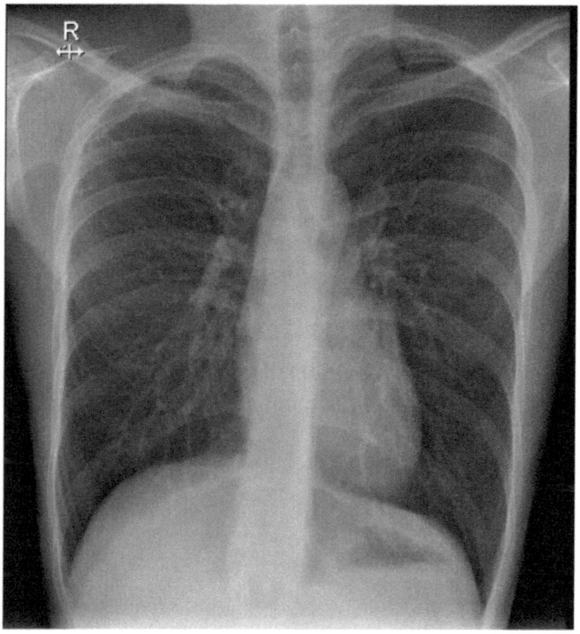

Fig. 23.5 Chest X-ray showed no more pneumothorax. (Image courtesy: Taufik Agung MD)

23.2 Discussion

Aspergillus infection rarely leads to recurrent pneumothorax. Moreover, recurrent pneumothorax patients, specifically those with chronic lung disease, should consider the possibility of an Aspergillus species infection in differential diagnosis [1]. This infection can occur without usually affecting the lungs, manifesting in individuals with a fully functioning immune system. The presence of Aspergillus infection in the lung can result in several respiratory conditions, including obstructive bronchopulmonary aspergillosis, mucoid impaction of the airways, tracheobronchitis, ulcerative bronchitis, pseudomembranous tracheobronchitis, invasive aspergillosis, or aspergilloma [2].

23.3 Epidemiology

Aspergillus spp. are widespread fungi that are obtained through the inhalation of spores in the air. Typically, Aspergillus airway colonization manifests in individuals with an underlying chronic respiratory condition, such as asthma, bronchiectasis, or cystic fibrosis. The consequences of chronic airway disease include cellular debris accumulation, excessive production of mucus, the formation of cavities, and bronchi dilation, playing a crucial role in capturing Aspergillus spores. Approximately more than 25% of asthmatic patients may experience

Aspergillus colonization, according to reports. Aspergillus infection rarely presents as recurrent pneumothorax and pleural aspergillosis [1]. Specifically, Aspergillus is an omnipresent fungus commonly encountered in soil, water, and decomposing organic material. It is recognized to induce a diverse range of respiratory ailments, such as allergic bronchopulmonary aspergillosis, parenchymal invasion, and mycetomas, which tend to develop in preexisting pulmonary cavities. Aspergillus fumigatus is the predominant saprophytic species, which frequently causes aspergilloma. Mycetomas have been observed in 10–15% of individuals with cavitating lung disorders who are not immunocompromised. Furthermore, mycetomas are often detected in areas where tuberculosis rates are decreasing, particularly in cases of severe sarcoidosis, pneumoconioses, bullous emphysema, bronchiectasis, lung abscesses, neoplasms, and pulmonary infarcts. The incidence of invasive aspergillus parenchymal infection in solid-organ transplant recipients is estimated to vary between 5–8%, significantly associated with a death rate ranging from 50–100%.

23.4 Clinical Manifestation

The predominant of mycetomas symptoms include cough and hemoptysis. The progression of the condition shows significant variability, and patients are often monitored without treatment unless experiencing hemoptysis. In cases of massive hemoptysis, surgical intervention is required, including the removal of the damaged lung or arterial embolization for patients who are not appropriate for surgery. Antifungal medications, namely itraconazole, voriconazole, or amphotericin B, are used when complete surgical excision is not feasible or the Aspergillus infection has progressed beyond the aspergilloma [3].

Based on previous investigations, there are no recent reports in the medical literature of pneumothorax caused by the rupture of mycetomas into the pleural space in patients who are not immunocompromised. Moreover, identifying the relationship is important since both pneumothorax and hemoptysis are clinical manifestations of a more severe progression of invasive fungal infections [3].

23.5 Diagnosis

Performing histological analysis of biopsy or autopsy samples allows for the identification of tissue invasion by a filamentous fungus, thereby confirming the presence of an invasive fungal infection. To definitively diagnose invasive Aspergillus, there is a need to obtain a positive culture of Aspergillus from the same specimen. This is due to the inability to identify the fungus only based on mycelium observed in tissue sections. Therefore, the significance of confirmed invasive aspergillus is considerable. In several cases, acquiring biopsy samples, particularly through transthoracic for pulmonary invasive aspergillus, is not often recommended due to low platelet counts or other medical risks [4].

Extensive analysis of tissue samples using the hematoxylin and eosin staining method should detect the presence of Aspergillus hyphae. However, additional staining methods such as period acid Schiff and Grocott's silver should be performed for increased accuracy. The hyphae of Aspergillus observed in tissue slices are typically slender, measuring 1–3 um in diameter, and include septa. This can be challenging to differentiate from other fungi, such as Fusarium and Scedosporium, which can contribute to infections [4].

23.6 Management

A lack of agreement exists on the appropriate treatment method for pleural aspergillosis. Conventional systemic antifungal medication and thoracic drainage, without the need for lung resection, have effectively treated some cases. Performing surgery for pleural aspergillosis is a complex task that presents technical challenges, particularly due to previous thoracic surgery on patients who typically require this intervention. The optimal results are commonly achieved by a mix of medicinal medication and surgical intervention [2].

23.7 Prognosis

Secondary pneumothorax caused by invasive Aspergillus is an uncommon occurrence and has a significant fatality rate. Progressive cavitary lung disease cases should be evaluated for possible Aspergillus infection to ensure adequate treatment [5].

Key Points

Pneumothorax can not only be spontaneous, primary, or tuberculosis-induced. Fungal infection can also cause pneumothorax. In such cases, surgery is the better option for diagnosis and therapy of pneumothorax.

Questions

1. The most common symptom of pneumothorax due to fungal infection:
   (a) Dyspnea
   (b) Night sweet
   (c) Loss weight
   (d) Hemoptysis
   (e) Chest pain
2. The following are preferred methods to diagnose pneumothorax caused by a fungal infection, except:
   (a) Biopsy
   (b) Galactomannan

    (c) Eosin staining.
    (d) Hematoxylin staining
    (e) Acid Schiff and Grocott's silver
3. Which of the following is true about pneumothorax due to fungal infection?
    (a) Aspergillus is a ubiquitous fungus found in air, water, and decaying matter.
    (b) The airway sequelae of acute airway disease are important for trapping aspergillus spores.
    (c) Aspergillus airway colonization usually occurs in patients with an underlying acute airway disease.
    (d) Recurrent pneumothorax and pleural aspergillosis may be rare manifestations of aspergillus infection.
    (e) In non-immunocompromised population, mycetoma has been reported to occur in 1–5% of patients with cavitating lung diseases.
4. The best therapy option for pneumothorax due to fungal infection:
    (a) Conventional systemic antifungal therapy
    (b) Thoracic drainage with pulmonary resection
    (c) Thoracic drainage without pulmonary resection
    (d) Combination systemic antifungal and thoracic drainage
    (e) Combination of medical therapy and surgical intervention
5. The systemic antifungal used if complete surgical removal is not possible?
    (a) Itraconazole
    (b) Clindamycin
    (c) Clotrimazole
    (d) Flucytosine
    (e) Terbinafine

Answer Keys

1. D
2. B
3. D
4. E
5. A

Acknowledgments Ersananda Arlisa Putri MD, Department of Internal Medicine, Respirology and Critical Illness Division, Universitas Indonesia, Dr. Cipto Mangunkusumo General Central National Hospital, Jakarta, Indonesia.

David Hutagaol MD DM, Department of Cardiovascular and Thoracic Surgery, Vascular and Endovascular Surgery Division, Universitas Indonesia, Dr. Cipto Mangunkusumo General Central National Hospital, Jakarta, Indonesia.

References

1. Zhang W, Hu Y, Chen L, Gao J, Xie L. Pleural aspergillosis complicated by recurrent pneumothorax: a case report. J Med Case Rep. 2010;4:180.
2. Ichikawa H, Doi R, Matsumoto K, Tomoshige K, Hirabaru M, Machino R. Spontaneous pleural aspergillosis in an immunocompetent young adult treated with minimally invasive surgery. Respir Med Case Rep. 2023;44:101869.
3. Gupta PP, Fotedar S, Agarwal D, Magu S, Saini K. Pneumothorax: a rare presentation of pulmonary mycetoma. Ann Thorac Med. 2007;2:171–2.
4. Barton RC. Laboratory diagnosis of invasive aspergillosis: from diagnosis to prediction of outcome. Scientifica. 2013;2013:459405.
5. Kao CT, Lee YJ, Salem A. Secondary spontaneous pneumothorax from invasive Aspergillus. Chest. 2021;160:A445.

Drugs Induce Acute Pancreatitis

24

24.1 Case Illustration

A 63-year-old male patient was brought to the emergency room by the family for control in the outpatient department (OPD) of Cipto Mangunkusumo Hospital for indications of Myelodysplastic Syndrome (MDS). Physical examination showed very low blood pressure and there was an increase in blood glucose level. After initial treatment, the patient was transferred to the emergency room. Five days before admission, there was a complaint of unusual drowsiness and difficulty communicating with family. Although the patient occasionally requests food, consumption could be half a portion of food and milk. Two days before admission, there was no appetite for food and eye contact was becoming inadequate. The patient was vomiting when attempting to eat, but there were no complaints of fever, cough, shortness of breath, one-sided weakness, lisp, spray vomits, or severe headache. The patient was hospitalized six days before admission and laboratory examination showed a thrombocyte of 1000 cell/mm^3 and hemoglobin 6 g/dl. Therefore, the patient was subjected to blood transfusion and was discharged after showing improved clinical condition. Six years before admission, the was diagnosed with MDS, alongside complaints of melena and occasional blood appearance. Laboratory examination showed very low thrombocyte and hemoglobin, leading to a bone marrow puncture that confirmed MDS. The patient routinely controls in the OPD of Cipto Mangunkusumo Hospital, to receive Sandimmune 50 mg twice daily and folic acid. Blood transfusion was also carried out once every two weeks.

Based on physical examination in emergency room, the patient appeared severely ill, with hypotension 69/49 mmHg, an increased pulse rate of 126 times/minutes, and eyes showed pale conjunctiva. On abdomen palpation, there was epigastric and upper right region tenderness. Laboratory examination showed various abnormalities, including Hyperglycemia (779 mg/dl), Amylase enzyme levels 1747 U/L, Lipase enzyme levels 6559 U/L, declining kidney function (ueam 109.1 mg/dL, creatinine 1.8 mg/dL, EGFR 39.2 mL/min/1.73 m^2). Other indications included

G. Singh, *Challenging Cases in Respirology and Critical Care*,
https://doi.org/10.1007/978-981-96-5002-6_24

absolute reticulocytes 16,100 μ/L, relative reticulocytes 0.44%, hemoglobin 10.4, Hematocrit 29.8, leukopenia 2400 cell/mm^3, thrombocytopenia 12,000 cell/mm^3, Diff Count (WBC 0.4, neutrophils 0, lymphocytes 40, monocytes 51.7, eosinophils 7.9), and normal chest X-ray (Fig. 24.1).

Based on the initial clinical and laboratory findings, the patient was diagnosed with septic shock due to acute pancreatitis. The patient was administered oxygen at 3 lpm through cannula nasal and several initiatives such as norepinephrine 4 mg in 0.9% NaCl 50 cc and novorapide 3.5 units/hour were planned to improve clinical condition.

The patient was hospitalized and received an abdominal CT-scan. The result showed cholelithiasis, increased hepatic and liver density, and suspected extramedullary hematopoietic appearance with a differential diagnosis of hemochromatosis. Additionally, minimal pleural effusion in bilateral hemithorax was observed, including calcified lymphadenopathy in the perihilar region of the liver (Fig. 24.2).

The next day, the patient lost consciousness and only responded to painful stimuli, requiring transfer to High Care Unit (HCU). Although consciousness was increased, inappropriate speaking of words was observed. Subsequent laboratory examination showed some improvements, namely hemoglobin 7.6 mg/dl, hematocrit 21.1, leukocytes 1330, thrombocyte 39,000, and Diff count (WBC 0.8,

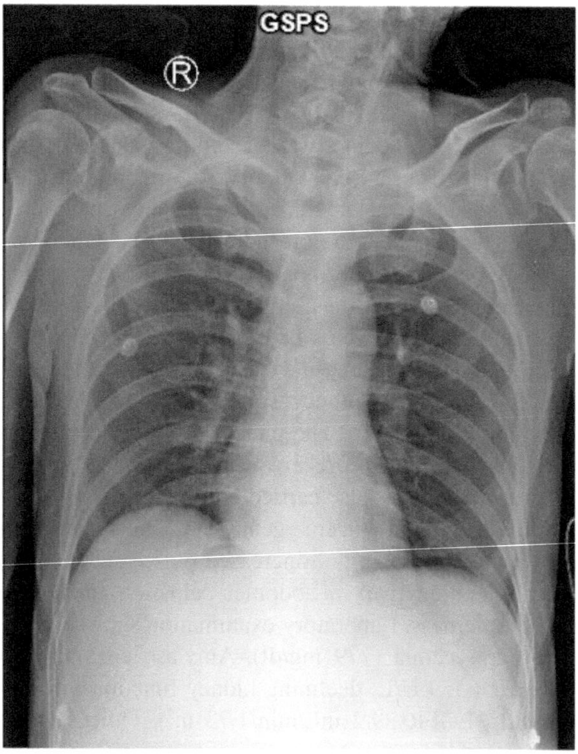

Fig. 24.1 Normal chest X-ray. (Image courtesy: Damayanti Sekarsari MD DM)

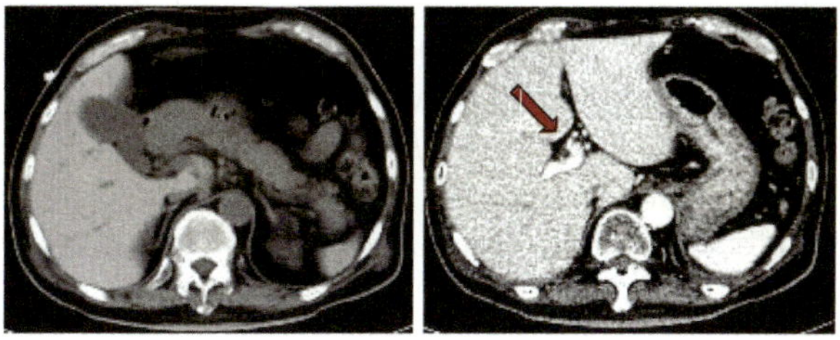

Fig. 24.2 Abdominal CT-Scan (red arrow) showed cholelithiasis. (Image courtesy: Mohammad Reynalzi Yugo MD)

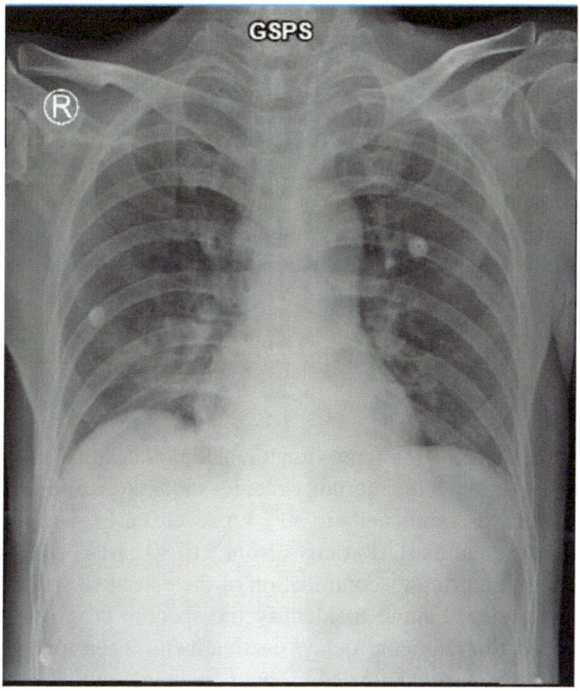

Fig. 24.3 The chest X-ray showed an infiltrate in the right lung, especially in the base. (Image courtesy: Taufik Agung Wibowo MD DM)

neutrophils 0, lymphocytes 52.6, monocytes 36.8, eosinophils 9.8) ANC 940. Others included albumin 2.4 g/dL, urea 126.3 mg/dl, EGFR 71.1 mL/min/1.73 m^2, procalcitonin 0.21 μg/L, lipase 157 U/L, amylase 100 U/L, and glucose 143 mg/dl. Additionally, chest X-ray examination was carried out to monitor lung condition, with results showing (Fig. 24.3) infiltration in the right lung.

Sandimmun treatment was temporarily stopped and the patient received Thrombocyte Packed Concentrate (TPC) and Packed Red Cell (PRC) transfusions. A subclavian central venous catheter (CVC) was inserted to facilitate access to several treatments. After discontinuation of Sandimmun for several days, clinical condition and ability to follow simple commands were improved. Additionally, there was bleeding from the mouth and nose, as well as fever, but abdominal pain was still present, as shown by Visual Analog Scale (VAS) 1. Laboratory examinations showed decreased enzyme amylase levels of 31 U/L and enzyme lipase levels of 24 U/L. The blood cultures were sterile, with a level of hemoglobin 8.1 mg/dl, hematocrit 23, leukocytes 890, thrombocyte 49,000, and ANC 450. The patient was planned to step down in the usual room and conduct another chest X-ray examination. The results showed that the infiltrate had decreased compared to the previous chest X-ray. The condition was improved and was diagnosed with drug-induced pancreatitis (DIP) due to sandimmun. Subsequently, the patient was advised to control in the OPD.

24.2 Discussion

Drug-induced pancreatitis (DIP) is an uncommon etiology of acute pancreatitis, with the majority of cases ranging from mild to moderate, including severe and fatal. Treating DIP includes discontinuing the responsible medication and providing supportive treatment. Cyclosporine is currently being studied for its potential correlation with acute pancreatitis, as an immunosuppressive drug under consideration. DIP is a frequently disregarded medical condition that can have catastrophic consequences, including considerable morbidity and mortality [1].

24.3 Incidence

Acute pancreatitis accounts for approximately 230,000 hospitalizations annually in the United States. Although the mortality rate for moderate acute pancreatitis is less than 1%, it can increase significantly to 30% for severe cases. The global prevalence of drug-induced pancreatitis (DIP) ranges from 5 to 80 cases per 100,000 individuals, with treatment requiring discontinuation of the causative substance and provision of supportive care. Failure to identify the specific drug responsible for the condition can lead to significant delays in treatment. Therefore, to prevent DIP, there is a need to have current knowledge about medicines with the most compelling evidence correlating their usage to the occurrence of pancreatitis [1, 2].

24.4 Clinical Manifestation

Individuals suffering from pancreatitis commonly show symptoms such as abdominal discomfort, nausea, and vomiting. These symptoms vary based on severity, as those with mild acute pancreatitis can simply experience slight discomfort after palpation. However, the discomfort is persistent, typically situated in the epigastrium, and commonly characterized as sharp and spreading to the midcentral back. Patients show restlessness and may adopt a forward-leaning posture, flexing knees towards the chest in an attempt to reduce the pain [2].

Jaundice is prevalent in pancreatitis and approximately 3% of severe acute cases may experience retroperitoneal hemorrhage, leading to the development of flank ecchymosis (Grey Turner sign) or periumbilical ecchymosis (Cullen sign). Severe acute pancreatitis patients can also experience symptoms such as fever, rapid breathing, low oxygen levels, and reduced blood pressure. Cognitive function changes are frequently observed in cases of acute DIP and are indicative of drug or ethanol exposure. However, it can also occur due to hypotension, hypoxemia, or the excessive release of toxic substances from the inflamed pancreas [2].

Complications of pancreatitis can lead to both local and systemic repercussions. Moreover, local complications include the buildup of fluid, pancreatic pseudocyst formation, necrotic collection, and walled-off necrosis. Secondary infection of the fluids and necrotic tissue contributes to the development of systemic inflammatory response syndrome and sepsis. Systemic consequences include splanchnic vein thrombosis, abdominal compartment syndrome, pseudoaneurysm, acute respiratory distress syndrome, and worsening of preexisting comorbidities such as coronary artery disease and chronic lung disease [2].

24.5 Diagnosis

Initial diagnosis of acute pancreatitis is required to examine drug-induced pancreatitis (DIP). Elevations in several biomarkers, such as serum lipase and amylase, are reliable indicators of pancreatitis. These biomarkers are primarily produced by pancreatic acinar cells and are the most frequently assessed. Additional diagnostic laboratory tests include serum trypsinogen, pancreatic proteases, C-reactive protein, interleukin-6, and interleukin-8. To diagnose DIP, there is a need to initially exclude other more prevalent causes, such as gallstone pancreatitis and acute pancreatitis caused by alcohol consumption. It is also essential to document a comprehensive medical history and the medications used by the patient. The medical history should prioritize the examination of past symptoms and any documentation of gallstones, excessive alcohol consumption, high levels of calcium in the blood, elevated triglycerides, and any history of physical injury. Recommendations are made to request serum amylase, lipase, lipid level, calcium level, and liver function tests. Abdominal and endoscopic ultrasounds are also crucial to assess the presence of gallstones and other potential obstructions, such as tumors located in the head of the pancreas. However, ERCP should be avoided following an incident of acute pancreatitis when there is no evidence of choledocholithiasis based on imaging or chemical tests [2].

Medications capable of inducing pancreatitis should be ceased or substituted with another from a distinct category. When pancreatitis subsides with the cessation of the medication, the potential of DIP becomes more probable. Establishing this connection is challenging due to the potential coincidence between the remission of the condition and the termination of the inciting substance. A definitive diagnosis can be reliably determined by administering the problematic medicine, which leads to the reappearance of pancreatitis symptoms (Table 24.1) [2].

Table 24.1 Severity and characteristics of acute pancreatitis [3–5]

Severity level	Key features
Mild	No organ failure
	Absence of local or systemic complications
Moderate	Temporary organ failure that resolves within 48 hours
	Presence of local or systemic complications without lasting organ failure
Severe	Persistent organ failure lasting more than 48 hours
Organ failure	
Organ	Defining features
Lung	P/F_2 ratio ≤ 300
Heart	Systolic blood pressure <90 mmHg (without vasopressor support)
	Unresponsive to fluid resuscitation or pH <7.3
Kidney	Serum creatinine ≥ 1.9 mg/dl
Complications	
Acute Peripancreatic fluid collections	Fluid accumulations adjacent to the pancreas
Pancreatic and Peripancreatic necrosis	Tissue necrosis, which can be sterile or infected
Pancreatic pseudocyst	Fluid-filled sac that develops due to pancreatitis
Walled off pancreatic necrosis	Organized collection of necrotic tissue, sterile or infected

24.6 Cyclosporin-Induced Acute Pancreatitis

Based on the Badalov classification, cyclosporine is categorized as a class III drug due to its potential to cause acute pancreatitis. This shows that there have been at least two documented cases in medical literature, but lack consistent data on the time between drug exposure and the appearance of symptoms or positive rechallenge [6].

Cyclosporine shows numerous adverse effects, such as nephrotoxicity, hypertension, dyslipidemia, and susceptibility to infections. In 1988, the National Kidney Foundation conducted a study, where 4 among 105 patients who were handled with cyclosporine after kidney transplant experienced severe pancreatitis. These patients showed elevated, moderate, and diminished cyclosporine trough levels at diagnosis. Moreover, there was improvement when the dose of Cyclosporine was reduced or completely withdrawn and replaced with another medication, indicating a strong recommendation for treatment. A further 1998 study conducted on rats showed that elevated dosages of cyclosporine worsen posttransplant pancreatitis, although lower levels did not have the same effect [7].

24.7 Management

In addition to evaluating the more common causes of acute pancreatitis, drugs should be considered. It is crucial that suspected drugs, such as Cyclosporin, be discontinued immediately to prevent ongoing pancreatic injury. The subsequent treatment should include the administration of intravenous fluids in a forceful manner, regular monitoring of vital signs such as oxygen saturation, and the use of a narcotic medicine supplied through a parenteral route to alleviate abdominal pain. Patients showing indications of organ failure, such as persistent low oxygen levels, low blood pressure unresponsive to intravenous fluids, impaired kidney function that does not improve with fluid injections, and alterations in mental state, should be promptly transferred to an intensive care unit for enhanced monitoring and treatment. Meanwhile, those experiencing severe abdominal discomfort, bloating, nausea, and vomiting should refrain from consuming food orally until the symptoms and overall clinical condition improve, a process that typically takes 3–7 days.

More severe cases of pancreatitis may require nutritional support, particularly for patients who are unable to eat for more than 7 days. Moreover, enteral nutrition should be given in preference to parenteral nutrition [8].

24.8 Prognosis

Drug-induced acute pancreatitis (DIP) is an uncommon condition that is challenging to identify due to the absence of specific clinical characteristics. The majority of cases range from mild to moderate severity, with the possibility of severe and fatal cases [6].

Key Points

Serial monitoring for pancreatic enzymes is necessary in long-term immunosuppressants therapy (such as Cyclosporin).

Questions

1. The worldwide incidence of drug-induced pancreatitis:
   (a) Around 5–80 per 100,000 adults
   (b) Around 5–80 per 10,000 adults
   (c) Around 5–60 per 10,000 adults
   (d) Around 5–60 per 100,000 adults
   (e) Around 230 per 100,000 adults
2. Clinical manifestations of severe acute pancreatitis are as follows, except:
   (a) Jaundice
   (b) Fever
   (c) Tachypnoea
   (d) Hypoxemia
   (e) Hypertension
3. Cyclosporin has many side effects including:
   (a) Autoimmune
   (b) Hypotension
   (c) Gout Arthritis
   (d) Pancreatitis
   (e) Hepatotoxicity

4. Which of the following is true regarding diagnosis of drug-induced acute pancreatitis:
   (a) Elevations in several biomarkers are indicative of pancreatitis
   (b) Endoscopic retrograde cholangiopancreatography should be performed after an episode of acute pancreatitis in the absence of imaging of choledocholithiasis
   (c) Abdominal ultrasounds should not be performed to evaluate for gallstones
   (d) Any drugs with the potential to cause pancreatitis should be continued or exchanged for a drug of a different class
   (e) Endoscopic ultrasounds should not be performed to evaluate for other obstructive possibilities such as tumors of the pancreas head
5. According to Badalov classification, what class is the drug Cyclosporine included in?
   (a) Class I A
   (b) Class I B
   (c) Class II
   (d) Class III
   (e) Class IV

Answer Keys

1. A
2. E
3. D
4. A
5. D

Acknowledgments Ersananda Arlisa Putri MD, Department of Internal Medicine, Respirology and Critical Illness Division, Universitas Indonesia, Dr. Cipto Mangunkusumo General Central National Hospital, Jakarta, Indonesia.

Nadia Ayu Mulansari MD DM, Department of Internal Medicine, Medical Hematology and Oncology Division, Universitas Indonesia, Dr. Cipto Mangunkusumo General Central National Hospital, Jakarta, Indonesia.

Rr. Dyah Purnamasari Sulistianingsih MD DM PhD, Department of Internal Medicine, Metabolic Endocrinology Division, Universitas Indonesia, Dr. Cipto Mangunkusumo General Central National Hospital, Jakarta, Indonesia.

Lie Khie Chen MD DM PhD, Department of Internal Medicine, Tropical Infectious Diseases Division, Universitas Indonesia, Dr. Cipto Mangunkusumo General Central National Hospital, Jakarta, Indonesia.

References

1. Alhaddad O, Elsabaawy M, Elfauomy M, Elsabaawy D, Mansour T. Updates in drug-induced acute pancreatitis. Egypt Liver J. 2020; https://doi.org/10.1186/s43066-020-00059-3.
2. Jones MR, Morgan Hall O, Kaye AM, David Kaye A. Drug-induced acute pancreatitis: a review. Ochsner J. 2014;15(1):45–51.
3. Walkowska J, Zielinska N, Tubbs RS, Podgórski M, Dłubek-Ruxer J, Olewnik Ł. Diagnosis and treatment of acute pancreatitis. Diagnostics. 2022; https://doi.org/10.3390/diagnostics12081974.
4. Mao L, Qiu Y. Intractable & rare diseases. Research. 2012;1:134–7.
5. Yen CM, Lin CL, Lin MC, Chen HY, Lu NH, Kao CH. Pneumoconiosis increases the risk of congestive heart failure. Medicine (United States). 2016; https://doi.org/10.1097/MD.0000000000003972.
6. Branquinho D, Ramos-Andrade D, Elvas L, Amaro P, Ferreira M, Sofia C. Drug-induced acute pancreatitis and Pseudoaneurysms: an ominous combination. GE Port J Gastroenterol. 2016;23:309–13.
7. Al-Najada E, Alobaidat A, Rabab'ah MM, Bani Salameh M, Alkhatib L. Post kidney transplant cyclosporine-induced acute pancreatitis. Cureus. 2022;14:e24519.
8. Balani AR, Grendell JH. Drug-induced pancreatitis. Drug Saf. 2008;31:823–37.

Heart Failure in Complex Black Lung Disease

25

25.1 Case Illustration

A 57-year-old male patient presented with severe chest pain persisting for a day prior to hospital admission. The chest pain increased with deep breathing and initially manifested mildly but progressively intensified. The pain radiated to the left arm and was not influenced by activity. The patient also reported coughing up blood every 2–3 days, with a volume of 5–10 cc. There was a weight loss of 15 kg in 8 months, although there was no report of fever, nausea, and sweating at night.

Six months before hospitalization, the patient complained of shortness of breath and went to a nearby hospital, where the patient was diagnosed with cardiovascular disease. An echocardiography examination was carried out and the results showed a 45% ejection fraction of the heart [classified as heart failure with preserved ejection fraction (HFpEF)]. The patient was then subsequently managed with cardiovascular disease treatment and routine control, and was advised for cardiac catheterization. A month before hospitalization, a recurrence of chest pain was reported, describing it as a heavy pressure on his chest, and despite taking nitrate 3 times, there was no relief. The patient then visited the Cipto Mangunkusumo Hospital and catheterization was performed. The results showed that 20% blockage was obtained, which did not warrant stent placement. During treatment, the patient also underwent several tuberculosis (TB) tests, but the results were negative. The patient was a private employee, works in a car spare parts warehouse, and has a side job in mining, with a smoking history of one pack a day for more than 30 years but has stopped now.

During the physical examination, the patient appeared severely ill. His conjunctiva was pale, and heart auscultation showed a diastolic murmur with a maximum punctum in the pulmonary valve. Laboratory examination showed various abnormalities, including a low level of hemoglobin 10.3 mg/dl, declining kidney function (blood urea 107 mg/dl, Creatinine 2.9 mg/dl, EGFR 23 mL/min/1.73 m^2), prothrombin time (PT) 11.4 sec, activated partial thromboplastin time (APTT) 35.2 sec, Troponin-T 42. Chest X-ray (CXR) showed pneumonia and cardiomegaly

G. Singh, *Challenging Cases in Respirology and Critical Care*,
https://doi.org/10.1007/978-981-96-5002-6_25

(Fig. 25.1). The electrocardiographic picture shows an inverted T in V2-V3 and a depressed ST segment in leads II, V5-V6.

Based on the initial clinical and laboratory findings, the patient was diagnosed with Unstable Angina Pectoris (UAP) using a differential diagnosis of Non–ST-Segment Elevation Myocardial Infarction (NSTEMI), Community-Acquired Pneumonia with a differential diagnosis of pulmonary TB with secondary infection and hemoptysis suspected pulmonary embolism.

The patient was subsequently admitted as an isolation inpatient and diagnostic tests were conducted, including Gen Xpert, Acid-Fast Bacilli (AFB), and culture using a sputum specimen. The results of the Gen Xpert MTB were not detected, the sputum AFB was negative, and the sputum culture showed gram-positive cocci. The patient is scheduled to be transferred to the regular inpatient unit.

In the following days, the patient complained of coughing up blood accompanied by blood clots. The patient also continued to experience shortness of breath and chest pain. Physical examination showed epigastric tenderness; the liver was palpable 2 fingers below the costal arch and edema in both lower extremities. Laboratory examination showed a low level of hemoglobin 10 mg/dl; a high level of leukocytes 16,160 cell/mm^3, a high level of thrombocytes 511,000 cell/mm^3, d-dimer 480 ng/

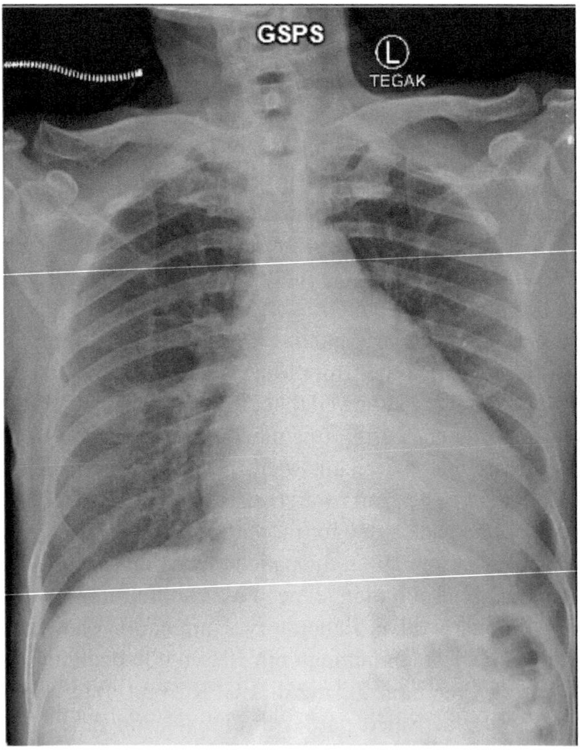

Fig. 25.1 Chest X-ray showed infiltrate and cardiomegaly. (Figure courtesy: Heltara Ramandika MD DM)

mL, negative galactomannan, calcium level 8 mg/dl, and magnesium level 1.75 mg/dl. Chest X-ray (Fig. 25.2) showed bilateral pleural effusions and infiltrates in the right lower lung have an increased impression compared to the previous examination.

Chest CT (Fig. 25.3) showed bilateral pleural effusion, specifically in the right lung, accompanied by comprehensive atelectasis subsegmental 9–10 right lung and 10 subsegmental left lung.

The patient underwent medical thoracocentesis, during which 600 cc of pleural fluid was obtained. Analysis of pleural fluid showed a transudative pleural effusion, negative adenosine deaminase (ADA), and no bacteria detected on the Gram stain. The following day, chest ultrasound examination was performed and the results showed a left pleural effusion (Fig. 25.4). Needle thoracocentesis and chest tube insertion (with water-sealed drainage (WSD) system) were then planned for the patient's Chest tube. WSD production of 750 cc of serous pleural fluid was obtained.

The patient also underwent a medical thoracoscopy procedure (Fig. 25.5), and the result showed recurrent post-thoracocentesis pleural effusion, parietal pleural nodules, and right and lower lobe pulmonary anthracosis. Pleural fluid obtained from medical thoracoscopy was analyzed in the laboratory and taken to the anatomical pathology department.

After several days of running the treatment, complaints of coughing up blood improved. During the physical examination, edema in the lower extremities has reduced, and WSD production has decreased gradually. Laboratory examination showed improvement, including hemoglobin 10.7 mg/dl, leukocytes 14,520 cell/mm^3, kidney function (blood urea: 72.8 mg/dl, creatinine: 2.2 mg/dl, EGFR: 32.1 mL/min/1.73 m^2), albumin 3 g/dl, sodium 136 mg/dl, potassium 4.4 mg/dl,

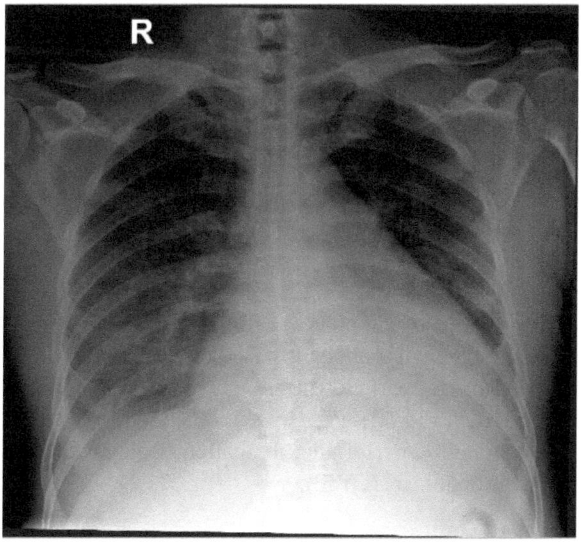

Fig. 25.2 Chest X-ray showed bilateral pleural effusions and infiltrates in the right lower lung have increased than previous examination. (Figure courtesy: Mohammad Reynalzi Yugo MD)

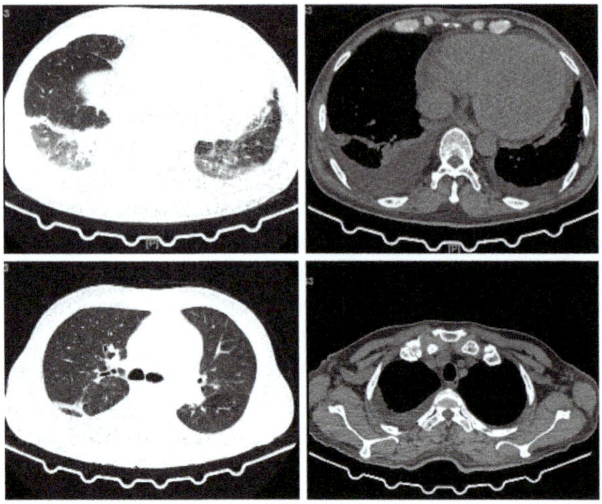

Fig. 25.3 Chest CT showed bilateral pleural effusion, and atelectasis subsegmental 9–10 right lung and 10 subsegmental left lung. (Figure courtesy: Mohammad Reynalzi Yugo MD)

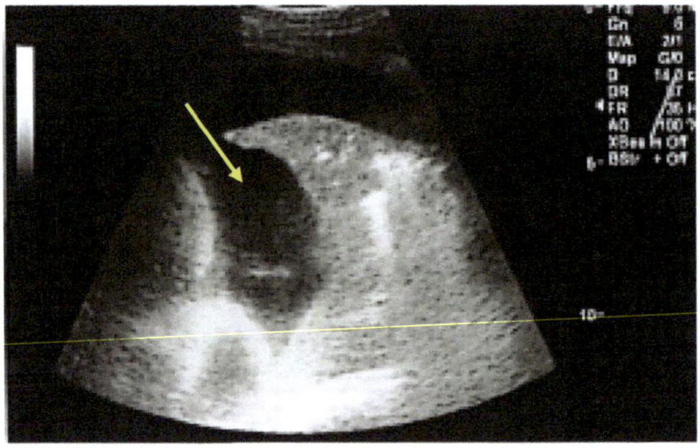

Fig. 25.4 The ultrasound examination showed left pleural effusion (*yellow arrow*). (Figure courtesy: Gurmeet Singh MD DM PhD)

chloride 99.5 mg/dl, Ca 9 mg/dl, Mg 3.2 mg/dl. Pleural fluid obtained from medical thoracoscopy showed transudate pleural effusion, negative for AFB, MTB not detected, and negative for malignant cells based on cytological and histopathology features (Fig. 25.6). Mineral particles in bronchoalveolar lavage fluid showed Mn BAL 18,2 μg/L, Fe BAL 1.756,10 μg/L, Cr BAL 66,03 μg/L, and Ni BAL 8,65 μg/L.

Based on the examination performed, the patient's diagnosis leads to anthracosis/coal worker pneumoconiosis (CWP).

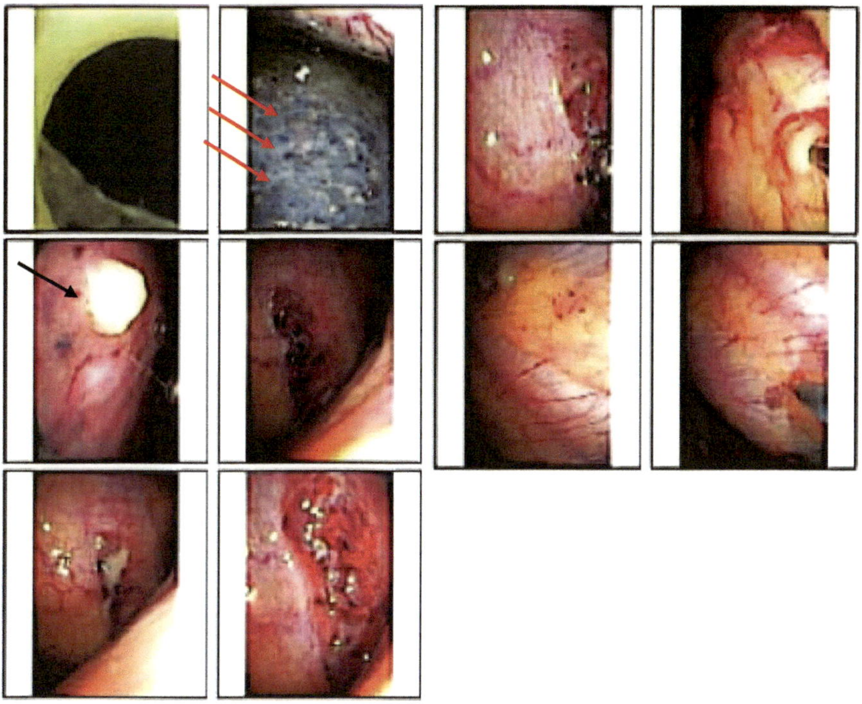

Fig. 25.5 The result of Medical Thoracoscopy showed blue black lung (*red arrow*), characteristic of anthracosis/coal worker pneumoconiosis (CWP). Nodular Lesion also visualize (black arrow). (Figure courtesy: Gurmeet Singh MD DM PhD, Ray Bryan Charles Rattu MD DM)

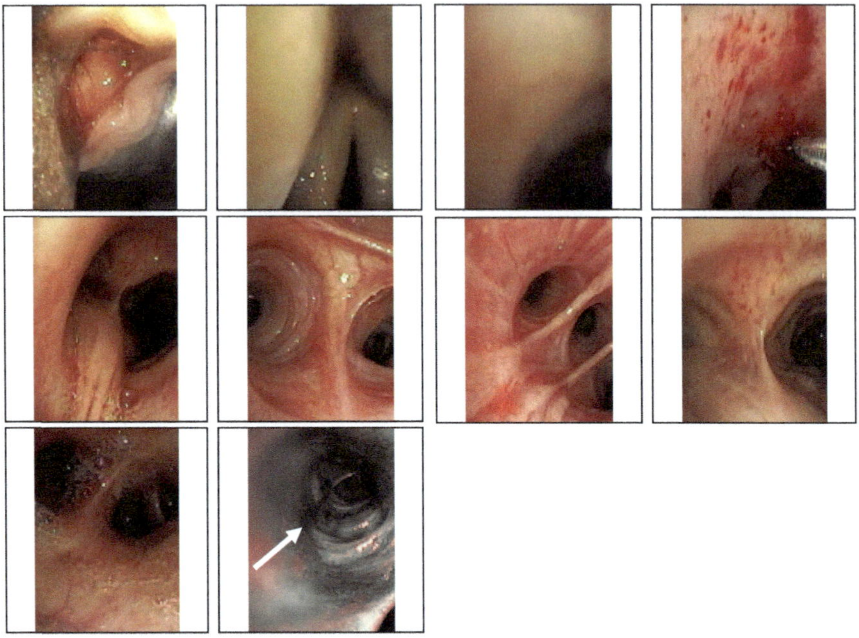

Fig. 25.6 The result of bronchoscopy showed black discoloration of bronchial mucosa (*white arrow*), suspected pneumoconiosis. (Figure courtesy: Herikurniawan MD DM)

25.2 Discussion

Anthracosis was confirmed via medical thoracoscopy, which demonstrated blue and black discoloration of the lungs and histopathological evidence of anthracofibrosis. The coexisting heart failure added complexity to the clinical picture. Pleural effusion, a hallmark of both anthracosis and HFpEF, was confirmed to be transudative through fluid analysis, aligning more closely with a cardiac etiology. However, the persistence of symptoms and the discovery of pleural nodules necessitated further investigation, ruling out malignancy and tuberculosis through cytological and microbiological studies. Chronic anthracosis and coal worker pneumoconiosis (CWP) are associated with a pro-inflammatory milieu, hypoxia, and secondary pulmonary hypertension, all of which place a burden on the right heart. The observed elevated d-dimer levels, recurrent pleural effusions, and pulmonary findings also raised suspicion for pulmonary embolism, further emphasizing the need for a thorough differential diagnosis in such cases. The interplay of anthracosis-induced pulmonary damage and cardiac dysfunction likely exacerbated the patient's clinical course. The patient's prolonged exposure to mining and automotive environments underscores the significance of occupational history in evaluating respiratory and cardiovascular conditions. Mineral particle analysis in bronchoalveolar lavage fluid revealed high levels of manganese, iron, chromium, and nickel, consistent with environmental exposure contributing to anthracosis. Such exposures can lead to chronic inflammation and fibrotic changes, compounding the risk of cardiopulmonary disease [3–5].

25.3 Prevalence

The prevalence of anthracosis in the general population has been approximately estimated due to the impossibility of conducting bronchoscopy, which is necessary for an accurate diagnosis of anthracosis, due to ethical reasons. The available data from extensive patient series who had bronchoscopy for unrelated causes showed that the prevalence of simple anthracosis ranges from 3.4% to 21%. The frequency of bronchial artery fistula (BAF) is comparatively lower in Western countries. Wynn et al. conducted a study where they recorded seven cases of BAF out of a total of 7000 bronchoscopies. Reports from other continents, such as North America or Africa, were equally limited, and occurrences of anthracosis in children are exceedingly uncommon. Anthracosis, which was historically common among coal workers, is now predominantly observed in farmers (40%) and rural residents (55–66%), according to recent data. The incidence of affected females in certain extensive studies has been equivalent to that of males. However, the aggregation of data shows that the prevalence of BAF in females is slightly higher than in males [6].

Currently, anthracosis affects more than 10% of miners who have been employed in or around mines for 25 years or longer. In central Appalachia, the prevalence of black lung disease among long-term miners is 20.6% [7].

25.4 Clinical Manifestation

Anthracosis usually presents with symptoms very similar to those of chronic obstructive pulmonary disease (COPD), except without a history of cigarette smoking. Cough and difficulty breathing are the most common symptoms reported in cases of BAF and anthracosis. The presence of TB does not alter the chronic symptoms, although it might lead to new weight loss or fever (25%). These symptoms should be distinguished from pneumonia, which occurs in 30% of individuals with bronchiectasis and TB [6].

Typically, a physical examination of lung shows wheezing, and less commonly, rales or reduced breath sounds. Several individuals with anthracosis exhibited normal results in the physical examinations. Anthracosis can lead to problems such as swollen mediastinal lymph nodes, resulting in vocal cord paralysis or broncho lithiasis. Additionally, numerous instances of these illnesses were recorded in correlation with TB [6].

25.5 Complication

Right heart failure can arise as a significant consequence of severe black lung disease. The presence of significant fibrosis in lung leads to elevated blood pressure in the pulmonary artery, responsible for transporting blood from the right side of the heart to lung. As a result, the elevated pressure causes the right side of the heart to grow and eventually leads to right-sided heart failure, also known as cor pulmonale.

Caplan syndrome is a rare complication that can occur in individuals with black lung disease. This illness is characterized by the presence of inflammatory nodules, known as rheumatoid nodules, in lung, in addition to a preexisting condition of black lung. Moreover, patients experience joint inflammation similar to that observed in rheumatoid arthritis. A previous study also observed a heightened susceptibility to lung cancer, specifically squamous cell carcinoma of lung, among individuals with simple black lung disease. Coal mine workers exhibit a higher prevalence of lung cancer, independent of the presence of black lung disease [8, 9].

25.6 Diagnosis

Anthracosis should be included in the differential diagnosis of conditions such as COPD, TB (excluding anthracosis), lung cancer, fungal infections (including mucormycosis and actinomycosis), and amyloidosis. An elderly nonsmoker with a history of chronic dyspnea or cough that worsens in winter may indicate the presence of anthracosis. Wheezing detected during the examination of lung suggests the presence of bronchial airway obstruction. The presence of obstructive lung illness in spirometry, along with lymph node or bronchial calcification (high attenuation), particularly in individuals who also exhibit a mass lesion (or atelectasis), significantly increases the likelihood of diagnosing anthracosis. Kim et al. identified smooth bronchial constriction with increased calcified lymph nodes as a valuable indicator for distinguishing between BAF and lung cancer. However, in all proposed scenarios, it is important to conduct bronchoscopy as the definitive method of diagnosis, and the specimens obtained from bronchoscopy should be submitted for TB examination. If a mass is detected in radiological examinations, it may be essential to perform an open lung biopsy, transthoracic lung biopsy, or advanced bronchoscopy procedures to eliminate the possibility of TB or cancer [6].

COPD is the primary differential diagnosis for anthracosis. Based on the available information, anthracosis should not be classified as a subtype of COPD, as it is caused by exposure to biomass rather than cigarette smoke. Progressive massive fibrosis should be taken into account as a potential alternative diagnosis. However, a history of occupational exposure to dust and a more widespread lung involvement can help distinguish it from pneumoconiosis [6].

25.7 Chest X-ray

Only 7% of participants had a normal chest X-ray report. The most commonly observed abnormalities in chest X-ray were nonuniform pulmonary infiltration, subsegmental atelectasis, and mass lesions. In many instances, chest X-ray showed the disappearance of anomalies when individuals with anthracosis were confirmed to have TB and received treatment using anti-TB drugs [6].

25.8 CT Scan

CT scan was more effective in detecting anthracosis and provided more precise radiological results. Initial findings indicate that 94% of cases exhibit mediastinal or hilar lymphadenopathy, with 57% of these instances showing calcification (high attenuation). Additionally, 94% of cases display bronchial constriction, with or without atelectasis. An investigation assessed the primary CT results and showed a notably greater occurrence and likelihood of lymph node calcification, bronchial wall calcification, bronchial stenosis, atelectasis, and mass lesion (14%) in individuals with black anthracotic fibrosis (BAF) compared to those without anthracosis. The majority of instances of bronchial stenosis exhibited a smooth appearance without the presence of endobronchial nodules (80%). Although infrequent, distal atelectasis was absent in a few cases. Additionally, 20% of BAF participants had bronchial wall thickening. Engagement can be either one-sided or two-sided, however, right middle lobe (RML), followed by the upper lobes, were typically identified as the most commonly affected sections. CT imaging showed no significant findings in 17% of individuals with uncomplicated anthracosis and 6% of those with anthracofibrosis. Pleural illness was detected in 25% of BAF participants. The occurrence of pleural involvement in BAF is infrequent, and data are scarce on this topic [6, 10].

25.9 Bronchoscopy

Bronchoscopy is the most reliable method for diagnosing anthracosis. It can be identified through imaging in various forms, including flat anthracosis, retracted anthracosis originating from an anthracotic lymph node near the bronchus, or protruded black staining of the mucosa, with or without bronchial constriction (BAF). Besides the presence of black lesions, one may see bronchial swelling accompanied by infiltration, erythema, and thickness, which might potentially lead to the complete blockage of bronchi. Anthracosis can manifest as either localized or diffused, unilateral or bilateral. Right middle lobe is the most commonly affected area, followed by the upper lobe bronchi, particularly at the bifurcation or input of the lobar or segmental bronchi. Tracheal involvement is infrequent and was observed in 3.8% of BAF individuals. In addition, bronchial washing may reveal the presence of unbound black particles, while performing a biopsy is typically challenging due to the firm texture of the mucosa. Hemorrhage during biopsy is a common occurrence, with a prevalence of 9%; however, it typically does not lead to any additional difficulties [6].

25.10 Medical Thoracoscopy

Medical thoracoscopy is a frequently used endoscopic procedure for the diagnosis and treatment of respiratory illnesses. As an intrusive procedure, it is mostly used for pleural effusions and pleural disorders that cannot be detected using noninvasive procedures. Furthermore, it has significant utility in the identification and management of specific medical conditions [1].

Thoracoscopy is a reliable and secure diagnostic technique in general medicine for identifying idiopathic anthracosis with pleural effusion. It can expedite the development of an effective therapeutic approach [11].

25.11 Management

Treatment in this case focused on addressing both cardiac and pulmonary components. Therapeutic thoracentesis and chest tube drainage provided symptomatic relief from pleural effusions, while optimized management of heart failure improved systemic symptoms. The clinical gradual improvement and laboratory parameters highlighted the importance of a multidisciplinary approach in managing heart disease associated with occupational lung disease. Early recognition and a systematic diagnostic approach are critical for distinguishing between overlapping conditions, optimizing treatment, and preventing complications [2].

25.12 Prognosis

The prognosis of black lung disease depends on the severity of the disease (simple or complex) and additional exposures to harmful substances. While simple black lung disease may have a sluggish progression over an extended duration, complex black lung disease can advance swiftly [7].

Key Points

Evaluation for occupational lung disease is beneficial to obtain a quick and accurate diagnosis, and to administer proper treatment in difficult to treat heart failure.

Questions

1. The following statements are true about the prevalence of anthracosis:
   (a) The frequency of simple anthracosis ranges from 3.4% to 21%.
   (b) Anthracosis was historically prevalent among coal workers, but recent studies report a higher prevalence among farmers, with 55% to 66% of cases being identified in this group.
   (c) Currently, anthracosis is present in over 10% of miners who have worked in or near mines for 35 years or more.
   (d) In some large studies, the number of affected males has been equal to the number of females.
   (e) The prevalence is higher in central Appalachia, where 10% of long-term miners have black lung disease.

2. One of the most serious complications of severe black lung disease:
   (a) COPD
   (b) Malignancy
   (c) Right Heart Failure
   (d) Massive Hemothorax
   (e) Secondary Pneumothorax
3. The gold standard for diagnosing anthracosis?
   (a) CT scan
   (b) MRI
   (c) Chest X-ray
   (d) Bronchoscopy
   (e) Thoracoscopy
4. The most frequent chest X-ray abnormality found in anthracosis:
   (a) Pleural effusion
   (b) Lung cavity
   (c) Consolidation
   (d) Interstitial lung edema
   (e) Subsegmental atelectasis
5. What is the empirical management of anthracosis:
   (a) Bronchodilators, antiviral, and antibiotics
   (b) Bronchodilators, corticosteroids, and antibiotics
   (c) Bronchodilators, anticholinergic, and antibiotics
   (d) Bronchodilators, anticholinergic, and corticosteroids
   (e) Bronchodilators, corticosteroids, and oxygen therapy

Answer Keys

1. A
2. C
3. D
4. E
5. B

Acknowledgments Ersananda Arlisa Putri MD, Department of Internal Medicine, Respirology and Critical Illness Division, Universitas Indonesia, Dr. Cipto Mangunkusumo General Central National Hospital, Jakarta, Indonesia.

Iwan Rivai Alam Siahaan MD PhD, Department of Occupational Safety and Health, Universitas Indonesia, Dr. Cipto Mangunkusumo General Central National Hospital, Jakarta, Indonesia.

References

1. Mao L, Qiu Y. Intractable & rare diseases. Research. 2012;1:134–7.
2. Yen CM, Lin CL, Lin MC, Chen HY, Lu NH, Kao CH. Pneumoconiosis increases the risk of congestive heart failure. Medicine (United States). 2016;95:e3972. https://doi.org/10.1097/MD.0000000000003972.
3. Simonneau G, Gatzoulis MA, Adatia I, et al. Updated clinical classification of pulmonary hypertension. J Am Coll Cardiol. 2013;62:D34–41.
4. Members AF, McMurray JJV, Adamopoulos S, et al. ESC guidelines for the diagnosis and treatment of acute and chronic heart failure 2012: the task force for the diagnosis and treatment of acute and chronic heart failure 2012 of the European Society of Cardiology. Developed in collaboration with the Heart Failure Association (HFA) of the ESC. Eur Heart J. 2012;33:1787–847.
5. Laney AS, Attfield MD. Coal workers' pneumoconiosis and progressive massive fibrosis are increasingly more prevalent among workers in small underground coal mines in the United States. Occup Environ Med. 2010;67:428.
6. Mirsadraee M. Anthracosis of the lungs: etiology, clinical manifestations and diagnosis: a review. Tanaffos. 2014;13:1–13.
7. Blackley DJ, Halldin CN, Laney AS. Continued increase in prevalence of coal workers' pneumoconiosis in the United States, 1970–2017. Am J Public Health. 2018;108:1220–2.
8. Nemakayala DR, Surmachevska N, Vaqar S, Ramphul K. Caplan syndrome. StatPearls [Internet]; 2024.
9. Garrison DM, Pendela VS, Memon J. Cor Pulmonale. StatPearls [Internet]; 2023.
10. Mirsadraee M, Asna-Ashari A, Attaran D, Naghibi S, Mirsadraee S. Bronchial anthracosis: a new diagnosis for benign mass lesions of the lung. Tanaffos. 2013;12:10–8.
11. Wang Z, Xu LL, Wu YB, Wang XJ, Yang Y, Zhang J, Tong ZH, Shi HZ. Diagnostic value and safety of medical thoracoscopy in tuberculous pleural effusion. Respir Med. 2015;109:1188–92.

GPSR Compliance

The European Union's (EU) General Product Safety Regulation (GPSR) is a set of rules that requires consumer products to be safe and our obligations to ensure this.

If you have any concerns about our products, you can contact us on ProductSafety@springernature.com

In case Publisher is established outside the EU, the EU authorized representative is:

Springer Nature Customer Service Center GmbH
Europaplatz 3
69115 Heidelberg, Germany

Batch number: 10732090

Printed by Printforce, the Netherlands